Perfect Health Diet

regain health and lose weight by eating
the way you were meant to eat

Paul Jaminet, PhD &
Shou-Ching Jaminet, PhD

SCRIBE
Melbourne • London

Scribe Publications Pty Ltd
18–20 Edward St, Brunswick, Victoria, Australia 3056
Email: info@scribepub.com.au

Published in Australia and New Zealand by Scribe 2013

This edition published by arrangement with Scribner, a division of Simon & Schuster, Inc.

Text design by Carla Jayne Jones
Printed and bound in Australia by Griffin Press

 The paper this book is printed on is certified against the Forest Stewardship
Council® Standards. Griffin Press holds FSC chain of custody certification SGS-
COC-005088. FSC promotes environmentally responsible, socially beneficial
and economically viable management of the world's forests.

National Library of Australia
Cataloguing-in-Publication data

Jaminet, Paul, 1963-

Perfect Health Diet: regain health and lose weight by eating the way you were meant to eat.

9781922070210 (pbk.)

Includes bibliographical references and index.

1. Diet. 2. Nutrition.

Other Authors/Contributors: Jaminet, Shou-Ching.

641.563

www.scribepublications.com.au

Dedicated
to the memory of
Annette Marie Jaminet,
Paul's mother, who died of cancer at age 33,
and
Tei-Kuang Shih,
Shou-Ching's father, who died of stroke at age 62,
and to the hope that
disease and premature death
will soon be eradicated.

Scribe Publications
PERFECT HEALTH DIET

PAUL JAMINET, PHD, was an astrophysicist at the Harvard-Smithsonian Centre for Astrophysics. Paul's experience of overcoming a chronic illness led the Jaminets to develop the views of ageing and disease presented in *Perfect Health Diet*.

SHOU-CHING JAMINET, PHD, is a molecular biologist and cancer researcher at Beth Israel Deaconess Medical Centre and Harvard Medical School, and director of BIDMC's Multi-Gene Transcriptional Profiling Core.

Contents

Foreword

In writing *The Primal Blueprint*, my goal was to improve the overall health of the general population — the folks who just want to be healthier, happier, stronger, fitter, and more productive. Most of the complaints, the aches and pains, and the concerns that your mother, your father, your friends, your grandparents, your coworkers, and you worry about aren't inevitable. Most health issues can be avoided with just a few simple tweaks to your lifestyle.

I try to help guide people toward these changes by showing them what's worked for me and countless others. I'm a generalist, and that's how I've always been. The world needs generalists. But the world also needs people who delve deeply into the medical and scientific literature, probing for knowledge that can address the specific illnesses and health issues reducing the quality of life — and life span — of people today.

Paul and Shou-Ching Jaminet, both trained scientists, are perhaps the finest examples of the type of experts we need. Their book and blog, *Perfect Health Diet*, represent the culmination of a half decade of rigorous research. They've combed the relevant literature for clues, hints, and knowledge they needed to address their own rapidly deteriorating health. What they found healed their ailments and changed their lives. And what began as a highly specific approach to their own health issues quickly became a more general, overarching approach to good health — for everyone. Anyone and everyone will benefit from their dietary recommendations, but the Jaminets' advice is particularly relevant for those suffering from health issues that traditional medicine has been unable to treat or improve.

If you're reading this book, you've likely had some personal experience with the failings of conventional medicine. Now, I don't want to sound antimedicine. I'm not. Conventional medical professionals are fantastic technicians and mechanics; they can patch you up, keep you alive, put in new equipment and take out old malfunctioning stuff. They wield an array of powerful drugs with specific applications, many of them helpful. They have an immense amount of technology at their behest. And yet many in the world of conventional medicine are missing the big picture — or at least a large part of it.

With Paul and Shou-Ching, you have the missing piece. They bridge the gap between the philosophical, broad-based, almost intuitive ancestral approach to health and the hardcore data hounds who need to see proof at every step. The authors are scientists through and through, an astrophysicist and a molecular biologist, who deftly wield the sceptre of cold, hard science while paying homage to the inescapable wisdom of traditional, ancestral, evolutionary health.

While we wait for the medical community to catch up and get with the big picture, we're lucky to have a pair of minds like the Jaminets' to read, absorb, and learn from in the meantime. This is the future of medicine, of health. It has to be, because it's the right way to do things, a way of thinking about food and nutrition that helps us to heal and live better lives rather than making us suffer.

If history is any indication, eventually we do get it right. A consensus forms and is broken; this process might repeat several times over many decades (or longer), but it eventually coalesces behind what is truly right.

We're reaching that moment. We started as a fledgling group of athletes, scientists, doctors, patients, parents, and sceptics who found something that seemed to work really, really well. And so we shouted it from our keyboards. We wrote books. People read our words, implemented the advice they advocated, and saw their health transform before their eyes. Now, I'm not sure we're quite yet out of the fledgling stage, but we're growing. You can't deny that.

This, the newest edition of *Perfect Health Diet,* is helping lead the charge. By reading this book, you are taking part in a new (yet ancestral), radical (yet reasonable) movement toward better health. For that, I thank you, and I look eagerly toward what lies ahead.

Mark Sisson
Author of *The Primal Blueprint,* publisher of Marksdailyapple.com

Preface

We are two scientists who ate poorly and ignored a gradual decline in our health. By age 40, we had developed disturbing health problems:

- Paul had neuropathy, memory loss, impaired mood, physical sluggishness, and rosacea.
- Shou-Ching had painful endometriosis, ovarian cysts, and uterine fibroids; hypothyroidism; allergies; constipation, acid reflux, and bloating.

Doctors were of little help. Nothing we tried worked; surgery made Shou-Ching worse. Medical professionals couldn't even offer a reason why we were experiencing these problems. Yet, every year, we were a little worse than the year before.

Then, in 2005, we tried Chinese herbal medicines: twigs, bark, seeds, and leaves prepared at home like a tea. They seemed to work, but we both developed allergic reactions to the medicine and had to stop.

That planted an idea: if medicines had no effect but a tea made from plants did, perhaps the path forward lay in what we were eating — in our diets.

Paul was then developing a new approach to economics, a theory of relationships and social networks (see relationshipeconomics.com). Through the economist Craig Newmark, Paul learned of the low-carb Paleo diet of the economist Art de Vany.

The Paleo idea is that we evolved for 2.6 million years eating hunted

Notes for this chapter may be found at www.perfecthealthdiet.com/notes/#Preface.

animals and foraged plants, and that these remain our most healthful foods. It is supported by evidence: robustly healthy Paleolithic skeletons were succeeded by unhealthy skeletons with cavity-riddled teeth after the invention of agriculture,[1] and some modern hunter-gatherers are entirely free of cardiovascular disease — for instance, the islanders of Kitava, on their diet of coconut, yams, taro, and fish.[2] We were persuaded to give the Paleo diet a try.

Paul became leaner and stronger. Shou-Ching's allergies and digestive problems cleared. Clearly there was something to this diet.

But new problems appeared. Paul developed a systemic fungal infection; over the next year his cognitive and neuropathic issues worsened, and after a year of very-low-carb dieting, he developed scurvy, which caused his weight to drop to a mere 66 kilograms.

The scurvy was a wake-up call: if we were malnourished in one nutrient, we were probably malnourished in others. As scientists, it was natural to us to turn to the biomedical literature for answers. Since the quality of our lives was at stake, we undertook to scour the literature, fine-tuning our diet to provide the optimal amount of each nutrient. This occupied the next five years.

In 2009, Paul traced his neurological problems to a chronic bacterial infection; a course of antibiotics cleared it. Our health kept getting better; we began to feel as though we were in our twenties again.

The Perfect Health Diet Is Born

Five years of arduous research had finally led us to a healthful diet. We were convinced that our work could help others and felt obliged to share what we had learned. So in June 2010 we started a blog and self-published a book spelling out our ideas and the reasoning and evidence that had led us to them.

Thanks to a glowing review (titled 'My New Favorite Book on Nutrition and Health') on the popular blog of the naturopathic healer Chris Kresser, we quickly gained hundreds of readers, many with chronic health problems. Soon they were sending us reports of health improvements.

Gradually the word spread. Over the next year and a half, readers reported recovery from a host of ailments: obesity, migraines, acid reflux, sleep disorders, mood disorders, depression, anxiety, borderline personality disorder, hypothyroidism, acne, dry eyes, traumatic brain injury, polycystic ovary syndrome, amenorrhea, infertility, allergies, constipation, bowel diseases, arthritis, high blood pressure, Raynaud's syndrome, and many more. Here are a few of our favourites:

- After years of yo-yo dieting and never finding a weight-loss diet that didn't make him ravenous, Jay Wright lost 36 kilograms in seven months on our diet without hunger. He reached his normal weight, 77 kilograms, and has maintained it for the last year without difficulty. A few months into his weight loss, Jay emailed us: 'THIS IS THE BEST DIET EVER!' He was at a restaurant eating a salad with balsamic vinegar and olive oil dressing, a 225-gram steak, and a baked potato with butter and sour cream, and drinking some water with lemon, and said to himself, 'I can't believe I'm eating this and still losing weight!'
- Kate Martins had had severe migraines for 15 years, plus anxiety. A host of prescription drugs, diets, and supplements had all failed. She tried the ketogenic version of our diet, along with our recommended supplements and intermittent fasting, and within a week her headaches had begun to disappear. Soon she was nearly headache-free, and her anxiety had disappeared. She wrote us, 'The PHD is strong brain medicine indeed!'
- Joan's sister had suffered from chronic fatigue syndrome and eczema her whole adult life. Ten days after starting our diet and supplement advice, Joan reported: 'Within 24 hours her eczema was much improved . . . Now 10 days later her eczema has completely cleared and her skin is looking good . . . Not only that, but some of her CFS symptoms have improved. Her constant headache is not as severe, irregular heartbeat episodes have almost completely stopped and she is tolerating slightly more physical activity . . . Her sense of despair and resignation has gone and you have given her hope of a better future. Words seem inadequate to express thanks for that.'
- Brian P. wrote to thank us for helping him lose 16 kilograms 'along with a general improvement in energy and "evenness".' He called our diet 'totally satisfying' and closed with this: 'I strongly suspect PHD played a pivotal part in my wife getting pregnant naturally, just prior to starting her next round of IVF.'

Perhaps the most touching story concerned two young boys with a genetic disorder, Neurodegeneration with Brain Iron Accumulation (NBIA). NBIA children typically lose the ability to walk around age three, cannot hold their heads upright, and have difficulty swallowing. Premature death occurs, usually in the teens. The last years are excruciatingly painful due to uncontrollable muscle spasms.

The mother of one of the boys wrote us:

My son, who is 6 . . . has been on the [ketogenic version of the Perfect Health] diet for less than one month and his hands have relaxed enough for him to regain his pointing ability (which had been lost).

Zach, the 12 year old on the diet, is much further progressed in the disease. Zach has been on the diet since late October, 2010 . . . The following are the improvements that have been noted by Zach's family and therapists: *Zach has begun holding up his head* even though his neck has been hyper extended backwards since he was nine, *he has begun pointing with his finger again* instead of the palm of his hand, *he is moving his right arm again* some, and the latest thing is that *he is now able to go from a lying position to a sitting position on his own* by hanging on to something or someone. He has not done this since he was 9 years old.

Both boys have begun smiling and laughing all the time.

Nothing is more gratifying than to receive an email like this!

A Strategy for Perfect Health

The book is designed to walk you through a strategy for achieving good health by seeking perfect heath. Our aim is to eliminate every nutrient deficiency, remove every dietary toxin, and eat nothing in excess.

This is a highly effective strategy for healing because most chronic diseases have many causes, each contributing a mite to the disease, but cumulatively causing great harm. Only when many causes are addressed can diseases be cured.

Not only does dietary perfection heal many diseases; we believe it is also the best strategy for healthful weight loss, for athleticism and fitness, as well as for longevity.

A Theory of Disease, Health, and Ageing

We believe that disease and ill health are largely caused by three factors:

- Nutrient deficiencies;
- Poisoning by toxins — most of them food toxins; and
- Chronic infections by bacteria, viruses, fungi, protozoa, and parasitic worms. These infections are fed by excess nutrition and flourish when immune function is impaired by nutrient deficiencies or circadian rhythm disruption.

Most people's diets are deficient in some nutrients, provide an excess of others (often ones that feed pathogens), and are rich in toxins. These dietary errors cause ill health.

Hippocrates, then, was right to declare, 'Let food be thy medicine.' Given the proper diet, the human body has amazing recuperative powers.

We believe that dietary therapy will work a revolution in medicine. Most of the chronic and degenerative diseases that afflict modern society cannot be cured until the diet is fixed. Much of what people consider 'ageing' is, in fact, infectious disease aggravated by a bad diet. Yet when the diet is healthful, the immune system may spontaneously defeat many diseases, and antibiotic drugs may work wonders.

About the Science in This Book

We want to help our readers to achieve perfect health and maintain it through a long life. We want to give hope to the diseased and weight loss to the obese. We want to persuade doctors and scientists, too, so that our medical revolution may arrive soon.

This is a science-rich book: we show our reasoning and evidence. It has to be, to persuade scientists and doctors. Chronic disease patients, too, are often sophisticated sceptics, keen to 'prove all things and hold fast that which is good'. We are both scientists and former chronic disease patients: we know what kind of book would have persuaded us to change our ways. We've tried to write that book.

Science is fascinating, and we have striven to make it entertaining. But we also want the book to be easy to read and helpful for people who just want to know 'What should I eat?'

Toward that end, we've tried to make it easy for casual readers to find practical guidance. The book is organised into five parts addressing practical issues: what foods to eat, what foods to avoid, how to be well nourished by food or supplements, and how to live a healthful lifestyle. Chapters conclude with prescriptive advice.

SCIENCE OF THE PHD

More esoteric science and interesting asides are placed in SCIENCE OF THE PHD boxes like this one. Casual readers may wish to skip or skim these boxes.

Readers can find further discussions at our web site, www.perfecthealth diet.com. We strive to answer any questions we receive there.

Best wishes, dear reader. May our insights help you to attain Perfect Health!

The Perfect Health Diet in Brief

The Perfect Health Diet is, by calories, a low-to-moderate-carbohydrate (20 to 35 per cent), high-fat (50 to 65 per cent), moderate-protein (15 per cent) diet. However, by weight, the diet is about 65 per cent plant foods, 35 per cent meats and oils.

DO eat:

- About 450 grams per day — roughly, four fist-sized servings — of 'safe starches': white rice, potatoes, sweet potatoes, taro, winter squashes, and a few others. Add up to another 450 grams of sugary plants — fruits, berries, beets, carrots, and such — and as many low calorie vegetables as you like. Be sure to include a bit of seaweed, for minerals. In total, you might eat 900 grams to 1400 grams of plant foods.
- At least 225 grams, probably not more than 450 grams, of fatty meats, seafood, and eggs. Once a week, eat salmon or other cold-water fish for omega-3 fatty acids.
- Eat 6 to 12 teaspoons of healthful cooking oils and fats per day — enough to make your food delicious but not oily. Butter, sour cream, beef tallow, duck fat, coconut oil, olive oil, and tree nut butters are the best fats. Use spices, including salt. Liberally use acids such as vinegar, lemon juice, and lime juice.
- Adjust the amount of food to fit your appetite, but keep these relative proportions of plant and animal foods. Adjust the proportions of fat, starch, and protein to make your food *as delicious as possible.*

Do NOT eat:

- Grains and cereals (including wheat, oats, and corn but excluding rice) or any products made from them (including bread and pasta). However, it is okay to eat gluten-free products made from rice flour, potato starch, and tapioca starch.
- Sugar, corn syrup, or products containing them (soda, sweets).
- Beans (such as soybeans, kidney beans, jack beans, or pinto beans) or peanuts.
- Omega-6-rich vegetable seed oils (such as soybean oil, corn oil, safflower oil, peanut oil, and canola oil).

AVOID:

- Milk, but DO eat fermented or fatty dairy products: butter, sour cream, ice cream, cheese, yogurt.

Finally, DO:

- Eat 'supplemental foods' such as beef liver, shellfish, kidneys, egg yolks, bone and joint broth soups, seaweed, tomatoes, and fermented vegetables to obtain crucial micronutrients. Supplement other nutrients as needed, especially magnesium, iodine, and vitamins C, D, and K.
- Practice intermittent fasting by restricting eating to an eight-hour window.
- Exercise in the morning; expose your skin to sunshine; avoid bright light and too much food at night; and get a good night's sleep.

The Perfect Health Diet Food Plate

For those who prefer graphic images, we created the Perfect Health Diet food plate shown on the opening page of the five parts of this book, including the page after this one. The body of the apple represents the components of a **meal;** the yin-yang symbol represents a **balance of plant and animal foods.** The leaves and stem represent pleasure foods that should be eaten in moderation. In the shadow of the apple are foods to avoid: grains except white rice; beans, peanuts, and other calorie-dense legumes; sugar and foods containing it, like soda; and vegetable seed oils.

Part I

....

An Evolutionary Guide to Healthful Eating

....

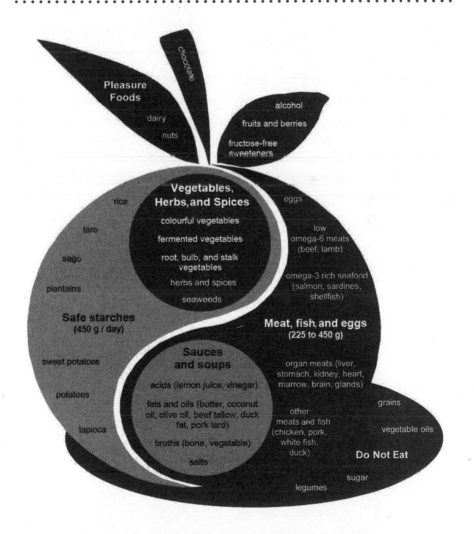

1

Why We Start with an Evolutionary Perspective

....

Why understanding the big picture is so crucial to your health.

....

An ancient Indian story tells of eight blind men trying to discern the nature of an elephant. Each felt a different part and reached a different conclusion about the nature of the elephant. The poet John Godfrey Saxe reported the outcome:

> *And so these men of Hindustan*
> *Disputed loud and long,*
> *Each in his own opinion*
> *Exceeding stiff and strong,*
> *Though each was partly in the right*
> *And all were in the wrong.*

Much the way experts quarrel about diet!

Why is it so hard to figure out the optimal diet?

Like the blind men in the fable, diet experts begin with no clear picture of what an elephant looks like and, after lifelong investigations, acquire only a partial grasp of the evidence. The biomedical database PubMed contains more than 22 million articles, and one million new papers are added each year. A typical scientist reads, at most, 1000 papers per year. No matter how

Notes for this chapter may be found at www.perfecthealthdiet.com/notes/#Ch1.

long a scientist's career, it's impossible to read more than 0.1 per cent of the literature. Most of this reading has to be in the scientist's specialty — a small part of the elephant.

Adding to the problem is the complexity of human biology. We need to get many nutrients, maybe hundreds, from our food. Food contains thousands of toxins. With so many different ways food can nourish or harm us and so many different ways to assemble foods into a diet, picking out which diet is healthiest is like answering a multiple-choice test that has a billion choices. It's easy to go wrong.

Looking at all this research is like looking at a disassembled jigsaw puzzle with no picture of the completed puzzle. It's hard to tell how to put the pieces together.

A Big-Picture View We Can Trust

What we really need is a big-picture view — a view of the whole elephant. We need a reliable guide to the optimal diet, a guide that gives us an approximation to the truth at the very beginning of our investigations. This approximate answer can be a lodestar that guides us through the labyrinth of details, preventing many a wrong turn.

This is where an evolutionary perspective comes in. We know that healthy people and animals are more likely to survive the vicissitudes of life and have children and grandchildren. This means that **evolution selects for healthful behaviours — including healthful eating.**

If we're looking for a human diet that evolution guarantees is healthful, the place to start is with the diets of the Paleolithic. The Paleolithic was so long — 2.6 million years — that **Paleolithic man became highly optimised for the Stone Age environment.** In the last 10,000 years, mutations have become much more common due to population growth,[1] but most beneficial mutations have not had time to become widespread. **The historical era has been a period of genetic diversification and emerging but incomplete adaptation to modern life.** That means if we want an environment, diet, and lifestyle that will be healthful for all of us, we have to look back to the Paleolithic.

SCIENCE OF THE PHD
Why We Share a Paleolithic Heritage

The Paleolithic began 2.6 million years ago with the invention of stone tools and ended 10,000 years ago with the invention of agriculture. The Paleolithic lasted 100,000 generations and was characterised by small populations, typically, tens or hundreds of thousands; at the end of the Paleolithic the human population was three million. The modern era has a large population — seven billion today — but evolution has had little time, less than 500 generations, to work its magic.

We can calculate how long it will take before every possible mutation appears in some person, somewhere. Every child has a similar number of mutations — about 175 new point mutations among the three billion base pairs of the human genome.[2]

- In the Paleolithic, with 10,000 children per generation, it would have taken 8000 generations, or 160,000 years, for each possible mutation to occur once.
- Today, with more than a billion children per generation, every possible point mutation now appears about 20 times per generation, or almost yearly.

We can also calculate the time required for a beneficial mutation to reach 'fixation', or universal presence throughout humanity. This time is on the order of $\ln(N)/s$, where N is the population size and s is the selection coefficient, a measure of how beneficial the mutation is in terms of expected number of children.[3]

- In the Paleolithic, a mutation that raised the probability of having an extra child by only 0.1 per cent would have reached fixation in 460,000 years. So a mutation with selective advantage of 0.1 per cent would have occurred within the first 160,000 years of the Paleolithic, then become

(continued on next page)

universal 460,000 years later — long before the Paleolithic
was over.

- In the modern era, a similar mutation would occur every
year but would require 200,000 years to reach fixation. The
modern era is less than 10,000 years old, however, so few
recently mutated genes have had time to become universal.
As a result, our genetic adaptation to the new environment of
modern life — agricultural foods, city living, the presence of
governments and complex institutions — is incomplete. And
human genetic diversity is greater than ever before.

Because mutations that would remove our adaptation to Paleolithic
diets have had little time to spread through the population, it is likely
that nearly everyone is extremely well adapted to Paleolithic diets. The
same cannot be said for modern diets.

2
The Paleolithic Diet

• •

- *Eat real food: recently living plants and animals.*
- *Eat mostly plants — but low-carb!*
- *Among plant foods, favour in-ground starches.*
- *Don't be afraid to eat fat! Hunter-gatherers flourished on a fat-rich diet.*

• •

The premise of 'Paleo' diets is that foods hunted and gathered by our Paleolithic ('Old Stone Age') ancestors represent the healthiest human way of eating, while agriculturally-produced foods may be dangerous to wellbeing.

There's solid evidence backing this idea. Direct evidence for the superiority of Paleolithic diets comes from archaeological studies of ancient skeletons. These studies tell us that until the modern era, with our reduced rates of infectious disease, the Paleolithic was the healthiest epoch of human history.

Studies of animals also show that 'wild' diets are the healthiest. For example:

- Thirty-two per cent of pet cats and dogs are obese,[1] but obesity is rare among wild wolves and tigers. It's not only pets: feral rats living in cities and eating discarded human food have grown increasingly obese in parallel with the human obesity epidemic.[2]

Notes for this chapter may be found at www.perfecthealthdiet.com/notes/#Ch2.

- Zoo-born elephants live only half as long as elephants living wild in parks such as Amboseli National Park, Kenya.[3] Zoo elephants also have much higher rates of obesity than wild elephants. Elephants make a great comparison animal, because they are rarely subject to predation in the wild.

What's the 'wild' human diet? Presumably, the diet obtained the same way wild animals obtain their food: by hunting and foraging in the manner of our Paleolithic ancestors.

READER REPORTS: a cure for IBS

I'm 62 and have suffered, along with anyone who gets near me, with IBS for the past 25 or so years, and have tried just about every supplement to alleviate the condition without success. Since starting the PHD my symptoms disappeared in less than a week — and haven't come back. As Billy Crystal would say, 'UN beWEEV abo.' Thanks so much.

— Jack Cronk

Paleolithic Health and Neolithic Decline

The tall stature and strong bones of Paleolithic skeletons indicate that Paleolithic humans were in remarkably good health. Paleolithic humans were tall and slender; cavities and signs of malnutrition or stress in bones were rare; muscle attachments were strong, and there was an absence of skeletal evidence of infections or malignancy.[4]

The adoption of farming in the Neolithic radically changed the diet, and with it came a dramatic loss of health. Farmers needed crops that yielded many calorie-rich seeds from each seed planted, so the harvest could feed the farmer's family for a year and supply seeds for sowing in the spring. This required a turn of the diet to grains and legumes — foods that, as we shall see, are toxic.

After the adoption of agriculture, stature lessened; smaller tendon attachments show that muscles weakened; bone and teeth pathologies, such as cavities and osteoporosis, became common; hypoplasias show that periods of malnutrition were common; and signs of infections and inflammation became common.

SCIENCE OF THE PHD
The Neolithic Decline

A large number of journal articles, anthropology PhD theses, and books discuss the collapse of health that is visible with the adoption of cereal-grain agriculture.[5] A few tidbits:

- Average height dropped, bottoming out at about 160 centimetres for men, 152 centimetres for women around 3000 B.C. — about 13 centimetres shorter than in the Early Upper Paleolithic.[6]
- Bones from the Neolithic site of Ganj Dareh in Israel, studied by the anthropologist Anagnostis Agelarakis, showed hypoplasias on the teeth, indicative of malnutrition when young; signs of ear infections and gum inflammation; broken or fractured bones; and arthritis. Those who survived childhood struggled to reach middle age.[7]
- Nine of 16 Bronze Age mummies — and seven of the eight of people who died after age 45 — in the Museum of Egyptian Antiquities, Cairo, had atherosclerosis.[8]

The drop in stature persisted throughout the agricultural era until modern times. Only in the 20th century, with rising wealth and the elimination of many infectious diseases, did humans regain Paleolithic stature.

So Paleolithic diets were quite healthful — agricultural diets, not so much.

We'd better look into what those healthy Stone Age hunter-gatherers were eating!

Paleolithic Plant Foods: savannah starches

Many people assume that our distant ancestors resembled chimps and gorillas — forest-dwelling apes who ate fruit. That's a mistake.

Our ancestors had a long association with open woodlands and tree-spotted grasslands. Where the fossils of human ancestors have been found, tree cover was generally less than 40 per cent, sometimes as low as 5 per cent.[9]

Fossils testify that our Paleolithic ancestors lived in open, grassy terrain. Fossil hominids lack the stiff spines and long powerful arms of forest-dwelling apes, and appear to have spent much of their time walking bipedally as grassland dwellers do.[10] Ape bipedalism has a long history. *Ardipithecus ramidus*, which dates from about 4.4 million years ago, spent a significant amount of time walking bipedally,[11] as did *Oreopithecus bambolii*, whose fossils date from ten to seven million years ago.[12] Another bipedal hominoid dates to 21.6 million years ago.[13] Very possibly the common human-chimp ancestor was a bipedal ape living in open terrain, and chimps and gorillas adapted to the forest after they diverged from the human line.

Not only did our hominid ancestors live in wooded grasslands — their food came from grasslands too. This has been proven by a clever method — 'isotope signatures' of fossilised bones. Combined with the structure of hominid teeth, this evidence tells us that our ancestors were eating savannah tubers, roots, and corms — foods similar to our modern potato and taro. They had invented the digging stick and were eating starch!

SCIENCE OF THE PHD
How We Know Paleolithic Hominids
Ate In-Ground Starches

Carbon comes in heavy (carbon-13) and light (carbon-12) forms, and grasses and sedges ('C_4 plants') incorporate relatively more carbon-13 than other plants. So the carbon-13 to carbon-12 ratio in a skeleton tells us what fraction of the creature's food was obtained from grassland plants or animals that ate grassland plants.[14]

There is considerable variability, but in general grassland plants

predominated in the diet of Paleolithic and earlier hominids. This
created a puzzle, known as the 'C_4 conundrum'. Hominids such as
Australopithecus africanus and *Paranthropus robustus* did not have the
right kind of teeth for eating grasses and were not thought to be major
hunters of grazing animals, yet their bones show that they got their
carbon from grasses. The resolution of the puzzle: those apes were
getting their dietary carbon from C_4 plant underground storage organs
— tubers and corms similar to the modern potato and taro.[15]

This emphasis on starchy roots, tubers, corms, and rhizomes continued
throughout the Paleolithic. Food residues from Upper Paleolithic sites dated
to 30,000 years ago show that the grinding of starchy roots and rhizomes into
flours and foodstuffs was a common practice.[16] Microfossils on Neanderthal
teeth from around 44,000 years ago show evidence of the consumption of
many roots and tubers, some of which show evidence of cooking.[17] Neanderthal consumption of starchy plants goes back at least 250,000 years.[18]

Modern hunter-gatherers who live in environments that lack starchy plants
all trade for starches produced elsewhere. The anthropologist Thomas Head-
land proposed that it would not be possible for humans to survive in forest
environments without such trade; this was debated as the 'wild yam question'.[19]

READER REPORTS: weight loss and improved energy

I am in the middle of the wardrobe crisis that I've been waiting to have
for ten years: all my clothes are too big. I don't mean a little loose;
I mean I perpetually look like I'm headed out to an M.C. Hammer
costume contest.

Over the past few months I've lost 25 pounds [11.3 kilograms].
That's a good thing, since the drop on the scale was a side effect of
lifestyle changes that have left me with more stamina and energy than
I had when I was 20.

It's not an exaggeration to say that the Perfect Health Diet changed
my life.

— Jennifer Fulwiler

A final line of evidence — genetics — supports the idea that our Paleo-lithic ancestors ate starches. Chimps have two copies of the gene for salivary amylase, the enzyme that digests starches. Humans worldwide average *seven* copies of the gene; aboriginal peoples eating low-starch diets, such as the rainforest-dwelling BiAka and Mbuti pygmies of the Congo Basin, average 5.4 copies.[20] A plausible interpretation is that our Paleolithic ancestors ate enough starch to reach five to six copies of the amylase gene and that subse-quent evolution since the Neolithic invention of cereal-grain agriculture has increased the amylase copy number a bit further.

Paleolithic Animal Foods

The Paleolithic began with the invention of stone tools about 2.6 million years ago. These tools were used to hunt animals, tear meat, and cut bones to reach the marrow. Bone marrow consumption is attested from 1.9 million years ago.[21] The pursuit of marrow, which is nearly all fat, shows that animal fats were a sought-after part of the early Paleolithic diet.

By 1.75 million years ago, ancestral *Homo* had spread to northern lati-tudes, where plant foods are relatively scarce. It is likely these northern hom-inids were eating a meat-based diet.

By 40,000 years ago, we can tell that Neanderthals (hunting herbivores such as mammoths) and humans (hunting many species with an emphasis on fish) were top-level carnivores. Upper Paleolithic humans weren't getting protein from plants — no beans for them! — and were higher-level carni-vores than wolves and arctic foxes.[22]

SCIENCE OF THE PHD
Isotope Signatures of Protein Sources

Nitrogen is found in protein and comes in heavy (nitrogen-15) and light (nitrogen-14) forms. Whenever an animal eats protein, it tends to incorporate nitrogen-15 in tissues and exhale or excrete nitrogen-14, so the ratio of heavy to light nitrogen increases by 3 to 4 per cent with every step up the food chain.

Unfortunately nitrogen-15 is unstable and is only preserved in bones and teeth from the last 50,000 years, so we have no idea how high on the food chain *Australopithecus* or *Homo habilis* were. But nitrogen isotope ratios show that both humans and Neanderthals were at the top of the food chain and getting nearly all their protein from animal food sources.

Another sign that Paleolithic humans were doing a lot of hunting is animal extinctions. The arrival of Paleolithic humans in Australia and the Americas was quickly followed by the extinction of large animal species. Earlier, in Eurasia and Africa, species such as mammoths and saber-toothed tigers were hunted to extinction.

Animal extinctions began at an early date. Between 1.9 million and 1.5 million years ago, *Homo erectus* appears to have caused the extinction of 23 of the 29 known species of large African carnivores.[23] The six species that survived were 'hypercarnivores', such as lions and leopards, which ate only meat; the 23 that went extinct were omnivores such as civets, which scavenged and ate a wide range of foods. It is thought that they went extinct because they were in direct competition — for scavenged carcasses — with hominids.[24]

Subsequent advances in human culture were often followed by new animal extinctions. The extinction of elephants from the Levant around 400,000 years ago was probably due to hunting by archaic humans.[25]

What Was the Proportion of Animal to Plant Food?

Anthropologists debate the relative proportions of plant and animal food in the diet of our Paleolithic ancestors. Unfortunately, for the earlier part of the Paleolithic there is no evidence that directly answers that question.

We do know that a great expansion of brain sizes occurred during the Paleolithic, and it was probably made possible by new calorie-rich food sources. There are two major theories:

1. Stone tools and cooperative hunting enabled our Paleolithic ancestors to obtain fatty animal foods.[26]

2. Control of fire enabled our Paleolithic ancestors to cook starchy plants, rendering them less toxic and more digestible. This greatly increased the calories obtainable from plant foods.[27]

The second theory has been popularised by Richard Wrangham in his book *Catching Fire: how cooking made us human.* However, most anthropologists favour the first. The use of stone tools coincided with the brain expansion; while the first known use of fire was one million years ago,[28] routine use of fire may have begun only 300,000 to 400,000 years ago,[29] and more sophisticated use of fire, such as heat treatment of tools, may have begun 164,000 years ago.[30]

So the foods driving the brain size expansion during the Paleolithic were probably fatty animal foods.

We do have solid evidence for the diets of modern hunter-gatherers, which probably closely resemble the diets of the Upper Paleolithic. They may be our most useful guide to what a 'Paleo diet' for modern humans should look like.

Modern Hunter-Gatherer Diets

The first attempt by an anthropologist to quantify the diets of modern hunter-gatherers was the 1967 *Ethnographic Atlas* of G. P. Murdock, which was corrected in 1999 by J. P. Gray.[31] This looked at 229 aboriginal groups still living in a way that resembled their traditional lifestyle.

The data were analysed by Loren Cordain and colleagues.[32] They found that hunter-gatherers obtained most of their energy from animal foods — meat, fish, and eggs:

- Forty-six hunter-gatherer groups obtained 85 per cent or more of their energy from meat, fish, and eggs, but no groups obtained 85 per cent of energy from plant sources. There were no vegetarian hunter-gatherers.
- One hundred and thirty-three hunter-gatherer groups obtained 65 per cent or more of their energy from meat, fish, and eggs; only eight groups obtained 65 per cent of energy from plants.

- The median group obtained 70 per cent of their energy from animal foods, 30 per cent from plant foods.

Plant foods contain both carbohydrates and fat. Tropical groups ate the most plant foods, and many of those plant foods, such as nuts, coconuts, and palm fruit, were rich in fat. So carbohydrate intake was well below 35 per cent for the overwhelming majority of groups.

The data in the *Ethnographic Atlas* are dated, and some researchers consider them unreliable.[33] Fortunately, detailed studies of the diets of authentic hunter-gatherers have been conducted very recently, and they confirm the results from the *Ethnographic Atlas*. On our blog, we looked at a study of nine hunter-gatherers — Onge of the Andaman Islands, Anbarra and Arnhem Aborigines of northern Australia, Aché of eastern Paraguay, Nukak of south-eastern Colombia, Hiwi of Venezuela, !Kung Bushmen of the Kalahari desert of southern Africa, Gwi Bushmen of Botswana, and Hadza of north-central Tanzania — by anthropologists Hillard Kaplan, Kim Hill, Jane Lancaster, and Ana Magdalena Hurtado.[34]

Every group ate a substantial amount of meat. Animal foods provided 50 to 85 per cent of calories. The !Kung ate the least meat, but still averaged 259 grams per day of meat.

Roots and other in-ground plants were the most important plant food. Seeds and nuts were a small contributor for every group but the !Kung, who ate mongongo nuts, a fatty food. 'Fruits' were more often fatty nuts than the sugary fruits we are familiar with; for instance, the Nukak ate the palm oil–rich fruit of the palm tree, and the Hadza ate a number of fatty fruits. Only the Gwi consumed a significant amount of sweet fruits, chiefly melons.

In eight of the nine cultures, roots were a much more important source of calories than fruits. Among the Gwi, fruits and roots provided an equal share of calories.

Measured by calories, the diets were generally low in carbohydrates and high in fat. **Seven of nine cultures** — the Onge, Anbarra, Arnhem, Aché, Nukak, Hiwi, and !Kung — **ate 10 to 20 per cent carbs.** For the Gwi San a majority of calories were carbs, and for the Hadza about 40 per cent of calories were carbs. For most groups, fat intake ranged from 40 to 70 per cent of calories.

Plant and Animal Food Balance

Although carbohydrates are a small part of calories for many hunter-gatherers, this does not mean they are unimportant. In fact, carbohydrates are a prized part of the diet among modern hunter-gatherers.

Indeed, the Mbuti pygmies of the Congo have two words for hunger: 'protein hunger' (*ekbelu*) and 'calorie hunger' (*njala*). In remote hunting camps on the Ituri plateau of the northeastern Congo, Mbuti generate very high hunting returns and dry large quantities of surplus meat for trade but have no access to starchy plants; in their camps they often complain of *njala*. Similarly, when the Maku hunters of the Amazon Basin run out of cassava in the forest, no matter how much meat they have, they 'have no food'.[35]

The natural inference is that a healthful diet needs a certain amount of plant foods to balance its animal foods. As we'll see, starchy in-ground plants are so calorie-poor that even obtaining a mere 15 per cent of calories from

READER REPORTS:
'drying out' from too few carbohydrates

I reached my weight loss goals by eliminating grains and limiting dairy to butter and cream and reducing fruit intake. That said, over the last month or so, I was wondering why my body seemed to be drying out from the inside out. I wanted to tweak my diet to optimum health and found your book. The information about the importance of mucin was helpful. What was missing in my diet were the carbs that you recommend. Sweet potatoes, white rice etc. Maybe less protein than I've been eating and more saturated fat . . .

I'm having better results every day. I am fascinated that I have a laboratory of my own body to put your ideas to a test and have them show positive results. Thank you both so much.

— Doris Hames, Atlanta, Georgia

carbs means consuming more plant foods than animal foods by weight. The Paleolithic diet may have been low-carb, but it wasn't low-plant.

Takeaway: the diet of the Paleolithic

The Paleolithic diet was a fat-predominant, low-carbohydrate diet. Calories came mainly from fat-bearing animal foods, but plant foods were an essential part of the diet and comprised most of the weight. Typically:

- Carbohydrates made up 15 to 20 per cent of calories, with excursions toward 50 per cent depending on food availability. Most calories came from fatty animal foods.
- Plant foods consisted predominantly of starchy in-ground carbohydrate sources such as roots, rhizomes, tubers, and corms, plus above-ground fat sources such as coconuts, palm fruit, and mongongo nuts. Sweet fruits were rarely a major part of the diet.

It was on a majority-fat, low-carb diet mainly composed of animal foods and in-ground plants that our ancestors evolved from a regional population of small-brained African apes numbering (probably) in the tens of thousands to a highly intelligent species at the top of the food chain and a global population in the millions.

As our Paleolithic ancestors who dominated the globe were characterised by tall stature and healthy teeth and bones, and their health deteriorated as soon as their diet was altered, we think it's safe to say that such a low-carb, high-plant, starch-, meat-, and fat-based diet is a healthful human diet.

3

The 'Cannibal Diet' of Fasting

· ·

Instead of 'You are what you eat,'
you need to 'Eat what you are.'

· ·

In Paleolithic times and often since, food was not always readily available. It would have been common to experience extended periods when food was scarce.

Hungry or not, it would have been necessary to hunt and forage — even, on occasion, to fight. Evolution would have selected human (and animal) biology to ensure that these tasks could be performed well even after days without food.

Indeed, we know that hunter-gatherers often went without food and functioned quite well. The Jesuit missionary Paul LeJeune, in his 1636 *Relation* of life among the Montagnais hunter-gatherers of Canada, described their attitude to involuntary fasts:

> I saw them, in their hardships and their labors, suffer with cheerfulness ... I found myself, with them, threatened with great suffering; they said to me, 'We shall be sometimes two days, sometimes three, without eating, for lack of food; take courage, *Chihiné*, let thy soul be strong to endure suffering and hardship; keep thyself from being sad, otherwise though wilt be sick; see how we do not cease to laugh, although we have little to eat.'[1]

Notes for this chapter may be found at www.perfecthealthdiet.com/notes/#Ch3.

Humans Must Have Been Well Adapted to Fasting

We know from accounts like LeJeune's that extended involuntary fasts were common among hunter-gatherer peoples.

Fasts would have been times of heightened mortality. During famines, the mortality rate from infectious disease is dramatically increased.[2] Also, hunter-gatherers are likely to pursue riskier food, increasing the death rate from accidents. These were common causes of death among hunter-gatherers. Among the modern Kitavans, infections — primarily malaria — and accidents — primarily drowning and falling from coconut trees while pursuing seafood and coconuts — are the leading causes of death.[3]

It's plausible to think that death rates from violence, too, would have been higher at times of food scarcity. Violent deaths were common among hunter-gatherers. Lawrence Keeley reported that at the first site he excavated, 'about 5 per cent of all human skeletons contain embedded arrowheads'[4] and estimated that in the late Paleolithic, violence accounted for 20 to 30 per cent of deaths. At the late Paleolithic cemetery at Gebel Sahaba in Egyptian Nubia, dating to about 12,000 to 14,000 years ago, over 40 per cent of those buried had stone projectile points associated with their skeletons. Several adults had multiple wounds (as many as 20), and many showed healed parry fractures of their forearm bones — a common trauma on victims of violence and proof that violence was not a once-in-a-lifetime event.[5] The risk of violence is illustrated by the death of Ötzi, the copper-age Tyrolean iceman. Ötzi was killed by an arrow; he was carrying a copper war ax, a flint knife, a bow, and 14 flint-tipped arrows; and he had the blood of four other persons on his arrowheads, knife, and clothing.[6]

It appears that Paleolithic people were often threatened with death at times of fasting and that **the ability to hunt, gather, fight, and survive infection during a long fast would have been strongly favoured by evolutionary selection.**

Nourishment During a Fast

During a fast, we cannibalise ourselves. Tissues throughout the body are broken down and their raw materials are released for other tissues to use.

The 'diet' of self-cannibalisation during a fast need not have been perfectly healthy, but it must have enabled near-maximal performance and been reasonably healthy.

We could reproduce this 'cannibal diet' by eating food identical in composition to the human tissues that are broken down during a fast. This diet, too, should be reasonably healthful, but also sustainable, as it wouldn't require any tissue loss.

So what nutrients do we obtain during the 'cannibal diet' of a fast?

The Composition of the Human Body

A relatively lean 70-kilogram 'reference man' is composed of 42 kilograms of water, 13.5 kilograms of fat, 10.6 kilograms of protein, 3.7 kilograms of minerals, and about 0.5 kilogram of glycogen (a storage form of glucose) in muscle and liver.[7]

If we just convert this to calories, allowing 9 calories per gram for fat and 4 calories per gram for protein or glycogen, we get the following macronutrient distribution:

Body Component	Mass (kg)	Energy (kcal)	Energy Fraction
Fat	13.5	121,500	73.2%
Protein	10.6	42,400	25.6%
Glycogen	0.5	2000	1.2%

However, this would be misleading. Fat and protein are complex molecules that are not burned for energy directly. **Both fat and protein actually contain some carbohydrate.**

The elemental forms of fat, protein, and carbohydrate that feed into energy metabolism — *fatty acids, amino acids,* and *glucose* — are not allowed to roam freely in the body because they are chemically reactive and would be toxic. Instead, they are found in more complex molecules.

The Composition of Fats and Proteins

Fat is present in the body as *triglycerides* and *phospholipids*. When these molecules are broken down for energy, 85 to 90 per cent of the calories is in the form of fatty acids, 10 to 15 per cent in the form of glucose assembled from their glycerol backbones. Protein also consists of complex molecules. Many of the proteins in the human body are 'glycosylated', meaning they are composed of sugars bonded to amino acids. In some there is more sugar than amino acids. For example, mucin-2, the main protein of digestive tract mucus, is 80 per cent sugar and 20 per cent amino acids by weight.

If we break down fats and proteins into their constituent fatty acids, amino acids, and sugars, the energy profile of a lean human body would look something like this:

Body Component	Energy (kcal)	Energy Fraction
Fatty acids	106,900	64.4%
Amino acids	37,300	22.5%
Carbohydrate	21,700	13.1%

This looks very close to the macronutrient mix eaten by Paleolithic hunter-gatherers!

We cannot get quite as much carbohydrate from eating animal foods as we can from self-cannibalisation during fasting, because carbohydrates and proteins degrade soon after the animal dies, releasing glucose, which cells consume through anaerobic metabolism. This process removes carbohydrates from meat. Nevertheless, proteins and fats in animal foods are hidden sources of dietary carbohydrate.

Eat What You Are, and Make Fasting Easy

Fasting means hunger and misery to most people. Never mind a three-day fast: just a four-hour fast between meals makes some people hungry and cranky!

Those who adopt a Paleo diet are often surprised and pleased to find that fasting has suddenly become easy and comfortable — not exactly pleasurable, but far from intolerable.

The reason this happens is that our body adapts to our diet. Different cellular machinery, enzymes, and vitamins are involved in metabolising glucose, fatty acids, and amino acids.

If our diet provides glucose, fatty acids, and amino acids in the same proportions that are released during the 'cannibal diet' of fasting, we'll be well prepared for a fast. Fasting will be easy.

But if we eat a very different diet, fasting can become hard. A high-carb diet will give us lots of machinery for metabolising carbs, but a dearth of machinery for metabolising fatty acids. When fasting starts and self-cannibalisation begins providing 65 per cent of energy in the form of fatty acids and only 13 per cent as glucose, cells won't be prepared to handle

---

READER REPORTS:
PHD and fasting for body recomposition

After 'standard' PHD (maybe too low carb PHD) for about six months I've been doing intermittent fasting for the past 3–4, and have had better success than before. (Success = weight loss without significant muscle loss.)

In my case I lift once a week, and on that day I drive carbs above 200g. I do 60–90g carbs on off days. Protein is consistent at 130–150g per day. All days are 16/8 IF.

By watching calories (1600 off day, 2000 workout), I'm now down 11 kilograms after nine months. I've taken a couple of multi-week 'diet breaks' in which I ate ~2000 calories per day making up the daily 400 calorie difference entirely in fat. It felt like a lot of food, but I didn't gain an ounce, and as soon as I resumed my 1600/2000 split I started losing immediately. During this time, I've maintained or increased my strength (as measured by weight and/or time-under-load).

So I am a fan. I've been lighter before, but never had this little fat mass.

— John Davi, Palo Alto, California

that mix. Instead, they'll be hungry for the much larger amounts of glucose they're used to getting.

The natural way of eating is to obtain macronutrients in similar proportions to the composition of our own tissues. The natural way to eat is to '**eat what you are**'. This will prepare the body for fasts and make hunger rare.

Takeaway

Obesity, like other diseases, has multiple causes. But whatever other factors may contribute to a weight problem, eating macronutrients in the proportions found in useful tissue will make weight loss easier.

Cells in lean tissue prefer to take in nutrients they can use as structural molecules; and they can only accept structural molecules in very specific proportions.

Eating food in the proportions of lean tissue allows all cells, not just adipose cells, to take up an energy excess. Potentially, excess calories may end up as useful tissue such as new muscle, rather than extra fat around the waist. Since muscle is the primary energy disposal tissue, while adipose tissue is where energy is stored, directing excess energy to muscle is more likely to lead either to muscle synthesis or successful elimination of the excess calories.

But if you eat in the wrong proportions, lean tissue will reject some of the excess energy and it will have to be stored as fat in adipose tissue. If pathologies subsequently inhibit the transfer of fat from adipose tissue to muscle for disposal, the fat will accumulate.

Do your body a favour: eat what you are. Make it easy for your body to build useful tissue, and you'll make it easy for useless fat tissue to melt away.

4

What Breast Milk Teaches Us About Human Diets

• •

Don't be afraid of fat.

• •

W hat is the perfect diet for a baby? We know the answer: **mother's milk.** Ideally, breast milk should be the sole food a baby consumes for its first four to six months of life, and a continuing part of its diet for some time thereafter.

How Perfect a Food Is Breast Milk?

The first six months of life are a perilous time for infants. Even today, with all of our progress in decreasing the infant mortality rate, among newborns it is higher than at any other age below 58 years.[1]

In prehistoric times, infants were in mortal danger. The infant mortality rate is 10 to 30 per cent among modern hunter-gatherers,[2] and in the Paleolithic it may have been even higher.[3] Given the high death rates among infants, any genetic change that improved infant survival would have been strongly selected by evolutionary pressure. Since the composition of breast milk is largely programmed by maternal genes, mortality was certainly subject to such selection. We can be confident that evolution would have optimised the composition of mother's milk to make it a **complete and perfect diet for infants.**

Notes for this chapter may be found at www.perfecthealthdiet.com/notes/#Ch4.
Notes specific to this Australian edition are indicated with †

Clinical Evidence That Breast Milk Is Best

Breast-fed infants experience many health benefits compared to formula-fed babies. The mortality rate from infectious disease is far lower in breast-fed babies. A study from Brazil found that non-breast-fed babies were 14.2 times more likely to die of diarrhoea and 3.6 times more likely to die of respiratory infections than exclusively breast-fed babies. Partially breast-fed babies were 4.2 times more likely to die of diarrhoea and 1.6 times more likely to die of respiratory infections than exclusively breast-fed babies.[4]

Some benefits of breast-feeding are long-lasting. In the Promotion of Breastfeeding Intervention Trial (PROBIT), children whose mothers had participated in a World Health Organization program that encouraged them to breast-feed had a substantially higher IQ at age six — 5.9 points higher — and better academic ratings from teachers than children whose mothers had not participated.[5] Another study found that breast-fed infants had IQs 8.3 points higher at age eight than formula-fed infants.[6] An Australian study found that breastfeeding for six months or longer leaves children less likely to suffer from mental-health problems later in life.[†]

The Composition of Human Milk

Along with water, the main constituents of milk are:[7]

- The sugar lactose (which is composed of the simple sugars glucose and galactose). Human milk typically has 70 grams of lactose per litre.
- Fats, typically 40 grams per litre.
- Human milk oligosaccharides — special sugars that, like fibre, are indigestible by humans but feed gut bacteria. Human milk typically has 15 grams of oligosaccharides per litre.
- Protein, typically 8 grams per litre.

Let's look at what these constituents tell us about the optimal diet for infants and adults.

Macronutrients

By calories, and excluding the contribution from milk oligosaccharides, human milk has a macronutrient profile of 54 per cent fat, 39 per cent carbs, and 7 per cent protein.[8]

Note the order:

- Fat provides the majority of milk's calories.
- Carbohydrate is the second largest calorie source.
- Protein provides the fewest calories.

This order holds in the milk of every mammalian species, not just humans. For instance, milk from cows is 52 per cent fat, 29 per cent carbohydrate, and 19 per cent protein.

This is similar to the pattern of Paleolithic diets, which were also majority fat, minority carbs and protein.

Fatty Acid Profile

Fats come in several kinds of *fatty acids*. The table below shows the fatty acid profile of human breast milk at day 16 after delivery.[9] We have organised the fatty acids into five groups:

- **Short-chain and medium-chain saturated fatty acids (SaFA),** which have no functional role in the body and are directed to the liver, where they are transformed into ketones that nourish the brain;
- **Long-chain SaFA** and **monounsaturated fatty acids (MUFA),** which are the primary fatty acids in cell membranes throughout the body;
- **Omega-6** and **omega-3 polyunsaturated fatty acids (PUFA),** which play special roles in the body by adding fluidity to cell membranes and serving as signalling molecules and sensors of oxidative stress.

Seventy-two per cent of breast milk fats are long-chain SaFA and MUFA. These fatty acids are the mainstays of cell membranes, the most abundant fatty acids in the body.

Fatty Acid Type	Share of Breast Milk Fat	Share of Energy
Short- and medium-chain SaFA	10.4%	5.6%
Long-chain SaFA	34.2%	18.5%
MUFA	37.6%	20.3%
Omega-6 PUFA	14.6%	7.9%
Omega-3 PUFA	3.1%	1.7%

Breast milk has relatively high levels of polyunsaturated fatty acids. These high levels support infant brain growth; infant brains are fast-growing, and the brain has very high levels of PUFA. Brain fatty acids are 15.4 per cent omega-6 and 11.7 per cent omega-3 — overall, 27.1 per cent PUFA.[10] The rest of the body has a much lower usage of PUFA.

This tells us that the optimal PUFA intake for adults, whose brains are no longer growing, is going to be less than the 9.6 per cent of energy devoted to PUFA in breast milk.

A (perhaps) surprising aspect of breast milk is its high content of short-chain and medium-chain fatty acids, which have no structural role in the human body. (Indeed, shorter-chain fatty acids are dangerous to bacteria, which incorporate them into cell membranes; membranes with shorter-chain fatty acids become leaky, potentially leading to cell death. This is why short- and medium-chain fatty acids can be used as antibiotics.) The short- and medium-chain fatty acids in breast milk are transformed in the liver into neuroprotective ketones that support growth of the infant brain.

SCIENCE OF THE PHD
Ketones for the Brain

Short- and medium-chain fatty acids are shunted to the liver, where they are converted to ketones — small water-soluble molecules that are building blocks for fats and can be metabolised for energy like fats. The ketones then diffuse through the body and are mainly taken up by the brain, where they are used for energy and as building blocks for the synthesis of cholesterol and saturated fat.

(continued on next page)

It turns out that ketones are essential to infant survival. Mice deprived of the ability to utilise ketones die within 48 hours after birth. Extra glucose can't save them.[11] In humans, major lipid components of the brain, such as cholesterol, are nearly all manufactured from ketones, and a mild elevation of ketones seems to be essential to infant brain function.[12]

The importance of ketones for the infant brain is relevant because, as we'll see later, ketogenic diets — diets that generate lots of ketones — are therapeutic for many brain and neurological disorders. Eating in a way that is mildly or occasionally ketogenic may help prevent diseases such as Alzheimer's dementia or Parkinson's.

Fibre

Human milk contains about 200 different 'human milk oligosaccharides' — special sugars that play a role similar to fibre in the adult diet. Milk oligosaccharides are indigestible by humans but feed beneficial gut bacteria while inhibiting pathogens from binding to the gut wall.[13]

Human milk contains up to 23 grams per litre of these oligosaccharides, providing babies with 10 to 17 grams per day.[14] Human milk has more of this 'fibre' than it does protein!

After feeding on these sugars, gut bacteria release short-chain fatty acids, such as butyrate, which provide about 3 per cent of a baby's total energy. These short-chain fats add to the ketogenic nature of the infant diet.

Probiotics

Breast milk contains lactic acid bacteria. These bacteria are thought to travel from the mother's intestine to her mammary glands inside white blood cells. They populate the infant digestive tract and can inhibit pathogenic bacteria from taking root there.[15]

Cholesterol

Human breast milk is rich in cholesterol. It always contains at least 100 milligrams per litre of cholesterol, and cholesterol levels reach 220 milligrams per litre in the afternoon and evening.[16]

A breast-fed baby's cholesterol intake is 100 to 200 milligrams per day. Scaled by body weight, this is ten times higher than the typical cholesterol intake of American adults.

SCIENCE OF THE PHD
How Cholesterol Phobia Spoiled Infant Formula

One would think the designers of infant formula would try to make an exact copy of human breast milk. Alas, they don't.

Infant formula is cholesterol-deficient. Formula typically has only 10 to 30 milligrams per litre of cholesterol, one-tenth the amount in human breast milk.[17]

This deficiency has consequences. Breast-fed babies reach normal serum cholesterol levels by age six months, while formula-fed babies are severely cholesterol-deficient at age six months.[18]

Cholesterol is important for neurological function and immunity, so this could be a reason why formula-fed babies have lower IQs and higher rates of infectious disease mortality.[19]

Cholesterol has been demonised for decades, based on a now-discredited hypothesis that dietary cholesterol might contribute to heart disease. It would have been best to ignore the experts and let evolutionary selection be our guide to what is healthful.

Differences Between Infants and Adults

Before we try to interpret what the composition of breast milk is telling us about diet, let's think about how infants differ from adults in their nutritional needs.

The major difference between infants and adults is that *babies have big brains.*

At birth, a baby's body is only about 5 per cent of adult size, yet the infant's brain already weighs fully 28 per cent of its adult weight. By age one, the infant brain weighs 75 per cent of its adult size, and by age six, 90 per cent.[20] So the infant brain is not only very large compared to its body; it also grows faster than the rest of the body throughout the first year of life.

The infant brain uses a lot of energy. At birth, the infant brain accounts for 11 per cent of body weight but fully 74 per cent of calorie consumption. By comparison, the adult brain accounts for just 2 per cent of body weight and 23 per cent of calorie consumption.[21]

Yet the brain has very different energy needs from the rest of the body. The brain does not utilise many fats for energy, because fats are transported into the brain too slowly to be burned routinely.

SCIENCE OF THE PHD
Why the Brain Doesn't Use Fats for Energy

The 'blood-brain barrier' is a name for the special behaviour of blood vessels feeding the brain. Normally blood vessels facilitate the passage of nutrients, including fats, into tissues behind them. But in the brain, blood vessels are more cautious.

One reason is that the body wants to prevent brain infections. Most pathogens have a fatty cell membrane. Even viruses, which aren't cells, are often 'enveloped' in a fatty container. Pathogens often spread from cell to cell using pathways taken by fatty particles. By limiting uptake through these pathways, the blood-brain barrier makes it hard for pathogens to enter the brain. (This is why brain infections are often preceded by an injury that breaches the blood-brain barrier.)

But keeping pathogens out has a cost: the brain can't take up fats very rapidly. Since fats come into the brain slowly, it would be risky to lose them. So they aren't routinely burned for energy. Instead, the brain relies on glucose and ketones for energy.[22]

If the brain uses much more energy in infants than in adults, and if the brain is reliant on glucose and ketones, that tells us that glucose and ketone needs are going to be much higher in infants than in adults. Infants need:

- More carbohydrate in their diet than adults do
- More short-chain and medium-chain fatty acids — the precursors of ketones — than adults do

If we are right in thinking that Paleolithic diets and the 'cannibal diet' of fasting are good patterns for the optimal adult diet, there's nothing surprising about the composition of breast milk. Here's a comparison:

Macronutrient	Paleolithic/ Cannibal Diet	Breast Milk
Carbohydrates	13–20%	39%
Short-chain and medium-chain fats	~3%	8.7%
Other fats	~60%	46%
Protein	15–25%	7%

Breast milk does indeed have more carbs and short-chain and medium-chain fats, and fewer long-chain fats and protein. The oligosaccharide content of milk, which after fermentation by gut bacteria provides another 3 per cent of energy as short-chain fatty acids, confirms the importance of ketogenic fats in the infant diet.

· ·

READER REPORTS: improved energy and health

The improvements I have seen since implementing this diet are numerous. My energy levels are much steadier throughout the day (as opposed to the constant 'peaks and troughs' I experienced whilst following a vegetarian diet for 4 years); my cravings for sugar have virtually disappeared; I have only suffered from one cold in the past 10 months as opposed to my usual 2 or 3; my weight is effortlessly stable; I never feel hungry despite switching from 6 small meals per day to just 3; the list goes on!

— Richard McBride

· ·

Takeaway: what breast milk tells us about the optimal diet

Breast milk tells us everything about the optimal infant diet, much about the optimal diet of children, and is supporting evidence for our view of the adult diet.

Regarding carbohydrates, it tells us that carbs should account for 39 per cent of calories in infants and then a gradually decreasing fraction of energy as children grow into adults. It doesn't tell us the optimal carb fraction for adults — we'll need more evidence — but we can be pretty sure that the 'cannibal diet' of fasting is too low in carbs, and the Paleolithic diet might have been too low in carbs. So optimal adult carb intake is probably above 20 per cent but probably not more than 35 per cent of total energy intake.

Breast milk probably gives us an upper limit to the optimal adult PUFA intake. Infants obtain about 9.6 per cent of their energy as PUFA, but they have a great need for PUFA to support the rapid growth of the infant brain. Adults, who have a stable brain size, need substantially less dietary PUFA.

Breast milk confirms that saturated and monounsaturated fats should be the largest source of calories at all ages. There's no good reason to be afraid of fats!

5
What Mammalian Diets Teach Us About Human Diets

· ·

*You can be healthy eating like a herbivore —
but not as a vegetarian!*

· ·

Shou-Ching's Buddhist friends used to try to persuade her to become a vegetarian by saying 'Look how strong cattle and horses are. Why not eat vegetarian and be as strong as they are?'

Of course, lions, tigers, and wolves are strong on carnivorous diets, so the argument wasn't very convincing.

Yet it raises an interesting question. Why are animal diets so varied? Can animal diets tell us anything about the optimal human diet? If not, why do scientists spend so much time studying mice and rats? Are scientists idiots? (Please don't answer that.)

If we told you that all mammals eat nearly the same diet, you might think we were crazy. The grassy diet of a lamb is nothing like the meaty diet of a lion.

But what if these dietary differences are illusory? Consider that:

- Cow's milk, indeed the milk of all mammals, has a similar macronutrient composition to human milk — with most calories as fat.
- All mammals have a similar body composition — their cells are

Notes for this chapter may be found at www.perfecthealthdiet.com/notes/#Ch5.

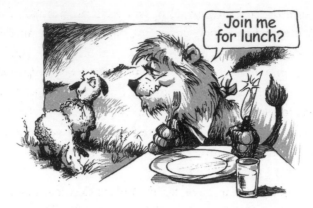

Lions and lambs don't eat the same diet . . . or do they?

composed of fatty membranes and proteins in roughly the same proportions — and 'cannibalise' themselves during starvation. So their fasting 'diet' must have a similar ratio of fat, protein, and carbohydrate.

These considerations tell us that *all mammals have similar macronutrient needs.* Why, then, do the foods they eat differ so greatly?

The Transformation of Food into Nutrients

To resolve this paradox, think about the process of digestion. **Food** is what is eaten; **nutrients** are what reach the body after digestion. The digestive tract converts food into nutrients:

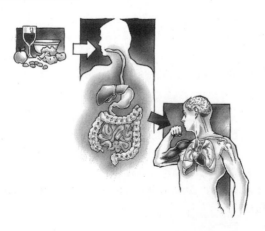

Conversion of food into nutrients isn't a simple process. The digestive tract doesn't merely break food down into its constituent nutrients; *it also transforms some nutrients into other nutrients.*

In most mammals, the most important digestive transformation is the fermentation of **fibre and carbohydrates** into **fats** — specifically, **short-chain fatty acids** such as propanoic and butyric acids — by gut bacteria. These short-chain fatty acids can be lengthened into saturated fatty acids that can be incorporated into tissue, or reduced to ketones that can be burned for energy.

Every mammal that eats a vegetarian or plant-dominant diet has sections of its digestive tract devoted to bacterial fermentation. There are two broad groups, foregut and hindgut fermenters. The ruminants — cattle, sheep, and goats — are foregut fermenters, and their digestive tracts begin with organs called rumens devoted to fermentation. In other species, such as gorillas, fermentation occurs in the latter part of the digestive tract, in the colon.

Let's look at various mammals to see what their diets look like *after* digestion.

Gorillas

The macronutrient composition of the diet of wild western lowland gorillas[1] is shown in the table below.

The Western Lowland Gorilla Diet

Macronutrient	Weight Fraction (g/100g)	Calories/g	Calories/ 100g of Food	Per Cent of Energy
Fats	0.5	9	4.5	2.3%
Carbohydrate (ex fibre)	7.7	4	30.8	15.9%
Protein	11.8	4	47.2	24.4%
Fibre	74	1.5	111	57.4%

It looks like a low-fat diet, doesn't it? Only 2.3 per cent of calories are in the form of fat.

But that is *before* food is transformed by the digestive tract.

Note the really large component of the gorilla diet: fibre. Fibre is fermented by gut bacteria. The bacteria get 4 calories per gram from fibre, but they give back 1.5 calories per gram in the form of short-chain fats to the gorilla. Even with such a low caloric density, the mass of fibre in the wild gorilla diet is so large — 74 per cent of the mass of food eaten — that those short-chain fats contribute fully 57 per cent of the gorilla's energy.

The Western Lowland Gorilla Diet *After* Transformation

Macronutrient	Per Cent of Energy
Polyunsaturated fat	<2%
Saturated and monounsaturated fat	58%
Carbs (ex fibre)	15.9%
Protein	24.4%

The fibre has been converted into short-chain saturated fatty acids, which can then be lengthened into saturated fats and desaturated into monounsaturated fats. So after transformation, SaFA and MUFA are 58 per cent of calories.

Polyunsaturated fats cannot be made from short-chain fatty acids, so they have to come from the original fat content of the diet, which was only 2.3 per cent. We haven't seen a fatty acid profile of gorilla foods, but PUFA content is surely less than 2 per cent of the diet.

As in Paleolithic human diets, the 'cannibal diet' of fasting, and breast milk for infants, a majority of calories are obtained as saturated and monounsaturated fats and a minority as carbs and protein.

Cattle, Sheep, and Goats

Ruminants have evolved special organs for bacterial digestion of plant foods. In these organs, bacteria scavenge every carb calorie, *leaving none for the animal.* As a by-product of carb digestion, the bacteria release volatile short-chain fatty acids. These fats are transported to the liver, which uses them for energy and for fabrication of sugars, ketones, and fats for the rest of the body.

Dr Richard A. Bowen summarises how cattle, sheep, and goats get their energy:

> Volatile fatty acids (VFA) are produced in large amounts through ruminal fermentation and are of paramount importance in that they provide greater than 70% of the ruminant's energy supply . . .
>
> Within the liver, proprionate serves as a major substrate for gluconeogenesis, which is absolutely critical to the ruminant because almost no glucose reaches the small intestine for absorption.[2]

After processing by the gut, ruminant macronutrient ratios are something like:

- 0 per cent carbs
- 18 per cent protein
- 70 per cent proprionate, butyrate, and other short-chain fatty acids
- 12 per cent long-chain fats

The liver then converts short-chain fatty acids to ketones, glucose, and saturated and monounsaturated fats to meet energy needs.

Once again, this is a fat-rich diet that is low in polyunsaturated fat.

Wolves, Dogs, and Cats

Most wild carnivores obtain nearly all their energy from animal flesh. Wolves, for instance, obtain about 5 per cent of calories as fallen fruit, but 90 per cent of calories or more come from animal flesh.

You might think this makes for a protein-rich diet, but carnivores favour the fattier parts of their prey. Barry Groves notes, 'This is particularly noticeable with hyenas whose jaws and teeth are designed to break the long bones and skulls to get at the bone marrow and brain within, which are very high in fat.'[3] Since carnivores seek out fatty parts of their prey and often abandon lean muscle meat for scavengers, it's fair to conclude that the animal portion of their diet is at least as fatty as the fat-protein ratio of the 'cannibal diet' during human fasting: 74 per cent fat, 26 per cent protein.

If the fats in their prey are 15 per cent polyunsaturated,[4] carnivore macronutrient ratios typically are:

- 5 per cent carbohydrates
- 23 per cent protein
- 61 per cent saturated and monounsaturated fats
- 11 per cent polyunsaturated fats

Cats typically eat no carbohydrates at all. In carnivores generally, the liver manufactures glucose from protein to meet the needs of neural and immune cells.

Mice

Rodents are omnivores that, in the wild, eat a lot of seeds. Seeds, like nuts, often contain substantial amounts of fat.

In the laboratory, mice are usually fed a chow that consists mainly of cereal grains, which are very high in starch. So the standard laboratory mouse diets are high-carb diets.

But what do mice really want to eat? When scientists let mice choose their own food from an unlimited supply of carbs, fats, and protein, most strains choose to get a majority of their calories from fat. In a study of 13 strains of mice, nine chose to get a majority of calories from fat. Only two chose to consume more carb than fat calories.[5]

When scientists allowed a wild-type mouse strain that develops obesity and diabetes on a 40 per cent carbs, 40 per cent fat chow to choose its own diet, it chose a diet of 5.6 per cent carbs, 82.5 per cent fat, and 12.0 per cent protein and 'proved highly resistant to the development of obesity and diabetes'. In the same study, transgenic mice genetically engineered to be even more prone to obesity and diabetes self-selected to a diet of 2.2 per cent carbs and 85.1 per cent fat and 'developed obesity [that was] . . . less pronounced than on a high-fat and high-carbohydrate Western diet . . . [and] did not become hyperglycemic; they showed decreased fed and fasted blood glucose levels'.[6]

We probably can't infer much from genetically mutated mice that avoided obesity by choosing 85 per cent fat diets. But it is telling that most strains of wild-type mice chose to get a majority of calories from fat and a minority from carbs and protein — the same pattern we've seen repeatedly in other mammals, in humans, and in breast milk of all mammalian species.

Summary: optimal mammalian macronutrient ratios

Wild mammals, no matter what foods enter their mouths, provide their bodies with very similar macronutrients:

- 0 to 16 per cent carbohydrates
- 15 to 25 per cent protein
- 56 to 77 per cent saturated and monounsaturated fats
- 1 to 11 per cent polyunsaturated fats

An equivalent diet for humans would have more carbs (to feed our larger brains) and less protein and fat. We might infer, then, that the optimal human diet is something like 20 per cent carbs, 15 per cent protein, 60 per cent saturated and monounsaturated fat, and 5 per cent polyunsaturated fat.

Why Humans Need to Consume the Optimal Mammalian Macronutrient Ratios

The digestive tract and liver transform food into the nutrients we need. The gut transforms fibre into short-chain fatty acids; the liver transforms nutrients into other nutrients.

What would happen to a creature that lost its ability to transform nutrients?

Exactly this has happened in humans: compared to apes and other mammals, *we've lost our guts.*

Here is a comparison of brain, liver, and gut sizes in humans and other primates:[7]

Organ	Per cent of Body Weight, Humans	Per cent of Body Weight, Other Primates (Scaled for Body Size)
Brain	2.0%	0.7%
Liver	2.2%	2.5%
Gut	1.7%	2.9%

Compared to other primates, humans have a 12 per cent smaller liver and a 40 per cent smaller gut. This means we have less ability to transform food with an improper nutrient mix into the nutrients we need to maintain health.

It gets even worse for us when it comes to transforming fibre into fat. In primates, this is done in the colon — the large intestine. The small intestine is where digestible nutrients — glucose, amino acids, and fatty acids — are absorbed. Here is the fraction of the gut devoted to small and large intestines in humans and apes:[8]

Species	Large Intestine	Small Intestine	Stomach
Gorilla	60%	14%	25%
Chimpanzee	57%	23%	20%
Human	17%	67%	17%

Humans with our small colons can obtain at most 7 per cent of energy from fibre[9] — much less than the 60 per cent of energy chimps and gorillas obtain from fibre. The highest fibre intake ever observed in any human culture is 86 grams (about 130 calories) per day — about 6 per cent of energy.[10]

The Paleolithic diet, it seems, was so close to our optimal nutrient needs that we ceased to need much of our digestive tract. Evolution got rid of 80 per cent of our colon volume and shrank our livers.

The implication is that like other mammals, we humans are best nourished when our digestive tracts deliver to our body a nutrient mix that is majority fat, minority carb and protein. Unlike other mammals, humans *lack the ability to transform foods* with the wrong nutrient mix into the right one. In particular, we lack the ability to ferment large amounts of vegetable matter into fat.

More than other animals, **we humans need to eat our natural diet** —
one that is majority fat, minority carbs and protein.

SCIENCE OF THE PHD
Human Dietary Variability

Is the same diet optimal for different people?

All mammals need the same nutrients, but the digestive tract
determines which foods will generate those nutrients.

If the optimal diet is determined by digestive tract differences, we
should expect the same pattern to recur in humans. All humans have
the same *nutrient needs*, but our optimal *food intake* may vary if our
digestive tracts differ.

In fact, there is evidence for variations in digestive tract structure
among human populations. Compared to Europeans, Africans have
slightly larger colons, suggesting a slightly more plant-focused
evolutionary diet and a greater ability to ferment fibre into short-chain
fats. Europeans have slightly smaller colons, suggesting a more animal-
focused evolutionary diet.[11]

We've previously mentioned the variation in the number of copies
people have of the gene for salivary amylase, which facilitates digestion
of starches. People globally average seven copies, but some people
have as many as 15 copies and some as few as two.[12] Higher amylase
copy numbers improve the quality of starch digestion and blood glucose
regulation.

Variability Due to Disease and Gut Microbiome

Everyone has a personal set of gut microbes. Gut microbes assist in the
digestion of food and alter immune function, so differences in gut flora
could lead to differences in the optimal foods.

Diseases and infections can also disrupt digestion, and this may
alter the optimal diet. We've long held the principle that 'All healthy
persons are alike; each unhealthy person is unhealthy in his own way.'[13]

(*continued on next page*)

In a way, the variability of diet with disease is good news: changes in the optimal diet can help us diagnose disease.

Conclusion

There is some dietary variability across persons, due to variations in digestive tract structure, genes for starch digestion, gut flora, and diseases. However, these variations are probably small. Fibre contributes only a few per cent of energy to the human diet, so it doesn't matter much if one person's colon is 20 per cent longer than another's. Similarly, nearly everyone has enough amylase copies to adequately digest starches.

So for the most part, the diet that is perfect for human health probably does not vary much across persons. There is certainly no reason to suppose that it varies with blood type or other nondigestive aspects of our biology!

The Three Mammalian Dietary Strategies

Although mammals thrive on similar macronutrient ratios, we can tease out a few differences among omnivore, herbivore, and carnivore diets.

Each diet has a different strategy for meeting the body's glucose needs:

- **Omnivores** eat enough carbohydrates to meet the body's glucose needs directly.
- **Herbivores** obtain little glucose from their diet but up to 70 per cent of their energy needs from short-chain fatty acids produced by bacterial fermentation. Short-chain fatty acids with even numbers of fatty acids may be transformed in the liver into ketones, which nourish neurons, reducing the body's glucose needs; fatty acids with odd numbers of carbons may be used to manufacture glucose.
- **Carnivores** obtain few or no carbohydrates from their diet and meet their glucose needs by manufacturing glucose from protein.

The fact that these three strategies are all evolutionarily successful shows that they can all produce superb health in mammals. There are some implications for human diets:

- **Most mammals satisfy their glucose needs by manufacturing glucose in the liver,** not by eating it. This suggests there may be a health advantage to keeping glucose intake a little below the body's needs and thereby keeping blood glucose levels low. *This is a clue to the benefits of low-carb diets.*
- **Mammalian short- and medium-chain fat intakes cover a huge range — 0 to 70 per cent.** This tells us that short- and medium-chain fats are safe for humans and that ketogenic diets, in which a large share of calories is obtained from short- and medium-chain fats — for instance, diets with a very high intake of coconut oil, which is 58 per cent medium-chain fat — may be a feasible human dietary strategy. *This is good because ketogenic diets are therapeutic for some diseases.*

We think it's fair to say that the solution to the optimal human diet was there all along — in the zoo! Mammalian diets are a reliable guide to the nutrient needs of the body and therefore to what we should be eating.

Takeaway

The basic structure of cells — a protein-rich intracellular compartment surrounded by fatty membranes — hasn't changed in billions of years. The need for cells to be able to obtain energy by cannibalising themselves hasn't changed in that time either. So it should come as no surprise that all mammals have similar macronutrient needs.

Mammals do need different foods — some are obligate herbivores, some obligate carnivores — but this is because they have different digestive tracts, not because their bodies have different nutrient needs.

All mammalian diets point to the same basic macronutrient ratio: a macronutrient ratio that is majority fat, minority carbs and protein. The typical mammalian diet is about 10 per cent carbs, 20 per cent protein, 65 per cent saturated and monounsaturated fat, and 5 per cent polyunsaturated fat.

Adjusting for our larger brain size, this suggests an optimal ratio for humans around 20 to 30 per cent carbs, 15 per cent protein, 50 to 60 per cent saturated and monounsaturated fat, and 5 per cent polyunsaturated fat.

Which is strikingly close to the Paleolithic diet, the cannibal diet of fasting, and the composition of breast milk adjusted for brain size!

6

The 'Tastes Great!' Diet

. . . .

Healthful food is tasty. Every meal should be delicious!

. . . .

'Nothing in biology makes sense except in the light of evolution,' said Theodosius Dobzhansky. Certainly this is true of our sense of taste. Why do some things taste bitter? We can sense the presence of toxins in food, and bitter taste makes us avoid them.

What makes food delicious? Why did evolution design our brain to enjoy certain food combinations?

The Compromise Between Efficiency and Health

Evolution undoubtedly selected for efficient food collection. The idea that easy-to-obtain foods will form the bulk of our diet has been dubbed 'optimal foraging theory'. ('Lazy forager theory' would have been a better name, we think; or 'path-of-least-resistance foraging theory'.) However, sometimes this idea is taken too far, to the inference that easy food-gathering is the sole determinant of our diet, as in this formulation by Michael Sheehan: 'human decisions are made such that the net rate of energy capture is maximized'.[1]

This is too extreme, because evolution also selects for *healthful eating*. It's not enough to merely seek energy; animals also need a host of nutrients in the right proportions. They need to avoid toxins. They need to seek out beneficial bacteria for the gut, as in probiotic foods, and avoid rotten foods that might cause disease.

The evolutionarily selected part of the brain that guides us toward healthful eating is called the *food reward system*. It teaches us to *like* and *want* foods that are good for us. Liking, or the pleasure in eating something healthful, rewards us for healthful eating; wanting motivates us to do extra work to obtain more healthful food.

Imagine you are one of our Paleo-era ancestors. Would you prefer a rotting carcass that you can capture in one minute, or fresh meat that requires 30 minutes to capture? If it's the latter, it's because your food reward system has overridden your 'lazy forager' system.

Can We Always Trust Our Food Reward Impulses?

It would be convenient if our likes and wants always led us to healthful eating. Unfortunately, that's not guaranteed.

In eating disorders, the food reward system is disturbed, so that sufferers want to eat in an unhealthful way.

But even in healthy people, the food reward system may lead us astray.

READER REPORTS: a need for carbohydrates

I was finally successful at adding back in some carbs. I am now able to eat half of a small sweet potato on a daily basis, while still losing weight! You were right, the weight gain — about 5 pounds [2.27 kilograms] — was merely a temporary 'hump' I had to get over before starting to go back down.
I was afraid I'd be stuck eating very low carb forever!

As a bonus, my eyes are no longer blurry, and my hair appears to have started growing back. When I put it in a ponytail, there is a thick halo of new fuzz where formerly my scalp was visible. I am surprised at how quickly these issues began to resolve — it has been perhaps a month, if not less.

— Melanie

Consider the case of sugar. We've already seen that in the Paleolithic, hunter-gatherers could easily obtain fatty meat by hunting but had a difficult time obtaining carbohydrates. Their diet was typically only 10 to 20 per cent carbs by calories. Suppose the optimal carb intake was 30 per cent of calories. Then the food reward system would evolve a want for carbs to try to induce Paleolithic foragers to do extra work to get their carb intake up to 30 per cent.

Our sense of taste is attractive for sweets but responds only weakly to fat; this may be evidence that evolution tried to enhance a strong want for carbohydrates but had no need to establish a similar innate attraction to fats.

But what happens in the modern world, where sugar is easily obtained? We still have our evolutionary want for carbs — sugar still tastes sweet — but we are no longer discouraged by the long, laborious search needed to find carbs in Paleolithic times. The 'food reward system' still encourages us to acquire carbs, but our 'lazy forager system' no longer discourages us.

The result, quite likely, is going to be that in the modern world we'll *overeat* carbs, especially sweet sugars.

Here is actual carbohydrate consumption as a share of calories from countries around the world, plotted against a measure of national income per person:[2]

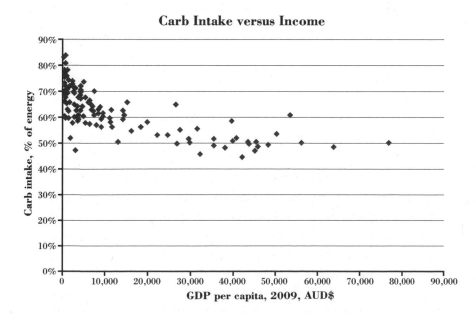

In very poor countries, people eat high-carb diets because grains such as wheat, corn, rice, and sorghum are all they can afford. As income increases, people buy more animal foods, and carb consumption goes down. However, at high income levels the drop in carb consumption levels off. When people can afford to eat whatever they want, they still consume 45 to 50 per cent of calories as carbs.

If our evolutionary reasoning based on the composition of breast milk was correct, the optimal carb intake is 39 per cent for infants and less — probably around 30 per cent — for adults. This indicates that people all over the world are overeating carbs.

We infer that the food reward system sometimes overshoots the mark. Evolution wanted Paleolithic man to eat more than 15 per cent carbs, so it made carbs tasty, sweet, and rewarding. In the modern world, where carbs are easy to obtain, the food reward system overrewards carbohydrate consumption and leads most people to eat more carbs than is optimal.

SCIENCE OF THE PHD
Is Obesity Caused by a Disconnect Between Our Brains and Our Food?

In November 2011, the television show *60 Minutes* did a fascinating report, 'The Flavorists', showing how the food company Givaudan makes industrial food enticing.

Flavourists at Givaudan go into orchards and fields to find natural flavours that can be chemically isolated and introduced into food to make it more pleasing. Among the flavours they've found: castoreum, which beavers secrete in urine to mark their territory. Castoreum tastes like raspberry and vanilla and is listed on labels as 'natural raspberry flavour'.

For decades, manufacturers have been learning how to make prepared foods out of the most inexpensive ingredients, not necessarily the most healthful ones, and improving the taste with chemically isolated flavouring compounds. This explains the long ingredient lists on packaged foods.

Many researchers believe that these industrial foods are contributing to the obesity epidemic. It's plausible: people stopped cooking at home and increased their intake of industrial foods at about the time the obesity epidemic started, in the 1970s; and since the 1970s industrial foods have increasingly diverged from natural foods.

A common view is that industrial foods promote obesity because they are 'hyperpalatable': so palatable that people will continue eating them even after they are full. (Have you ever been at a restaurant and said, after the steak and potatoes, 'I can't eat another bite,' but then found room for dessert? The meat and potatoes were palatable; the dessert was hyperpalatable.) Junk food is often designed to be hyperpalatable: eat one nacho cheese–flavoured Dorito, and before long you've eaten the whole bag and headed out to the store for more.

Here is how one recent review phrases the idea that modern food is *too rewarding:*

> Food reward, not hunger, is the main driving force behind eating in the modern obesogenic environment. Palatable foods, generally calorie-dense and rich in sugar/fat, are thus readily overconsumed despite the resulting health consequences.[3]

Another review concludes:

> These findings collectively suggest that obesity can arise when animals or humans are confronted with foods whose palatability/reward value greatly exceeds that to which they are genetically adapted.[4]

Though these ideas have a solid experimental basis — nothing makes rats fatter than a 'cafeteria diet' of hyperpalatable junk food — we believe that an equally important factor is that industrial food is *malnourishing.*

The brain's appetite regulation mechanisms evolved to make the body well nourished. Evolution has produced sophisticated mechanisms optimising every human activity. It has surely generated a mechanism for sensing the nutritional status of the body, promoting appetite when nutrients are needed, and suppressing appetite when the body is well nourished and food unnecessary.

(*continued on next page*)

If this is so, the fact that tasty foods are available need not by itself lead to chronic overeating. Hyperpalatable but nourishing foods might cause temporary overeating, but would be followed by subsequent undereating. Chronic overeating occurs only if the tasty foods are malnourishing and fail to satisfy bodily needs. Unfortunately, too many modern industrial foods are severely lacking in many of the nutrients contained in real food — plants and animals.

Whatever the reasons commercial foods promote obesity, there's a simple solution: *don't eat non-nourishing industrially manufactured foods.* Until packaged foods manufacturers start assembling their products out of real foods — edible plants and animals — good health may demand avoidance of their products. That means shopping around the edges of the supermarket to obtain fresh plants and animals and cooking at home.

The good news: if we eat natural foods, our reward system will be a reliable guide to what is good for us, just as it was in the Paleolithic.

READER REPORTS: a delicious and satisfying diet

I'm never hungry on the PHD and I'm really enjoying all the food I CAN eat, while not missing the food I can't eat.

— David S.

I have been eating the PHD for a while, and it has really reduced any sort of cravings and tendency to mow down, even if the food is really yummy.

— Wyatt

So the food reward system is not a perfect guide to what we should eat. But it is a very good guide. When we look at nutrients that were easily obtained in the Paleolithic, we find that the food reward system guides us very accurately to the optimal amount.

Protein is a good example. Let's consider it.

Protein Consumption

How much protein should a person or animal eat?

Well, dietary protein has two uses in the body:

- It can be used to make human proteins.
- It can be converted to glucose or substitute for glucose as an energy source.

The amount of protein that should be eaten is the amount that will satisfy both needs. For the sake of argument, let's say that 200 calories of protein is needed to satisfy the body's protein needs and 600 calories of carbohydrates will satisfy the body's carb needs. Therefore:

- If the amount of carbs eaten is greater than 600 calories, we should 'want' 200 calories of protein.
- If the amount of carbs eaten is less than 600 calories, we should 'want' 200 calories of protein for protein synthesis needs, and enough additional protein to make up the deficit in carb intake. When carb intake is below 600 calories, every reduction of carb intake should lead to a corresponding increase in protein intake.

This pattern has been tested in rats. Rats were fed chow with various combinations of protein and carbs to see when they would stop eating. Here is what happened.[5]

When carbohydrate was abundant, the rats kept eating until their protein intake was 4.6 grams. They would consume extra carbohydrate and extra calories until they got precisely that amount of protein. Rats never ate more than 4.9 grams of protein when carbs were abundant.

When carbohydrate was scarce, the rats ate extra protein. The less carbohydrate was available, the more protein they ate.

We've fit the data with two lines. Once the rats obtained about 12 grams of carbohydrate, they ceased to care about dietary carbohydrate at all; they just kept eating until they'd obtained 4.6 grams of protein, then stopped eating. However, below 12 grams of carbohydrate, the rats ate extra protein, presumably so that they could manufacture glucose to replace the missing carbs.

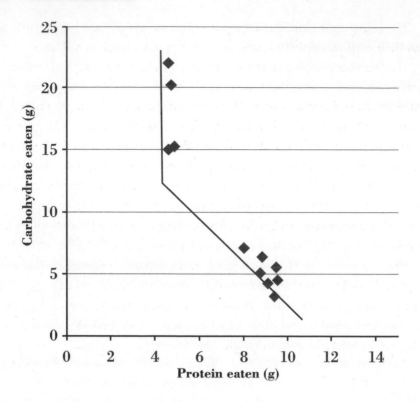

SCIENCE OF THE PHD
On a Low-Carbohydrate Diet, How Is Glucose Replaced?

The rats' ideal carb and protein intake looks to be about 12 grams of carbs and 4.6 grams of protein. As carb intake decreases below 12 grams, protein intake increases. On a zero-carbohydrate diet the rats would eat about 12 grams of protein.

If protein utilisation stays constant at 4.6 grams, only 7.4 grams of protein are used to manufacture glucose to replace the missing 12 grams of carbohydrate; only about 60 per cent of ideal glucose intake is replaced with protein. Reductions in glucose utilisation and displacement of glucose with ketones made from fat account for the other 40 per cent.

The rats seem to know exactly the right amount of food to eat to meet both their carb and protein needs. A similar pattern holds in humans.[6]

The fact that at high carb intakes, protein intake is fixed and independent of carb intake has some interesting implications. It means that *protein is a dominant determinant of appetite.* Both rats and people want to get a particular amount of protein, and they keep eating until they've gotten it. This is why so many popular weight-loss diets, from Atkins to the Dukan Diet, are high in protein. When people try to eat high-protein diets, they find that their appetite disappears as soon as they have eaten the amount of protein that the food reward system seeks. They end up eating less. For a while, this appetite suppression causes rapid weight loss. Those few weeks are often enough to get dieters excited and telling their friends, 'This new diet really works!'.

Unfortunately, we do need other nutrients beside protein, and after a while the brain realises that the body needs some missing nutrients. Appetite is upregulated in order to get those missing nutrients. So lean-meat diets only suppress appetite and promote weight loss for so long. We do not recommend them as a long-term weight-loss strategy.

Salt Consumption

Another nutrient that the food reward system manages is salt.

Salt is a highly rewarding nutrient, in animals as well as humans. Indeed, animals will dig caves deep into mountains in order to mine salt. Kitum Cave reaches 700 feet into Mount Elgon in Mount Elgon National Park, Kenya, and it's thought to have grown to its current size through the efforts of elephants to scrape salt from its walls.[7] Gorillas chew on rotted wood for reasons that once mystified scientists. It turns out they do it for sodium.[8]

The American Heart Association urges consuming less than 1500 milligrams of sodium per day, but hardly anyone in the world complies with that.[9] A survey of 33 countries found that despite vast differences in cuisine, people consistently take in about 3700 milligrams of sodium a day.[10] That's the amount in 1.6 teaspoons of salt.

We have biological evidence for how much salt we need. When the body's sodium levels become low, levels of the hormones renin and aldosterone rise in order to conserve sodium. A significant increase in these hormones occurs when salt intake drops below 1.5 teaspoons per day.[11]

So it looks as though biology and food reward are both sending us the same message: we need about 3.7 grams of sodium per day, equivalent to the amount in 1.6 teaspoons of salt.

This was confirmed recently in a careful study reported in the *Journal of the American Medical Association* that measured salt intake via sodium excretion in urine and followed subjects for five years to assess their death rates. The mortality rate was lowest when sodium intake was in the range of 4 to 6 grams per day. Sodium intake below 3 grams per day significantly raised the mortality rate, as did sodium intake above 7 grams per day.[12]

SCIENCE OF THE PHD
The Experts' Faulty Advice to Avoid Salt

For years, people have been warned to avoid salt. The American Heart Association advises consuming less than 1.5 grams per day of sodium. (The Australian Heart Foundation and the New Zealand Ministry of Health have more sensible guidelines, recommending less than 6 grams and 4 to 6 grams respectively.)[†]

The hypothesis — it is little more than that — is that eating more salt can lead to a slight rise in blood pressure, higher blood pressure is associated with heart disease and strokes, so maybe eating more salt will cause more heart disease and strokes.

Too often, experts dole out such advice based on unproven hypotheses without ever looking at the evidence from evolutionary selection. In fact, evolution selected for a certain salt intake. Antisalt advice was not supported by reliable studies: as recently as summer 2011, before the JAMA study was released, a Cochrane review found that no long-term studies on the effects of salt intake had yet been performed and the short-term studies that had been performed had found no clear benefit from reducing salt intake.[13]

The JAMA study indicates that those consuming less than 2 grams per day of sodium raised their five-year cardiovascular mortality risk by 37 per cent. Anyone following the American Heart Association's advice would have raised his or her mortality risk by even more.

Flavour Combinations

Flavour combinations are highly rewarding. Desserts usually combine carbs with fat, for instance.

Try this experiment. Take a baked potato and put butter, vinegar, and salt on it. It will taste delicious. Now eat the baked potato by itself, butter by itself, vinegar by itself, and salt by itself. You may have trouble finishing the meal.

It looks as though evolution designed the food reward system to get us to eat foods in combination. Does that make sense?

It does, because combining foods *increases their nourishment* and *reduces their toxicity.*

For good nourishment, we need a balanced diet — a diet that includes a broad range of nutrients. No single food has a broad enough range of nutrients. It's easiest to achieve balance if we combine a diversity of plant and animal foods at every meal. The food reward system encourages us to do that.

Toxicity is another problem with unbalanced diets. A famous rule of toxicology — Paracelsus's rule — is that 'the dose makes the poison'. Small amounts of a toxin will be harmless, but large amounts can be very dangerous. Many foods are like this: a small amount of bok choy is healthful, but 900 grams a day of raw bok choy can be deadly. Recently a Chinese woman needed four weeks in the hospital to recover from that amount.[14]

So the food reward system encourages us to mix and match foods, eating only a modest amount of any one food.

Food combining is beneficial for starchy carbohydrates. You may have heard of the 'glycemic index', a measure of how high blood glucose levels rise after eating a food. In general, blood glucose levels below 140 milligrams per decilitre are safe, but glucose becomes increasingly toxic above that level; and higher-glycemic-index foods are more likely to increase blood glucose to a dangerous level.

But the glycemic index is radically reduced when foods are combined:[15]

- Fat reduces the glycemic index. Putting butter on French bread lowers its glycemic index from 95 to 65.
- Fibre reduces the glycemic index. Adding a polysaccharide fibre

to cornstarch reduced its GI from 83 to 58; to rice reduced its
GI from 82 to 45.

- Acids, such as vinegar, reduce the glycemic index. The amount
of vinegar in sushi rice is sufficient to dramatically reduce its
glycemic index. Pickled foods, which are sour due to lactic acid
released by bacteria, reduce the glycemic index of rice by 27 per
cent.

Sauces in traditional cuisines typically combine an acid, such as lemon
juice or vinegar, and a fat, such as olive oil or coconut milk. These sauces
beneficially reduce the glycemic index of a meal, lowering its potential to
induce hyperglycemic toxicity. (They are also nourishing in their own right.)

Takeaway: eat delicious, nourishing foods

The food reward system evolved to make us healthy, and the evidence from
food combining, salt intake, and protein intake is that it does, in fact, induce
us to eat in the optimal way. For these foods and others, following our innate
taste preferences is the healthiest course.

So eat tasty, delicious meals. Delicious food is good for your health!

There is a concern among some researchers that eating tasty food may
encourage people to overeat.

We believe this concern is valid in the case of non-nourishing junk food.
On a junk food diet, the body will crave nourishment and the brain will
keep sending you back for more food until the body has been nourished.

However, we believe that most people will have no tendency to overeat
on a Paleo-style diet composed of real foods — plants and animals. Real
food nourishes and satisfies. However enjoyable a Paleo meal may be, it's
unlikely you'll feel a desire to continue eating and eating.

So go ahead, eat a steak and potato! It's good for you.

Strategies for Limiting Overeating

If you do find that eating tasty, delicious food causes you to overeat, there are well-attested methods for reducing caloric intake:

- *'Hara hachi bu'* is an ancient Confucian principle: eat until you are 80 per cent full. Step away from the table before you are stuffed.
- Intermittent fasting is a proven technique for calorie restriction, which has many health benefits. Skip either the first or last meal of the day — breakfast or dinner — to extend the overnight fast to 16 hours. You'll find this is easy to do on a low-carb Paleo-style diet.
- During your fast, eat a spoonful of an MCT oil or coconut oil. The psychologist Seth Roberts, in *The Shangri-La Diet*, found that eating such 'tasteless calories' in isolation suppresses appetite.

There are also healthful ways to increase calories expended, such as exercise or exposure to cool temperatures. All of these methods for balancing caloric intake would be more healthful than avoiding delicious food.

7

The Way We Were Meant to Eat

Evolutionary evidence has gotten us far enough that we can see the outlines of the Perfect Health Diet. Let's summarise the PHD (for Perfect Health Diet) macronutrient profile:

Macronutrient	PHD Recommended Intake as Per cent of Energy
Carbohydrates (not including fibre)	20–30% for adults, 30–40% for children
Protein	7% for infants, 10–20% for adults
Carbohydrates plus protein	30–50% for adults, 46% for infants
Fats plus fibre	50–70%
Polyunsaturated fats	2–5%
Fibre	1–3%

Other dietary guidelines:

- Eat real food — plants and animals.
- Make your food as delicious as possible.
- Stop eating when you are 80 per cent full; engage in intermittent fasting, just as Paleolithic people did.

We have a pretty good idea, now, what the optimal human diet will look like. This evolutionary diet will be our lodestar as we look at the science in more detail.

But before we do that, let's consider one question. How important is it to eat the way we were meant to eat? Does it really matter if we deviate from our natural diet?

It's Important in Gorillas

For many decades, zoos have fed gorillas something very different from their evolutionary diet.

The natural gorilla diet consists of fibrous, low-calorie vegetation and wild fruits. About 57 per cent of calories comes from fibre, which is converted to short-chain fatty acids. Only 16 per cent of the natural gorilla diet reaches the body as carbs.

But the standard zoo diet for gorillas, which includes biscuits and sweet domesticated fruits, reversed those percentages. Only 14 per cent of calories come from fibre and over half from carbs.[1]

The result? Over one-third of zoo gorillas die of heart disease. Even at young ages, many zoo gorillas show evidence of health problems such as obesity, high blood pressure, high cholesterol and triglyceride levels, fibrosis of the heart, and unnatural behaviours including regurgitation and reingestion ('R&R') of food and plucking and eating their own hair.

After Brooks, a 21-year-old gorilla, died of heart failure at Cleveland Metroparks Zoo in 2005, the zoo and Case Western Reserve University biologists looked to see if the gorillas' diet could be improved.

The biscuits were replaced with 4.5 kilograms per day of vegetables: endive, dandelion greens, romaine lettuce, green beans, and alfalfa hay. The zoo's remaining gorillas, Bebac and Mokolo, each lost 29.5 kilograms, their abnormal behaviours of R&R and hair plucking were eliminated, and their cardiovascular biomarkers improved.[2]

Australians Deviate from the Evolutionary Diet Just as Gorillas Did

The macronutrient ratio eaten by the typical Australian is 45 per cent carbs, 32 per cent fat, 18 per cent protein, and 5 per cent alcohol.[3]

This is similar to the 50 per cent carbs, 30 per cent fat, 15 per cent protein, and 5 per cent alcohol diet that is recommended by the Australin government.[4]

It is also similar to the composition of a McDonald's large cheeseburger meal, with French fries and a soft drink.[5] Yes, the 'standard Australian diet' (or SAD) and the Australian government's dietary recommendations are, in terms of their macronutrients, indistinguishable from fast food.

Zoo gorillas had to switch about 40 per cent of calories from carbs to fat to match the ratio that evolutionary evidence says is best. Australians would have to shift about 30 per cent of calories from carbs to fat to do the same.

Just like gorillas, one-third of Australians die of cardiovascular disease.

Would Australians benefit, just as zoo gorillas did, from eating the way evolution equipped us to eat?

The experience of Perfect Health Dieters has been that, in humans as in Bebac and Mokolo, cardiovascular risk markers dramatically improve within weeks of adopting the diet. Often, improvements to blood pressure and lipid profiles are the first things new PHD'ers notice. Reversal of atherosclerosis and of all components of metabolic syndrome have been reported.

Onward

We've now completed our big-picture evolutionary view of the natural human diet. It should give us confidence to ignore dieticians who tell us to avoid salt, fat, and tasty food.

From here we have two missions:

- to understand what foods we should be eating
- to understand in detail how food interacts with the body in health and disease, so that we can use biological science to further refine our way of eating

Part II looks at the foods that should provide the bulk of our calories: safe starches, other healthful plant foods, meat, fish, eggs, and healthful oils.

Part II

What to Eat for Energy

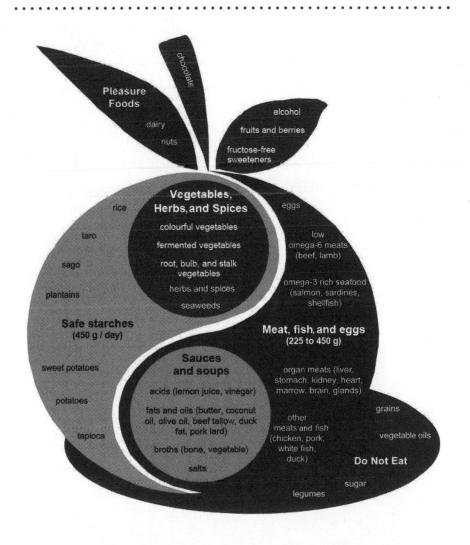

8

An Economical Approach to Nutrition

In Part I, evolutionary evidence got us close to the optimal diet. Now we need to close in on its precise nature. *Nutritional biology* will get us there.

You'll recall that food only directly affects the digestive tract; it's quickly broken down into nutrients that nourish the body:

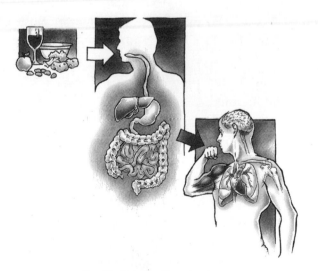

Foods enter the digestive tract;
nutrients leave the digestive tract and enter the body.

Notes for this chapter may be found at www.perfecthealthdiet.com/notes/#Ch8.

The natural way to investigate diet is to study the impact of foods on the digestive tract *and* the impact of nutrients (and any toxins that survive digestion) on the rest of the body.

Nutrients Are Not Food

Even though we'll be talking for a number of chapters about nutrients, one thing should be clear: nutrients are no substitute for food — edible plants and animals.

Michael Pollan has made this point eloquently: 'Food rules,' he says, and it is disastrous to pursue 'nutritionism' — the idea that collections of nutrients can replace natural foods.

Plentiful evidence supports this position. For example, laboratory mice and rats are fed either 'chow', which consists of seeds, grains, beans, and alfalfa — foods similar to what rodents eat in the wild — or a 'purified-nutrient diet', whose ingredients are:

> Casein, L-Cystine; Corn Starch, Maltodextrin 10, Sucrose; Cellulose; Soybean Oil, Lard; Mineral Mix; DiCalcium Phosphate, Calcium Carbonate, Potassium Citrate; Vitamin Mix, Choline Bitartrate; FD&C Red Dye #40.[1]

Purified-nutrient diets are protein, starch and sugar, fibre, fat, vitamins, and minerals. Nothing more. They are missing a host of biological compounds found in plants and animals.

Rodents that eat purified-nutrient diets are usually in worse health than rodents that eat chow. Often, purified-nutrient diets make rodents fat. (When you see a 'high-fat diet' reported in the news, it means a purified-nutrient diet that is 30 to 60 per cent fat by calories.)

Most likely, purified-nutrient diets are unhealthy because *they are malnourishing.* Research versions of purified-nutrient diets are clearly nutrient-deficient, since extra choline,[2] extra zinc and copper,[3] or extra zinc, chromium, and selenium[4] relieve the health problems they induce. More fundamentally, food is full of nutrients that we don't know we need. We share a common biology with plants and animals, and their tissues contain premade biological compounds that are valuable to us and that we may not be able to construct in adequate quantities from purified nutrients.

It's curious: when humans want to lose weight, they often start eating meal replacement bars and weight-loss shakes composed of purified nutrients — the very kind of diet that makes rodents fat!

Packaged food products, too, often have a long list of ingredients quite similar to the ingredients in purified-nutrient rodent diets. In the last 50 years, a large share of our food consumption has shifted from natural foods prepared at home to industrial foods manufactured from purified sources. It may be no coincidence that the obesity epidemic began around 1970, the time when packaged foods became a large part of our diet.

In place of this misguided 'nutritionism', Pollan suggests a few simple rules: 'Eat food. Not too much. Mostly plants.'[5]

We agree with Pollan's food rules — we'll elaborate on why at the end of Part II — but the most important is the first: 'Eat food.'

Although Pollan's rules are valid, we need to delve deeper. Look at how sparse Pollan's rules are. They don't tell us *which* foods to eat or in what proportions to eat them. A raw vegan diet and a meat-and-vegetables low-carb diet could both be diets of 'food; mostly plants'. To understand which foods to eat, we need help from nutrition.

READER REPORTS: success from eating 'real food'

I've been following your PHD for over a year now. You can add me to the list of your success stories as I lost 15 pounds [6.8 kilograms], have no 'cravings', and eliminated GERD, heart palpitations, panic attacks and other annoying pains. It still amazes me that something as simple as eating 'real food' as the majority of my diet can have such a profound impact on my health.

— Shelley, Pennsylvania

Nutrients Are Guides to Foods

Our strategy is this: *let nutrients guide us to the best foods.* In Part II, we will study our nutrient needs and then work backward to find foods that provide them. If we eat foods that have the nutrients we know we need, it's likely we'll get healthful amounts of the unknown nutrients too.

Studying diet at the level of nutrients has two great advantages:

- It takes advantage of the science of biology. Our bodies are composed of cells, and the nutrient needs of cells can be studied in test tubes; but cells cannot be fed foods, as they have no digestive system. So if we didn't think in terms of nutrients, we would lose the information from all those test-tube studies and from molecular biology.
- There are fewer nutrients than foods, so nutrient-body interactions are simpler than food-body interactions.

Studying how nutrients impact health, rather than how foods impact health, gives us more information and fewer variables. It's far more likely to be successful at figuring out the best diet than thinking in terms of foods or food categories, such as 'red meat' and 'whole grains'.

But even though studying nutrients is easier than studying foods, it's still complex. We need to approach nutrition the right way.

The Puzzle of the Perfect Diet

The perfect diet should:

- provide a sufficiency of every nutrient
- deliver a minimum of toxins and no excess of nutrients that might feed pathogens or promote cancer or obesity

That way, all possible benefits from nutrients are obtained, and none of the detrimental effects from toxins or nutrient excess are experienced.

What makes nutrition complicated is that there are many nutrients —

perhaps over 100 — which need to be obtained in the right proportions. Proportions matter, because nutrients cooperate with one another to make us healthy. A cell that was all fatty membranes and no protein, or all protein and no fatty membranes, would be dead.

That nutrients need to be in proportion makes it hard to figure out the optimal amount of each. If a study shows that vitamin A is harmful, does that mean people should reduce their vitamin A intake? Or does it mean that the study population was vitamin D–deficient and vitamin A and D need to be in proportion, so the proper thing to do is to keep vitamin A intake the same and increase vitamin D?

It's easy to leap to false conclusions when nutrient interactions are important. Often, nutritional scientists do just that. That's why they so often have to reverse past advice.

These reversals are confusing, and not only to those who just want to know what to eat. They're confusing to scientists, too. We know this from personal experience!

Economics Can Help Our Understanding of Nutrition

Fortunately, another discipline can help us to think sensibly about nutrition: economics.

Like the human body, an economy is built through cooperation. Nutrients cooperate to make a healthy body in much the same way that factors of production, such as people, resources, and machines, cooperate to make a productive economy.

The most important concept we can borrow from economics is that of *declining marginal benefits:*

- In economics, this means that the first worker a business hires does the most important work. The next labourer does the next most important work. And so on — each additional worker does less valuable work, until it doesn't make sense to hire another.
- In nutrition, this means that the greatest benefit comes from the first bit eaten of any nutrient. Each additional bit provides less benefit than the bit before. Eventually, the benefit from additional amounts approaches zero.

Declining marginal benefits apply to toxins as well as nutrients. It implies that the first bit eaten of any toxin has low toxicity. Each additional bit is slightly more toxic than the bit before. At high doses, the toxicity of each bit continues to increase, so that the toxin is increasingly poisonous.

Increasing marginal toxicity of toxins was first noticed by the medieval physician Paracelsus, who formulated the toxicologist's rule: the dose makes the poison. At low doses, toxins are not dangerous; but at high doses they can be deadly.

At very high doses, most nutrients become toxic or harmful. We can draw for most nutrients a 'marginal benefit curve' that looks like this:

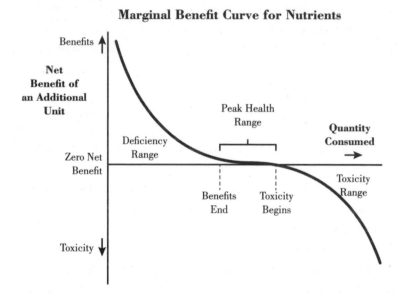

Marginal Benefit Curve for Nutrients

As the quantity consumed goes up, marginal benefits decrease and go to zero at a point marked in the figure by the phrase 'Benefits End'. As the quantity consumed increases further, marginal benefits turn negative at the point in the figure labelled 'Toxicity Begins'. A 'good calorie' or 'nutrient' at low doses becomes a 'bad calorie' or 'poison' at high doses.

There is an optimum quantity of most nutrients, located over the range in the curve where the marginal benefits are close to zero. This range, which we call the **peak health range,** encompasses doses for which all the benefits of the nutrient are captured, but none of the toxicity.

If we were to translate this *marginal benefits curve* into a *total benefits curve,* plotting all the benefits received — in other words, how healthy a person is — against how much of the nutrient has been consumed, it would look like this:

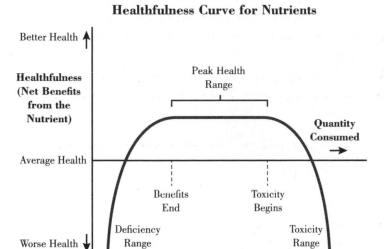

Healthfulness Curve for Nutrients

At low intakes, health is poor because of nutritional deficiency disease. At high intakes, health is poor due to toxicity. Health is maximised in the peak health range.

One interesting lesson these curves teach us: the same nutrient can be a 'good' nutrient (if it is relieving a deficiency) or a 'bad' nutrient (if it is aggravating an excess). If omega-6 fats are bad, it is because we eat too much of them; if omega-3 fats are good, it is because we eat too little of them.

The perfect diet is the one that gets *every* nutrient into its peak health range. It is defined by a single principle: **eat so as to gain all possible benefits and no toxicity from food.**

READER REPORTS: addressing autism through nutrition

My [autistic] son's gastrointestinal issues have been improving from the addition of probiotics and better nutrition. He is also starting to say a lot more words this summer. He is asking for things with words for the first time. I can't say what helped him since there are so many variables interplaying [including intensive ABA therapy] but I am happy to see improvements in language. Our pediatrician was shocked and excited about his improvements. Many thanks again for your help and kindness!

— Erik

Macronutrients and Foods for Energy

Part II looks at **macronutrients** — nutrients that can be burned for energy. (We'll look at micronutrients — nutrients that can't be burned for energy — later.)

Macronutrients fall into five categories:

- **Proteins,** which are digested into *amino acids.*
- **Carbohydrates,** which are digested into elemental *sugars:* glucose, fructose, and (in the case of milk sugar) galactose.
- **Fats,** which are digested into several varieties of *fatty acids* with different biological effects:
    - **Short-chain and medium-chain fatty acids** are directed to the liver and redistributed to the body as ketones (a water-soluble energy source, similar to alcohol) or other lipids;
    - **Long-chain saturated fatty acids and monounsaturated fatty acids** are the main structural fats of the body, composing over 80 per cent of cell membrane fatty acids;
    - **Omega-6 and omega-3 polyunsaturated fats** have both structural and signalling functions. They are

chemically fragile and act as 'sensors' of danger that stimulate various protective responses. In small quantities, they enter into cell membranes, making them slippery and fluid. (When you next buy fresh salmon, let the oil get on your hands and see how slippery it makes them!)

- **Fibre,** which is digested by gut bacteria and transformed into short-chain fatty acids.
- **Alcohol,** which may also be metabolised for energy.

We'll aim to find the peak health range for each macronutrient and then work backward to the foods we should eat to provide our body with energy. Let's start with protein.

9
Protein

· ·

- *Optimal protein intake is achieved by eating about 225 to 455 grams per day of meat, fish, and eggs.*
- *More protein is needed on low-carb diets and by athletes in training.*
- *Children, especially infants, shouldn't eat too much protein.*
- *People trying to lose weight shouldn't eat too little protein.*
- *Lower protein intake may promote longevity; higher protein intake promotes strength.*
- *For longevity and muscle both, try intermittency: high protein intake after workouts, low protein intake on rest days.*

· ·

Except for some protein-deficient vegans and misguided bodybuilders, almost everyone eats a healthful amount of protein. As we mentioned earlier, the food reward system of the brain takes a special interest in protein; people are hungry for protein when they need it, find it bland and unpleasant when they don't, and naturally gravitate to an optimal protein intake.

So we could make this a very short chapter: *let your appetite guide you to your optimal protein intake.* But then you might feel we hadn't earned the price of the book. As there are interesting links between protein intake and disease resistance, ease of weight loss, athleticism and strength, and longevity, let's take a few pages to explore.

Notes for this chapter may be found at www.perfecthealthdiet.com/notes/#Ch9.

The Deficiency Range

The body has no protein reserve except muscle and lean tissue; all dietary protein is put to functional use or metabolised for energy.

At healthful protein intakes, the body has an excess of protein that is metabolised for energy, releasing nitrogen-bearing amine groups that are converted to urea, ammonia, or uric acid, and excreted.

Traditionally, the minimum healthful protein intake has been estimated by assessing nitrogen balance. Nitrogen balance means that protein losses are exactly matched by protein intake, so that the quantity of functional protein is unchanging.

Generally, after a change in dietary protein, the body achieves nitrogen balance within a few days.[1] It does this by altering the amount of protein that is metabolised for energy.

If protein intake is too low, nitrogen balance cannot be achieved and functional proteins are lost. If allowed to persist, this loss of functional protein can become quite dangerous. Death from total fasting, which occurs after 60 to 70 days in adults and after five days in neonates, is caused by loss of protein.

In deficiency, proteins are lost first from the liver and visceral organs such as the kidneys and gut. The liver loses up to 40 per cent of its proteins on a protein-deficient diet.[2] Protein loss can significantly impair the function of these organs. Take rats given a low dose of aflatoxin daily — after six months all rats on a 20 per cent protein diet were still alive, but half the rats on a 5 per cent protein diet had died.[3] On the low-protein diet, rats lacked sufficient liver function to cope with the toxin.

That's not all. Protein deficiency:

- impairs all organs,[4] especially the kidneys[5]
- harms immune function, resulting in higher risk of infection[6]
- makes the gut permeable, increasing the risk of infectious invasion[7]
- in children, stunts growth and harms the brain and brain function[8]

Good reasons, we think, not to become protein-deficient!

The amount of dietary protein needed to avoid deficiency varies. Protein needs are increased during infection, wound healing, carbohydrate restriction (since protein is converted to glucose to avert a glucose deficiency), and endurance exercise (one reason long-distance runners have trouble maintaining muscle mass). So it is not possible to name a specific amount of protein that is safe for everyone.

The Australian recommended daily intake (RDI) for protein — 0.8 gram per kilogram of body weight per day — is designed to bring 97.5 per cent of Australians into nitrogen balance. That seems a fair estimate to us of the minimum safe protein intake — the low end of our peak health range. The RDI corresponds to a dietary protein intake of 46 grams (184 calories) per day for women and 64 grams (256 calories) per day for men.[9]

For simplicity, let's call this 200 calories per day, or 10 per cent of energy. Women can tweak that number downward a bit, men upward.

The Toxicity Range

There are two main sources of toxicity from protein: ammonia waste from protein metabolism and toxins produced by gut bacteria that ferment protein.

Toxicity from Nitrogenous Waste

Excess protein is metabolised for energy or converted to glucose. Either way, nitrogen is released. The nitrogen forms ammonia, a toxin, which is disposed of by conversion to urea, a safe molecule.

However, the body's ability to convert ammonia to urea peaks with a protein intake of 230 grams per day (920 calories per day), indicating that at that protein intake, marginal nitrogen is going entirely into ammonia.[10] The protein intake at which levels of ammonia become significant is lower, somewhere in the range of 600 to 800 protein calories per day.

Ammonia toxicity can be quite serious. The explorer Vilhjalmur Stefansson, who spent the winter of 1906 living with Inuit on the Mackenzie River delta near the Arctic Ocean, told of the danger of 'rabbit starvation'. That occurred in spring, when lean rabbits were the only available food. When protein intake exceeds 45 per cent of calories (approximately 900 calories), nausea and diarrhoea begin in days and death can follow in weeks.[11] Rabbit starvation was reproduced in the Bellevue All-Meat Trial.[12]

Toxins from Gut Bacteria

Protein is not food for us alone; gut bacteria can ferment protein.

Although fermentation of carbohydrates by gut bacteria is usually beneficial, fermentation of protein is not: it generates toxic compounds, including amines, phenols, indoles, thiols, and hydrogen sulfide, which make a foul-smelling stool.[13]

It seems likely, therefore, that high protein intakes are suboptimal for gut health. A few other factors increase fermentable protein: some proteins, such as soy, egg white, and pasteurised milk casein, are hard to digest and are more likely to reach the colon. Also, when large amounts of protein are eaten at one sitting, a smaller fraction may be absorbed, leaving more to be fermented in the colon.[14]

Summary

Based on ammonia toxicity in adults, we suggest 600 calories per day, or 30 per cent of energy, as the beginning of the toxicity range for protein. Large men might be okay on a bit more than 600 calories, but we wouldn't push it.

Toxicity may begin at lower protein doses due to fermentation of protein by gut bacteria. This is most likely in those with poor protein digestion, perhaps due to low stomach acid levels.

Infants, especially pre-term infants, experience negative effects at much lower intakes of protein. Human breast milk is only 7 per cent protein. Pre-term infants fed with 20 per cent protein had more fever, lethargy, poor feeding, and lower IQs at three and six years of age.[15] A slight increase in the protein content of formula, from 7 per cent to 9 per cent, is enough to make babies overweight at age two.[16]

Pregnant mothers also should limit their protein intake to less than 20 per cent of calories to avoid risks to their baby both perinatally and in later life.[17] Excess protein can cause neural tube defects in developing embryos.[18]

Summary: the peak health range

The peak health range for protein is, in healthy adults with good digestion eating sufficient carbs, fairly broad: about 200 to 600 calories per day, or 10 to 30 per cent of energy.

As a rule, 15 per cent of energy as protein is close to optimal for any adult eating sufficient carbs. This works over a very broad range of intakes. Athletes in training who burn 4000 calories per day will flourish on 600 calories of protein. Korean centenarian women consume only 1247 calories per day and are healthy on a mere 41 grams of protein per day, or 13 per cent of energy.[19]

On low-carb diets, protein needs are increased, but the ability to dispose of nitrogen is not, so the peak health range narrows. On a zero-carb diet, the peak health range for protein may be as narrow as 550 to 600 calories per day.

Children, especially infants, and pregnant women also have a narrower peak health range, but it lies at lower protein intakes. Infants shouldn't be given more protein than the 7 per cent found in breast milk.

Finding a Place Within the Peak Health Range

Depending on your personal goals, you may wish to skew protein intake toward the high or low end of the peak health range.

Weight Loss

The food reward system has a strong appetite for protein. This means that when protein is a small fraction of food, people eat more food, at least in the short term.

Controlled trials have found that people consume the same number of total calories on 15 per cent protein and 25 per cent protein diets, but on 10 per cent protein diets they consume additional calories.[20]

This suggests that those seeking to lose weight should eat at least 15 per cent protein — more if calories are restricted. Otherwise, their protein appetite will lead them to consume additional calories, inhibiting weight loss.

Strength Gains

For athletes seeking to add strength, there may be benefits to high protein intake.

From one point of view, this is a bit surprising. The amount of protein needed to build muscle is modest. The protein content of muscle is 16.4 per cent,[21] so adding 11.8 kilograms of muscle per year requires only 5 grams (20 calories) of protein per day to be incorporated into tissue.

But protein has hormonal effects. Abundant protein signals to the body that resources are readily available and it's a good time to invest in muscle growth, fertility, and reproduction.

Exercise itself leads to muscle breakdown, and exercise followed by fasting leads to loss of muscle. (The actor Christian Bale's recipe for becoming cadaverously skinny — 183 centimetres, 55.3 kilograms — in *The Machinist* was overtraining combined with undereating.[22]) It is the combination of exercise *and* subsequent overfeeding that grows muscle. Overfeeding should begin in the first two hours after exercise, and muscle growth continues to be promoted by overfeeding in the 48 hours following exercise.[23]

Overfeeding for muscle growth should not be focused exclusively on protein. A balanced diet, with evolutionary macronutrient ratios, is the best strategy for muscle growth. When total calories are kept constant, but protein intake is varied, controlled trials find that higher protein intake leads to only slight, statistically insignificant muscle gains.[24] On the other hand, consuming more calories, whatever the source, leads to substantial muscle gain.[25]

The exception to this rule is low-protein diets. When protein is scarce, extra intake of certain amino acids — notably leucine, a branched-chain amino acid — will prevent muscle breakdown and stimulate muscle growth. Leucine supplementation increases muscle growth in piglets on a low-protein diet by 61 per cent and prevents muscle loss in people on low-protein diets.[26]

To maintain a lean body composition while overfeeding for muscle growth, the trick is to have rest days with reduced calorie consumption. A good rule of thumb is to overeat by 20 to 25 per cent of calories in the immediate aftermath of training and to undereat by 20 to 25 per cent on rest days.

Longevity

In animal studies, protein restriction extends life span.[27] Experiments with individual amino acids have shown that reduced intake of methionine, which is ubiquitously present in food proteins, extends life span by reducing oxidative stress on mitochondria.[28] Excess methionine can also promote atherosclerosis.[29]

SCIENCE OF THE PHD
Protein Restriction, Autophagy, and Longevity

One mechanism by which protein restriction extends life span is by promoting a recycling process called autophagy.[30]

Proteins generally become useless after a time: they fold into the wrong shape, or they glycate with sugar and no longer work. Similarly, organelles such as mitochondria become damaged and dysfunctional.

These 'junk proteins' and dysfunctional organelles gather in cells until a cleanup mechanism, autophagy, is triggered. When resources are scarce, cells turn on cleanup crews — lysosomes and proteasomes — that digest junk, recycling their components. This cleanup improves cellular health. Autophagy is necessary for protein or calorie restriction to extend life span.[31]

Autophagy also protects against infections. Autophagy digests bacteria and viruses along with cellular junk and is essential to intracellular immune defence.[32]

Takeaway

Protein intake of 200 to 600 calories per day seems to be the peak health range if sufficient carbs are eaten. For weight loss, 300 calories or more is desirable. Within the peak health range, protein intake should scale with total calorie consumption; 15 per cent of energy is a good number.

Meat and fish are the best sources of protein, since (as we'll see later) plant proteins are often toxic.

So how much meat and fish should we eat? Most meats have about 400 protein calories per 450 grams:

Beef	Salmon	Mussels (cooked)	Shrimp	Chicken	Pork Loin
369	360	432	380	378	390

There are a few exceptions to this rule: bacon, if uncooked, has 210 protein calories per 450 grams, due to its high fat content; but it has 700 protein calories per 450 grams if fried to a crisp. Eggs have 230 calories per 450 grams. But 400 protein calories per 450 grams is a good rule of thumb.

Therefore, the peak health range for protein of 200 to 600 calories is satisfied by eating 225 to 680 grams of meat, fish, and eggs per day.

Athletes and very-low-carb dieters will benefit from eating in the upper half of that range, but most people will want to consume 200 to 400 calories of protein, or *225 to 450 grams of meat, fish, and eggs per day.*

10
Carbohydrates

· ·

- *Carbohydrates should comprise 20 to 35 per cent of calories, except for those on therapeutic ketogenic diets (a bit less) or athletes in training (a bit more).*
- *About 85 per cent of dietary carbs should digest to glucose, 15 per cent to fructose; therefore, starches should be preferred to sugars.*
- *Starches should be eaten with fat, vinegar, and vegetables to minimise their hyperglycemic toxicity. Starches are meal foods, not snack foods!*
- *Avoid added sugars. When you do indulge, keep to the 85 per cent glucose guideline by using rice syrup or dextrose in place of honey or sucrose.*

· ·

Few nutrients have inspired as much controversy as carbohydrates.

Mainstream dietary guidelines have been based on common practice. Cultures all over the world obtain 50 per cent of energy from carbohydrates. Can they all be wrong?

Among hunter-gatherers, the carb fraction of the diet tells us more about food availability than about how many carbs are healthiest. The islanders of Kitava are healthy on a diet that is 69 per cent carbs,[1] and the Inuit maintained low rates of cardiovascular disease on diets that, before the arrival of trading posts selling flour, ranged below 5 per cent carbohydrates.[2]

Notes for this chapter may be found at www.perfecthealthdiet.com/notes/#Ch10.

This suggests that a wide range of carbohydrate intakes may be compatible with good health.

The discovery by Dr Robert Atkins that low-carb diets are effective for weight loss and by Dr Richard Bernstein and others that they are beneficial for diabetes sparked the modern low-carb movement. Low-carb ketogenic diets are a standard therapy for epilepsy. Is a diet that is therapeutic for obesity, diabetes, and epilepsy also desirable for healthy people?

To answer this, we'll have to look to biology for guidance.

Two Kinds of Carbohydrates

Plants store carb calories in two ways: as starches and as sugars.

Starches digest entirely to **glucose.** Sugars come in several forms, but the most common is sucrose, which digests to equal parts **glucose and fructose.**

Since it's the nutrients — *glucose* and *fructose* — that affect the body, biology will tell us how much glucose and fructose we should eat. From that we'll work backward to our optimal intake of starchy and sugary plants.

Let's start with fructose.

Optimal Fructose Intake

. . . .

Fructose intake should be below 25 grams (100 calories) per day.

. . . .

Fructose has two major defects as a calorie source:

- **It is chemically reactive.** Fructose rapidly reacts with proteins to form 'advanced glycation end products' (AGEs) that disrupt normal functions. Fructose is seven times more likely than glucose to cross-link with proteins.[3] AGEs cross-link collagen for stiff joints and aged skin, damage DNA, hasten ageing,[4] stiffen blood vessels to cause high blood pressure, and cause kidney disease.[5]

- **It is a useless macronutrient.** Fructose has no structural role in the human body. The digestive tract shunts fructose to the liver via the portal vein and, at the levels of fructose contained in natural foods, virtually 100 per cent is absorbed on that first pass through the liver — essentially, no fructose reaches the general circulation. In the liver, fructose is converted to glucose, glycogen, lactate, and fat.[6] It's telling that the first thing the body does with fructose is convert it into something else.

If evolution designed human biology to shield the body from fructose, we have to question whether fructose is healthful for the tissues that are exposed to it — the gut, portal vein, and liver.

And if fructose is rapidly converted to glucose and fat, we wonder whether it may be better to eat the glucose and fat in the first place.

So perhaps the place to start is by looking at why it might be beneficial to eat any fructose at all.

Benefits of Fructose

At first glance it seems unlikely that fructose would have benefits. Dietary fructose survives only briefly before it is transformed into other macronutrients, usually glucose.

We know of two possible benefits to the consumption of small amounts of fructose:

- **Athletic performance.** When liver glycogen levels are low, athletic performance is hindered. Fructose and galactose are directed entirely to the liver, whereas glucose is taken up by the whole body; so one might expect that a bit of fructose might aid glycogen replenishment. So it does: the most rapid glycogen replenishment occurs with a mix of 70 per cent glucose, 30 per cent fructose or galactose.[7] Such a mix of sugars is helpful for athletes who need quick recovery (for several performances on the same day), or for endurance athletes trying to replenish glycogen during a race.
- **Catalysis of glycemic control.** The liver manages blood glucose levels and may do it better when given small doses of fructose. Small, 'catalytic' doses of fructose — less than 10 grams,

typically about 3 grams, per meal; roughly the amount in one fruit or two servings of vegetables — improve the glycemic response to starchy meals.[8] In a clinical trial, diabetics experienced better glycemic control with higher consumption of fruit — HbA1c levels were reduced by 0.5 per cent.[9]

For a sedentary adult, it is the assistance to glycemic control that matters. Benefits from fructose will be fully realised by consuming in the vicinity of 15 to 25 grams of fructose per day (assuming 3 to 8 grams of fructose per meal and two or three meals per day, plus a fruit snack or dessert).

We therefore estimate the level of fructose intake at which benefits end to be 25 grams, or 100 calories, per day.

Fructose Toxicity

At high intakes, fructose can be quite harmful. We'll discuss the harms of fructose in Part III, but here's a brief list:

- In the gut, fructose promotes gut permeability and poisoning of the body by endotoxemia.
- In the liver, fructose promotes fatty liver disease and metabolic syndrome.
- Fructose disposal generates uric acid, which can cause gout or kidney stones.
- If the liver can't dispose of fructose quickly enough and the blood level becomes elevated, it promotes cancer.[10]
- High doses of fructose clearly promote obesity in clinical trials and in animal studies.

Given the known dangers of high fructose consumption, it seems prudent to minimise fructose intake.

So let's consume at most 100 calories of fructose per day.

Determining Optimal Carbohydrate Intake

Glucose is the 'good carb' — the sugar that circulates in the blood and is used to construct essential molecules such as glycosylated proteins and phospholipids.

For glucose, as for all other nutrients, our strategy is to find the peak health range — the intakes at which benefits have ended and there is still no toxicity. Now, glucose is unlike many other nutrients in that the body can manufacture glucose from protein to relieve a deficiency and can convert glucose to fat to eliminate an excess. This means that the body can cope with a very wide range of carb intakes. But it also gives us an easy way to find **the amount of glucose that the body really wants.**

Consider this: if we plot *carbohydrates eaten* against the amount of *glucose utilised by the body,* the two curves will look like this:

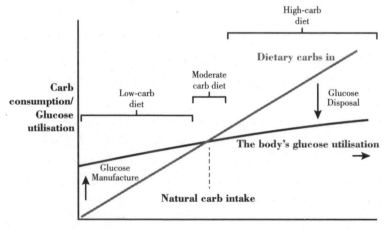

At low carb intakes, the body will manufacture glucose from protein, a process called gluconeogenesis. The body's glucose utilisation will be higher than the dietary intake.

At high carb intakes, the body will dispose of excess glucose, perhaps by converting it to fat. The body's glucose utilisation will be lower than the dietary intake.

In the middle, there will be a **natural carbohydrate intake** at which the two curves cross. At this natural level, *the carb calories eaten exactly equal the body's glucose utilisation.* The body neither manufactures additional glucose from protein nor disposes of excess carbohydrate by conversion to fat.

Let's call a diet with this natural level of carbs a 'moderate-carb diet', a diet with significantly fewer carbs a 'low-carb diet', and a diet with significantly more carbs a 'high-carb diet'.

It's surely healthful to consume our natural carb intake. If some level of glucose utilisation other than our natural carb intake were healthiest, evolution would have selected for either gluconeogenesis or disposal pathways to be invoked, so that the body's glucose supply would be shifted toward its optimal level. The curves would cross at a different point.

We can't have the same confidence about other carb intakes. Low carb intakes risk reduced glucose utilisation and loss of some benefits. High carb intakes risk creating toxicity from excess glucose before its disposal. This risk will be greatest in the metabolic diseases, such as diabetes, but possibly present at a low level even in healthy people.

READER REPORTS:
natural carbohydrate intake for reduced appetite

I had a mental adjustment period before accepting white rice. I had cut starch out of my diet for so long. I found including 400 calories of white rice and/or potatoes reduced my cravings for something sweet. My calories naturally lowered without hunger. I was also able to start intermittent fasting, something that was impossible for me to do before introducing the starch.

— Sarah Atshan

The Body's Natural Carbohydrate Intake

A fasting person's daily glucose production has been measured at 8 micromoles per kilogram per minute, which for typical adults equals 120 to 160 grams, or 480 to 640 calories, per day.[11] If most of the body's optimal glucose needs are met during fasting, we can estimate the natural carb intake at about 160 grams, or 640 calories, per day.

We can get to a similar number by adding up the body's specific uses of glucose.

Glucose has three main uses in the body: it combines with proteins to form structural molecules called glycoproteins; it is an alternative fuel that cells can burn instead of fats; and it is a precursor for killing compounds ('reactive oxygen species' or ROS) made by immune cells.

Glucose in Structural Molecules

Wet sugar is sticky and highly reactive. It likes to combine with proteins and can do so in many ways. The human body has 20,000 genes, 200,000 proteins, but two million glycoproteins, or compounds built up by combining proteins with sugars.

Interactions between cells are mediated by glycoproteins. Evolution of these sticky glycoproteins made multicellular life possible.

Some sugar compounds are highly abundant in the body:

- **Mucin** is one of the main components of mucus and protects the gut and airways from pathogens and foreign matter. It is also a key part of tears and saliva.
- **Hyaluronan** lubricates joints and helps provide the scaffolding that shapes cells into tissues. **Glucosamine** and **chondroitin sulfate** are similar sugar-rich compounds important in connective tissue.

The production of hyaluronan alone consumes 5 grams, or 20 calories, of glucose per day;[12] more than a litre of mucus is produced per day.[13] It is not known how much glucose is consumed in production of all two million glycoproteins, but our guess is about 200 calories per day.

Glucose as Fuel for Neurons

One often hears that glucose is the body's 'primary fuel'. This is quite mistaken.

It is true that all human cells can, if need be, metabolise glucose. But mitochondria, the energy producers in most human cells, prefer to burn fat. So in the body, fat is the preferred and primary fuel, except in specialist cells that lack mitochondria (red blood cells) or ready access to fat (neurons); or when oxygen is limited, as in muscle cells during intense activity.

Use of glucose as a fuel is dominated by neurons. The brain and nerves require about 20 calories per hour, waking or sleeping. These 480 daily calories can be provided by either glucose alone, or by a mix of glucose and ketone bodies (which are derived from fats or protein). So daily glucose consumption by the brain and nerves will be somewhere between 150 and 480 calories, depending on ketone availability.

Glucose for Muscle Glycogen

In addition to the cells such as neurons and red blood cells that routinely consume glucose, muscles consume glucose in the form of glycogen during intense exertion. Glycogen is made of long chains of glucose compounded with a pyrophosphate group and is energy-rich because it can readily donate phosphate groups to restore adenosine triphosphate (ATP).

Muscle glycogen usage is a small drain on glucose for sedentary people, but can be a substantial drain for athletes. Here's a guide to how much glucose is used during exercise.

First, total calorie expenditure in one hour of various forms of exercise for a 73-kilogram man is:[14]

Bicycling, <16 kph	Basketball	Ballroom dancing	Golfing, carrying clubs	Running, 13 km	Swimming laps	Tennis	Walking
292	584	219	314	861	423	584	204

Heavier athletes and elite athletes working at high intensity will use more calories. Elite runners, swimmers, or cyclists may exceed 1000 calories per hour.

The fraction of calories utilised as glycogen or fat depends on intensity, as indicated by breath rate and pulse. Breath frequency and pulse increase when cells need more oxygen, and when oxygen is scarce, cells switch over from fat to glycogen. When oxygen usage is 25 per cent of maximum ('VO$_2$ max'), carbs provide only 7.5 per cent and fat 92.5 per cent of energy. When oxygen usage is 65 per cent of maximum, carb and fat utilisation are equal. When oxygen usage is 85 per cent of maximum, carbs account for 75 per cent of energy, fat 25 per cent.[15]

Multiplying these percentages by total calorie expenditure, we can see that highly trained runners or cyclists working at 70 per cent of maximum oxygen utilisation will utilise about 500 calories of glycogen per hour.[16] Most athletes will use less. A person who goes walking, bicycling, or dancing at low intensity uses very little carbohydrate.

SCIENCE OF THE PHD
Carbohydrate Loading for Endurance Athletes

When endurance athletes run out of muscle glycogen, it is known as 'hitting the wall'. Endurance athletes can maximise stored muscle glycogen by 'carb loading'. About three weeks before an event, the athlete adopts a zero-carb diet and continues to train intensively, depleting muscle glycogen. This causes muscle cells to enlarge their glycogen storage reservoirs. A few days before the event, the athlete begins to eat starch. About 3000 calories of starch is needed to fill muscle glycogen reservoirs. Caffeine aids the process.[17]

Glucose as a Killing Agent

Glucose, when metabolised for energy, readily produces reactive oxygen species (ROS). These dangerous molecules can damage or destroy cells.

The destructiveness of ROS has been put to use by the immune system. Immune cells produce abundant ROS from glucose whenever they need to kill pathogens such as bacteria and fungi.

Under normal circumstances the immune system probably isn't doing a lot of killing and doesn't consume much glucose. However, people with certain infections may need extra glucose.

Endogenous Glucose Production

Against these glucose needs must be set the glucose that is produced routinely by the body as a consequence of the metabolism of fats.

Fats are stored in the body as either phospholipids, which consist of two fatty acids joined by a glycerol backbone to a phosphate group, and an organic molecule such as choline or inositol, or triglycerides, which consist of three fatty acids and a glycerol backbone. Phospholipids make up cell membranes, whereas triglycerides are a storage form of fats.

When fatty acids are consumed for energy, the glycerol backbones are released. Two glycerols make one molecule of glucose. Recycling of glycerol from fats helps to meet the body's glucose needs, since fats in food enter the body already attached to glycerol backbones.

A typical triglyceride provides about 12 per cent of calories as glycerol, 88 per cent as fatty acids. Consuming 2400 calories per day on the Perfect Health Diet, with 65 per cent of calories derived from triglycerides or phospholipids, will generate about 200 calories per day of glucose from the glycerol in food fats.

Summary: the body's natural carb intake

Although the precise magnitude of the various quantities is uncertain, it appears that the body's natural daily glucose consumption is about 480 calories for brain and nerves (decreasing to as little as 150 calories if ketones are available), 200 calories for glycoproteins such as hyaluronan and mucin, 100 calories for muscle glycogen and immune, intestinal, and kidney cell use, offset by about 200 calories of glucose produced in the course of fat burning.

For sedentary healthy people, then, the natural carb intake is about 600 carb calories per day. Ketogenic dieting can decrease glucose needs by up to 300 calories. Athletic activity increases glucose needs by up to 500 calories per hour of training. Illness or wound healing may also increase glucose needs.

READER REPORTS: more benefits from eating at the natural carbohydrate intake

I have had for the last several years, not exactly numbness, but a strange burning sensation in feet and/or legs only at night — not every night, but frequently — which would wake me. If I moved my legs a bit it would go away. It started after being VERY low carb for over six months. It has dwindled significantly, perhaps completely. I have been eating 200 calories safe starches for three and a half months now. Chalk up another one for PHD!

— Ellen

I had been a low carber for several years and over that time have suffered 4 painful bouts of kidney stones. Your post on kidney stones on a low-carb diet was eye opening. My urologist did various tests and I ended up with having high levels of uric acid and oxalates. Incorporating your PHD, I dramatically brought down my uric acid levels. I hope this and the other benefits of your PHD will help prevent future stones.

— George

I've been following the Perfect Health Diet for about a year now after 10 years of low carb and very low carb. It's a very easy diet; I've never eaten healthier and never felt better and more satisfied, and I'm happier — my mood is so much better, I have more energy and I have much less anxiety and am no longer anxious about food and what to eat, which is an incredible accomplishment for me. And my fiancé is much happier too — he notices the huge improvement in my mood and doesn't want me to ever go back to low carb — not that I would want to!

— Connie Warner

Let's define a moderate-carb diet as a nonketogenic diet that delivers the natural carb intake. A moderate-carb diet has about 600 carb calories per day, plus however much is needed to support athletic endeavours.

The Peril of Glycemic Excursions

Another factor affecting the healthfulness of carbohydrate consumption is the degree to which blood glucose levels fluctuate.

Blood glucose levels should remain in a stable range, between about 85 to 105 milligrams per decilitre. After eating carbohydrates, the blood glucose level should rise no higher than about 140 milligrams per decilitre and should return to the normal range within a few hours.

When blood glucose levels move outside the healthy range, significant health problems can follow. Indeed, mortality rates are lowest when both fasting blood glucose and two-hour postmeal blood glucose levels are between 81 and 108 milligrams per decilitre; both lower and higher blood glucose levels are associated with an increased risk of death.[18]

Hyperglycemia — blood glucose levels that are too high — is common in diabetics and leads to organ damage[19] and heightened mortality rates.[20] Even in nondiabetics, postprandial (after meal) surges in blood glucose cause nerve damage[21] and greatly increase the risk of stroke[22] and cancer.[23] To avoid these risks, it's important to keep postprandial (postmeal) blood glucose levels below 140 milligrams per decilitre.[24] Failing to do so may poison the nerves, little by little, every day.

How to Avoid Hyperglycemic Toxicity

So how can we avoid high blood glucose levels after consuming carbs? There are two poor strategies and one good one.

Lowering Carbohydrate Intake Doesn't Work

You might think that the answer is to consume very few carbs. But this would be naive!

It turns out that on low-carb diets, much of the body becomes insulin resistant — meaning that it doesn't respond to insulin signals and so doesn't take in glucose after meals. This happens so that glucose will be directed to the liver, where it can be stored in glycogen and released later for use by the brain.

This 'physiological insulin resistance' is a protective response of the body that assures that the brain gets the benefit of a limited supply of glucose. But it has a paradoxical effect: because the rest of the body is refusing to take up glucose and the liver takes it up slowly, a meal of carbohydrates is followed by higher postprandial blood glucose levels in low-carb dieters than in high-carb dieters.

In short, low-carb dieting can *increase* the risk of postprandial hyperglycemia.

Eating Sugar Instead of Starch Is Not Smart

The glycemic index is a measure of how high blood glucose levels rise in response to a fixed amount (usually 200 carb calories) of a food. Starches, which digest entirely to glucose, generally have a higher glycemic index than sugars, because half the calories in sugar are from fructose, which doesn't circulate.

So one might think that replacing starches with sugars would reduce posprandial hyperglycemia and perhaps improve health.

However, that's not what the evidence shows. Sugars, probably due to fructose toxicity, are more dangerous than starches. A review of the literature comparing starches and sugars as carb sources concluded:

> From the literature reviewed in this paper, potential beneficial effects of intake of starchy foods, especially those containing slowly-digestible and resistant starches, and potential detrimental effects of high intakes of fructose become apparent.[25]

Starches are also better than sugars when it comes to weight loss. According to Dr Richard Johnson:

> [S]tarch-based foods don't cause weight gain like sugar-based foods and don't cause the metabolic syndrome like sugar-based foods . . . Potatoes, pasta, rice may be relatively safe compared to table sugar. A fructose index may be a better way to assess the risk of carbohydrates related to obesity.[26]

The Best Strategy for Glycemic Control

What, then, is the best way to minimise the risk of postprandial hyperglycemia?

The glycemic index is defined so that pure glucose has a GI of 100. A GI of 55 or less is considered to be low; fruits and vegetables typically have a GI in this range. The risk of hyperglycemic toxicity after eating 200 calories of a low-GI food is minimal. So if we can eat with a GI below 55, our diet should be safe. Fortunately, this can be done with any starch. The trick is to prepare the starch properly and to eat it as part of a meal, in combination with other foods.

Here are some ways to reduce the GI of starchy foods:

- **Cook them gently.** When starches are cooked in boiling water (as with home-cooked rice or boiled potatoes), their GI is fairly low, around 50 to 60; but when they are roasted at high temperatures, their GI often approaches 100.[27]
- **Avoid industrially prepared foods.** To speed foods through factories, industrial foods are often processed at very high temperatures, raising their glycemic index. Commercial puffed rice or instant rice has a GI almost double that of home-cooked rice.[28]
- **Eat starches with fat.** Fat greatly slows down the speed at which starches are digested, substantially reducing the peak blood glucose following a meal.[29] Dairy products — milk, butter, and sour cream — are especially helpful.[30] Put some butter on your potato!
- **Eat starches with vegetables.** Including fibre in a meal significantly reduces the GI of accompanying starch.[31] Vegetables are a natural way to add fibre to a meal.
- **Eat starches with acids, especially vinegar.** Vinegar, pickle juice, and many other acids reduce the GI of starches.[32]

The effect of all these measures is to lower the GI of starchy foods by more than 50 per cent. If starchy foods are cooked gently and eaten as part of a meal that includes vegetables, fat, and an acidic sauce, even diabetics can expect a low risk of postprandial hyperglycemia.

· ·

READER REPORTS: managing diabetes

I'm type I diabetic. I had my HbA1c checked at my doctor's office as routine bloodwork. It was excellent for a diabetic — 5.7. This is the lowest HbA1c result I've ever had in my 11 years as a diabetic, and I attribute much of that to the Perfect Health Diet which I've been following now for almost 9 months. The addition of fats has helped me immensely in controlling my blood sugar (for example, when I add butter to a baked potato, I usually only need to take half the amount of fast-acting insulin as I would've taken if eating the potato plain).

Additionally, though I haven't been overweight at all, I did lose about 10 pounds [4.5 kilograms] and my body does appear more toned. I know the diet here is helping me a lot and I've been feeling more energetic lately and less moody, which my husband is VERY HAPPY about!!

— K.H., Virginia

I am a type II diabetic. I switched from the Atkins Induction diet to the Perfect Health Diet. I have been eating rice, potatoes, bananas, and other safe starches ever since, as well as fermented dairy products, such as plain, whole milk yogurt. I have also slowly lost another seven pounds [3.2 kilograms]. Note that since following the Perfect Health Diet, my fasting blood glucose reading has gone down. So not only am I losing weight on the Perfect Health Diet, my blood glucose levels have actually improved.

— Newell Wright

· ·

Low-Carbohydrate Diets May Be Better than High-Carbohydrate Diets

In our survey of mammalian diets, we noted that in many mammals carbs are almost completely lost during digestion. Ruminants meet their glucose needs by manufacturing glucose from odd-carbon short-chain fatty acids; hypercarnivores meet glucose needs by manufacturing it from protein. This suggests that *low-carb diets, in which glucose is manufactured rather than eaten, are healthful,* or at least that animals readily evolve an ability to flourish on low-carb diets.

Yet the reverse phenomenon, natural high-carb diets, is unheard of. Many mammals eat plant-based diets, but **no mammal eats a high-carb diet.** Every mammal whose food is rich in carbs has a digestive tract that transforms some or all of the carbs into fatty acids before allowing them entry to the body.

This calls into question the healthfulness of high-carb diets. If they are healthful, why don't animal digestive tracts allow hefty amounts of glucose to enter their bodies?

What about in humans? Is there clinical evidence for health dangers from high-carb dieting?

Dietary Carbohydrates and Heart Attacks

A mammoth long-term U.S. study, the Nurses' Health Study, enabled evaluation of the effects of different levels of carbohydrate intake on the nurses' health.[33] The researchers followed 98,462 women who completed a diet questionnaire in 1980, splitting the women into ten equal-sized groups based on the fraction of calories they obtained from carbohydrates. For simplicity, we'll just compare the bottom and top deciles:

- The high-carb decile obtained 58.8 per cent of calories from carbohydrates and 26.9 per cent from fat.
- The low-carb decile obtained 36.8 per cent of calories from carbohydrates and 39.9 per cent from fat.

Now, in general, the low-carb decile did not take good care of their health. They were more likely to smoke (26 per cent smoked, compared to 17 per cent of the high-carb decile) and to avoid exercise (the low-carb decile got 20 per cent less exercise than the high-carb decile). They also drank a lot of coffee.

But the rate of coronary heart disease cases was 0.131 per cent in the high-carb decile and 0.092 per cent in the low-carb decile. The high-carb group smoked less and exercised more, but their chance of a heart attack was 42 per cent higher!

Dietary Carbohydrates and the
Atherogenic Blood Lipid Profile

It's well known that a bad blood lipid profile — high triglyceride levels, low HDL levels, and high levels of 'small, dense' LDL — is a risk factor for heart disease.

What's less commonly appreciated is that the bad blood lipid profile is almost entirely determined by excess carbohydrate consumption.

A series of studies by the group of Dr Ronald Krauss grouped people by the carbohydrate fraction of their diet and measured their blood lipids, classifying them as 'atherogenic' or 'nonatherogenic'. This was the result.[34]

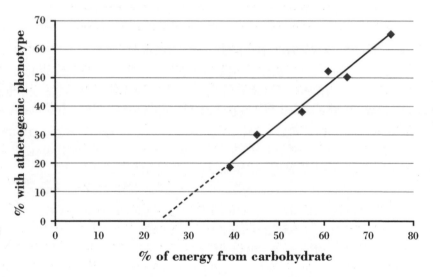

Percentage of people with atherogenic blood lipid profiles
as a function of carbohydrate fraction of the diet.

A fit to the data suggests that atherogenic lipid profiles should disappear with carb consumption of 25 per cent of energy. For a diet of 2400 calories per day, this corresponds to 600 carbohydrate calories per day — precisely the natural carb intake!

Our conclusion: if you want a good lipid profile with low triglyceride levels, high HDL levels, and negligible 'small, dense' LDL levels, eat a moderate-carb diet, not a high-carb diet.

SCIENCE OF THE PHD
The Disposal of Excess Carbohydrates

Excess carbohydrates are eliminated by two pathways: glucose oxidation for energy and conversion of glucose to saturated fat by a process called *de novo lipogenesis* — in roughly similar amounts.

In one study, five men were fed a diet of 3740 calories glucose, 425 calories of protein, and 82 calories of fat per day and monitored for four days. They gained about 1.8 kilograms over the four days, and their resting energy expenditure rose by 57 per cent over the four days as metabolism was upregulated to get rid of the excess carbohydrate. On the first day most of the excess carbs went into glycogen stores and elevated glucose oxidation; but by day four at least 170 grams per day of fat were being synthesised from dietary glucose — equivalent to 1530 calories per day and disposing of nearly half of dietary glucose.[35] Nearly all the fat-to-glucose conversion occurred in adipose tissue and skeletal muscle, less than 2 per cent in the liver.

That particular study fed its subjects an energy excess and an 88 per cent carb diet. What of diets with normal caloric intakes and carb levels typical of the American diet, which is around 50 per cent carbohydrates, 35 per cent fat, and 15 per cent protein?

That can also be measured, though it takes longer than four days. In a six-month study, it was found that 20 per cent of the saturated fat in adipose tissue had arisen from glucose-to-fat conversion.[36] This level of fat synthesis suggests that perhaps 10 per cent of carbohydrates eaten had been converted to fat during the course of the study.

Insofar as excess carbohydrates are converted to saturated fat, it would seem more healthful and less stressful to eat saturated fat to begin with.

Optimal Plant Foods

Now we have enough information to select the plant foods that will provide our carbs.

Our goal is to get about 600 carb calories per day — our natural carb intake. Of those, 100 calories may come from fructose and 500 calories from glucose. So our plant foods should provide 200 calories of sugar (which is half fructose), and 400 calories of starch (which is all glucose).

Let's look at some good ways to meet these targets with starchy and sugary plant foods.

Safe Starches

In Part III, we'll look at some **unsafe starches:** cereal grains and beans. They are unsafe because they contain toxins after normal cooking.

Fortunately, there are a number of **'safe starches'**, starchy plants that contain minimal toxins after cooking. These include white rice, potato, taro, tapioca, sago, winter squashes, sweet potatoes and yams, plantains, and some others.

Here are some of our safe starches with their calorie counts. We've arranged them from low to high in fructose fraction — so pure starches are at the top, foods with more sugar at the bottom.

Plant Food	Glucose (cal/450 g)	Fructose (cal/450 g)	Fructose Fraction
White rice	521	0	0%
Taro	531	5	1%
White potato	351	13	4%
Butternut squash	173	18	9%
Sweet potato	180	39	18%
Plantain	398	127	24%

They range from about 200 to 530 calories per 450 grams. So to get 400 calories per day, we want to eat about 450 grams of safe starches daily.

A fist-sized quantity of safe starches typically weighs about 115 grams. So **four fist-sized servings per day of safe starches — one or two per meal — is the proper quantity of safe starches.**

Healthful Sugary Plants

The number of safe starches is limited, but a much wider array of plants can provide a bit of fructose for its beneficial catalysis of glycemic control.

In the table below, we've ranked a number of sugary plant foods — mostly bulbs, roots, fruits, and berries — from high to low in their potassium-to-fructose ratio. Potassium is a beneficial nutrient, so we should eat plants with a **high potassium-to-fructose ratio** in order to maximise potassium intake.

Nutritional Content of Sugary Foods

Fruit, Berry, or Sugary Vegetable	Glucose (cal/450 g)	Fructose (cal/450 g)	Potassium-to-Fructose Ratio (mg/g)
Tomato	23	25	173
Sweet potato	180	39	104
Carrot	69	43	98
Onion	45	32	81
Beet	73	73	76
Cantaloupe	67	74	66
Raspberries	36	44	62
Papaya	77	77	60
Banana	210	110	59
Strawberries	40	49	57
Peach	79	71	49
Plum	106	70	41
Orange	75	80	38
Pomegranate	124	124	35
Watermelon	40	72	28
Grapes	132	149	23
Pineapple	86	93	21
Mango	134	134	21
Pear	57	120	18
Apple	64	126	15
Blueberries	90	91	15

The healthiest sugary plants, based on potassium-to-fructose ratio, are tubers (such as sweet potatoes), roots (carrots), and bulbs (onions, beets). Tomatoes don't have many calories but are a terrific source of potassium, placing them atop the list. Melons, berries, bananas, peaches, plums, citrus fruits, and pomegranates rank highest among the fruits. Modern breeds of pears and apples, which have been bred for sweetness, rank the lowest. (Heritage breeds of those fruits are more healthful.)

Combining Starchy and Sugary Plants

As a rule, the sugary plants have fewer calories than the starchy plants. So even though we want twice as many calories from starches than sugars, we'll eat roughly similar weights of the two types of plant foods.

To illustrate some food combinations that would add up to 500 glucose and 100 fructose calories, let's use bananas and beets as our sugary foods and white rice, white potato, butternut squash, and sweet potato as our starchy foods. Some combinations that work include:

- 270 grams of white rice and 365 grams of banana
- 365 grams of white rice and 545 grams of beets
- 450 grams of white potato and 320 grams of banana
- 545 grams of white potato and 455 grams of beets
- 1 kilogram of butternut squash and 180 grams of banana
- 1.2 kilograms of butternut squash and 270 grams of beets
- 1.2 kilograms of sweet potato

A rough rule of thumb is: to eat **a moderate-carb diet,** combine **450 grams per day** of safe starches, such as white rice, white potato, winter squashes, taro, or sweet potato, with **450 grams per day** of sugary plant foods, such as beets or fruits and berries. Add as many low-calorie vegetables as you like.

About 450 grams of sugary plants equals about three beets, three bananas, or three large peaches per day. Let's generalise that as **three or four fruits or sugary in-ground plants per day.**

Processed Foods

As a general principle, it's more healthful to eat whole foods, such as rice or potatoes, than to eat purified nutrients such as rice flour, potato starch, or rice syrup (which is rice flour predigested into sugars).

Eat Vegetables, but Don't Count Them as Carbohydrate Sources

We recommend that you eat vegetables to taste — as many or as few as you like — but don't count them as a source of carb calories. Why?

Most vegetables have 80 calories per 450 grams or less, divided more or less evenly between glucose and fructose. (For example, our table of sugary foods includes onions, with 77 calories per 450 grams, and tomatoes, with 48 calories per 450 grams.) But the digestive tract and the immune cells that line the gut use glucose during digestion. For each 450 grams of plant food consumed, approximately 40 calories of glucose may be consumed by the gut. Vegetables have less glucose than that, and some of their fructose may be intercepted by gut bacteria or converted to fat. So the net contribution of vegetables to the body's glucose balance is virtually nil.

Since our target of 600 carb calories is designed to satisfy the glucose needs of the body, it's inappropriate to count vegetables, which provide only enough glucose for their own digestion.

However, if you do choose to eat purified starches and sugars or foods made from them, such as baked bread, muffins, cookies, or pizza dough, here are our guidelines.

- **Use 'safe starch' flours:** rice flour, potato starch, tapioca starch. Many commercial gluten-free flours and products, such as Country Life bread, Domino's gluten-free pizza, rice noodles, and rice crackers, use safe starches.
- **Use sweeteners that digest into glucose.** Glucose-only sweeteners include rice syrup, tapioca syrup, and dextrose powder. These can be used by themselves for a 100 per cent glucose sweetener or mixed with honey or sugar to produce an 80 per cent glucose sweetener.

The Perfect Health Diet Is Mostly Plants

At the start of Part II, we said we agreed with Michael Pollan's 'Food Rules'. One of his rules was 'Eat mostly plants.'

It's now apparent why we agree with that one:

- As we saw in the 'Protein' chapter, optimal protein intake for most people will be around 300 calories per day, which works out to *less than 450 grams of animal foods* — meat, fish, and eggs — per day.
- As we see in this chapter, optimal carb intake from our recommended plant foods requires eating about 450 grams of safe starches, plus 450 grams of sugary plant foods, plus as many vegetables as you like. So eat *900 grams to 1.3 kilograms of plant foods* per day.

By weight, the diet is 65 to 75 per cent plants — 'mostly plants'.

Meal Preparation

How plants are prepared and eaten is important:

- Starches should be cooked gently — preferably by boiling or steaming — and eaten as part of a meal in combination with fat, vinegar or other acidic flavourings, and vegetables.
- Fruits can be eaten raw and are excellent snack foods. They don't need to be combined with meal ingredients to control their glycemic index.

On our 'PHD Food Plate', the body of the apple represents our recommended meal design. Along with a safe starch, the food plate recommends a meat, a sauce made from fat and an acid such as vinegar, and vegetables. We think you'll find this meal design is not only healthful — it is delicious!

11
The Dangerous Fats: PUFA

. . . .

- *Americans eat five times more omega-6 fat and less omega-3 fat than is optimal.*
- *You want to be at the top of a food chain whose base is green plants and algae; so eat fish, shellfish, and ruminants (beef, lamb, goat).*
- *Eat tropical plants but not their seeds.*
- *Ruthlessly purge high-omega-6 foods — especially seed, bean, and grain oils such as soybean oil, corn oil, canola oil, and safflower oil — from your diet.*

. . . .

We'll start our exploration of fats with the so-called essential fatty acids, omega-6 and omega-3 polyunsaturated fatty acids (PUFA). Polyunsaturated fatty acids are named for their multiple carbon double bonds; monounsaturated fatty acids have one double bond and saturated fatty acids have none.

Omega-6 and omega-3 PUFA are considered to be 'essential' because, unlike saturated fatty acids (SaFA) and monounsaturated fatty acids (MUFA), they cannot be manufactured from glucose. They must be obtained from food.

Omega-3 fats originate in green leaves and algae, while omega-6 fats mostly come from seeds. Since seeds yield much more oil than leaves and can be grown cheaply, industrial food producers prefer omega-6-rich seed oils such as soybean oil, corn oil, canola oil, and safflower oil. As our diets

---

SCIENCE OF THE PHD
'Essential' Does Not Mean 'Good'

Omega-6 and omega-3 polyunsaturated fats are termed 'essential' fatty acids. But this word does NOT imply these fats are desirable!

'Essential' is a scientific term; it means that the human body cannot manufacture these fats from other foods, so any omega-6 or omega-3 fats in the body must be obtained from diet. It says nothing about how many are needed. In fact, it implies that *they are rarely needed:* if dangerous deficiencies had ever developed, the body would have evolved a way to make them. The body's most important lipids can all be manufactured from carbohydrates and protein.

---

have shifted to industrial food, Australians have doubled their consumption of omega-6 fatty acids since the 1960s, while Americans have more than tripled their consumption since 1909, with most of the increase since the 1960s.

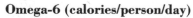

Omega-6 (calories/person/day)

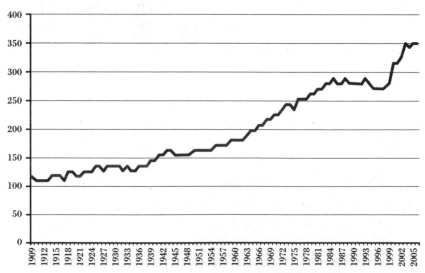

This shift to high-omega-6 diets is perhaps the most important dietary change of the last 50 years and may have caused the obesity epidemic. So it's important to understand the optimal intake of these fats.

Dangerous Partners: PUFA in the body

PUFA are dangerous compounds. The problem is their carbon double bonds, which are quick to react with oxygen. Think of PUFA as firecrackers, reactive oxygen as an open flame: a cell is like a home filled with firecrackers and lit candles. There is potential for things to go wrong.

Here is an index of the 'peroxidisability' of various fatty acids: [1]

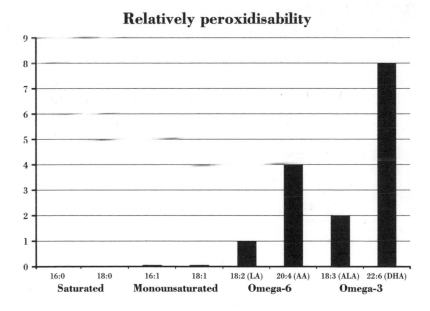

Relatively peroxidisability

Peroxidisability is zero for saturated fats and almost zero for monounsaturated fats, but high among polyunsaturated fats.

Lipid peroxidation is extremely dangerous, for two reasons: [2]

- It is a cascading process; as in an avalanche, peroxidation of one PUFA leads to peroxidation of many more.
- Peroxidation of PUFA generates highly toxic compounds, such as aldehydes, which mutate DNA, oxidise LDL, and turn proteins into advanced lipoxidation end products (ALEs).

Due to the abundance of PUFA in the body, their extreme fragility, and the highly toxic nature of their peroxidation products, PUFA peroxidation is a central factor affecting health and longevity.

Peroxidative damage to mitochondria causes serious health problems:

- Damage to mitochondria in skeletal muscle — the chief disposal organ for excess omega-6 fats — leads to rapid fatigue and decreased physical endurance. These in turn lead to reduced physical activity and contribute to obesity.[3]
- Damage to liver mitochondria leads to liver disease.[4]

Peroxidative damage to LDL particles creates oxidised LDL, a major factor in atherosclerosis.

The rate of lipid peroxidation appears to be a dominant factor controlling longevity in animals. The more PUFA animals have in their membranes, the shorter their life span. Here is how the 'peroxidation index' of membranes relates to life span across a number of animal species:[5]

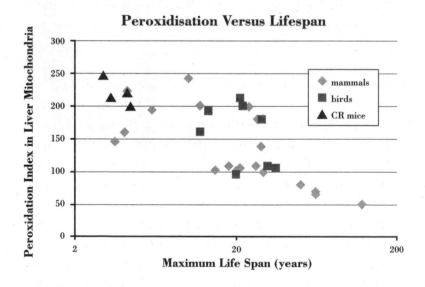

The lower the peroxidation index, the longer the maximum life span.

If PUFA are so dangerous, why do our bodies keep them around? There are two main reasons:

SCIENCE OF THE PHD
Life Span Extension with a PUFA-Restricted Diet

No other factor accounts for variations in life span as well as the rate of lipid peroxidation. A study of the reasons why rats live at most five years, while pigeons live up to 35 years, concluded:

> The only substantial and consistent difference that we have observed between rats and pigeons is their membrane fatty acid composition, with rats having membranes that are more susceptible to damage.[6]

Diet can modify the peroxidation index. In mice, calorie restriction extends life span and lowers the peroxidation index. The reduction in peroxidation index and the increase in life span exactly track the interspecies relationship.[7]

This is exciting, because it suggests that dietary interventions that reduce polyunsaturated fat content of membranes can extend human life span.

- Some biological processes function best in flexible PUFA-rich membranes. Saturated fats, which lack carbon double bonds, are rigid, which is why beef fat (which is full of saturated fat) is white and solid at room temperature. PUFA bend and twist at their double bonds and are liquid, flexible, and slippery. (Next time you have fresh salmon, get some of the oil on your hands and feel how slippery it is.) Neurons and retinal cells, in particular, need PUFA-rich membranes. Cold-water fish such as salmon and arctic char have a lot of PUFA in order to maintain flexible membranes at cold body temperatures.
- The body uses the fragility of highly unsaturated fatty acids (HUFA) — PUFA with four or more double bonds — to sense

when something is awry. For instance, infections and immune activity generate oxidative stress, and the body uses oxidated HUFA to sense and regulate the local level of oxidative stress. Oxidation of omega-6 HUFA detects infections and stimulates an inflammatory immune response; oxidation of omega-3 HUFA detects excessive inflammation and tamps it down. The body carefully regulates the amount of HUFA in membranes to preserve the integrity of this signalling.

The Peak Health Range for Omega-6 Fats

As we did with carbs, we'll let biology guide us to the optimal intake. You'll recall that when carb intake is too low, the body manufactures glucose from protein; when carb intake is too high, the body converts carbs to fat. The neutral carb intake, where the body neither manufactures nor destroys glucose, is the optimal carb intake.

Something similar happens with PUFA. Omega-6 and omega-3 fats cannot be manufactured, but the body can regulate PUFA abundance in tissue by controlling whether they are burned for energy and can regulate HUFA levels in membranes by controlling whether PUFA are lengthened and desaturated into HUFA.

Omega-6 Benefits End:
the bottom of the peak health range

On omega-6-deficient diets, omega-6 fats are conserved and rarely oxidised for energy.[8] Reduced oxidation of omega-6 fats indicates that dietary omega-6 intake is too low.

Another sign of PUFA deficiency is a failure of the body to achieve optimal levels of HUFA in membranes. This failure to achieve optimal HUFA levels causes dysregulation of immune function and generates the clinical symptoms of omega-6 or omega-3 deficiency. When dietary PUFA intake increases from zero, PUFA are rapidly converted to membrane HUFA until the membrane HUFA levels reach their optimum. From that point, membrane HUFA levels plateau; cells resist adding more HUFA to their membranes. Additional dietary PUFA are burned for energy.

Only a small amount of dietary PUFA is necessary to prevent a deficiency:

- Judged by the dietary omega-6 intake at which tissue levels of arachidonic acid (an omega-6 HUFA) plateau, omega-6 deficiencies are eliminated by 1 to 2 per cent of calories as omega-6 fats if the diet has no omega-3 fats,[9] and by just 0.3 per cent of calories as omega-6 fats if the diet has over 1 per cent omega-3 fats.[10] Thus, a little omega-3 fat in the diet reduces the requirement for omega-6 fat.
- Omega-3 fat deficiency can be relieved, bringing DHA in the liver to normal levels, by eating as little as 0.2 per cent of calories as omega-3 fats.[11]

Thus, the peak health range for PUFA can be entered by consuming as little as 1 per cent of energy as PUFA (0.5 per cent each of omega-6 and omega-3). Even on unbalanced diets, 2 per cent of energy as PUFA will achieve optimal membrane HUFA levels.

Omega-6 fats constitute 2 per cent or more of most natural foods, so on plant-and-animal-food diets it is impossible to become deficient in omega-6 fats, unless some medical condition such as cystic fibrosis prevents fat digestion. Absolute omega-3 deficiencies are also rare.

SCIENCE OF THE PHD
The Rarity of PUFA Deficiency

It is so difficult to induce PUFA deficiencies that it took decades to prove a human need for PUFA.[12] The only known cases of omega-6 fat deficiency have occurred on purified-nutrient diets, such as infant formula or intravenous feeding, not on natural diets of plant and animal foods.

The need for PUFA was originally discovered in the 1920s by feeding rats lifelong fat-free diets. On zero-PUFA diets, rats grew more slowly.

In humans, the main symptom of an omega-6 deficiency is a dry,

(continued on next page)

scaly skin rash. In the 1940s and 1950s, it was common to feed infants a fat-free milk formula: skim milk with sugar. After some months, the infants developed eczema that could be cured by giving them lard, which is about 10 per cent PUFA. Other possible effects of an omega-6 deficiency are impaired growth of infants, susceptibility to infection, and slow wound healing.[13]

Evidence showing that PUFA deficiencies were possible in adults came from the period when intravenous nutrition did not provide fats.[14]

- Two cases of omega-6 deficiency arose in 1969 and 1970 in people who had much of their intestines surgically removed and who were placed on fat-free intravenous feeding for months.
- A case of omega-3, but not omega-6, deficiency arose in a girl who in 1982 underwent a series of surgeries after a gunshot wound in the abdomen. After five months of intravenous feeding with safflower oil as the only fat — which has abundant omega-6 but negligible omega-3 — she developed an omega-3 deficiency, characterised by episodes of numbness, tingling, weakness, inability to walk, leg pain, psychological disturbances, and blurred vision.

Although deficiency of omega-6 fats in general is almost impossible, it is possible to achieve a deficiency of omega-6 HUFA, such as arachidonic acid, under oxidative stress. High levels of immune activity generate oxidative stress, and if the diet is deficient in antioxidants, depletion of AA may follow, generating classic omega-6 deficiency symptoms such as eczema.

Our reader JC's sister, whose story is on the following page, had just this condition.

Omega-6 Toxicity: the upper end of the peak health range

As omega-6 intake increases above optimal levels, the body begins to preferentially oxidise omega-6 fats ahead of other fats. This is an effort to dispose of excess omega-6.

READER REPORTS:
eczema and chronic fatigue syndrome

You will remember 12 days ago I asked you about my sister who has CFS and was taking 100 mls a day of safflower oil to keep eczema under control.

You wrote: 'My guess is that there is a high level of oxidative stress which is diminishing AA levels, and the safflower oil makes more arachidonic acid and relieves the problem. So the strategy I would try first is (a) supplementing antioxidants . . . and (b) treating any infections. Also, get serum 25OHD levels tested and normalize vitamin D/A/K status.'

Your advice was spot on and the results have been miraculous. She started supplementation with zinc, copper, selenium, vitamins C, E, D and K and NAC. Within 24 hours her eczema was much improved and she began reducing the safflower oil. Now 10 days later she is down to 10 mls of safflower oil and is confident she can discontinue it completely in a few days. Her eczema has completely cleared and her skin is looking good.

An interesting note: prior to starting the antioxidants she craved the safflower oil and could hardly wait for her next 'dose'. That has been replaced with feeling nauseous even at the thought of the oil. Obviously her body no longer needs it.

Not only that, but some of her CFS symptoms have improved. Her constant headache is not as severe, irregular heartbeat episodes have almost completely stopped and she is tolerating slightly more physical activity. Needless to say she is absolutely delighted and wants me to pass on her deepest gratitude to you. Her words are, 'It's a miracle.' Proverbs 13:12 springs to mind. 'Hope deferred makes the heart sick, but a longing fulfilled is a tree of life.' Her sense of despair and resignation has gone and you have given her hope of a better future. Words seem inadequate to express thanks for that.

— JC

On nearly all modern diets, omega-6 fats are preferentially oxidised. An ingested omega-6 fatty acid is three times more likely to be burned for energy than an ingested saturated fatty acid.[15] Moreover, omega-6 fats are not completely oxidised to carbon dioxide and water; rather, most omega-6 fats are partially oxidised and then reassembled into cholesterol and saturated fat.[16] This increases the number of omega-6 fats that can be disposed within the limits to mitochondrial energy production and transforms the dangerous and useless omega-6 fatty acids into safer and more useful cholesterol and saturated fatty acids. The crossover point — the 'natural intake' level at which omega-6 fats are equally likely as saturated and monounsaturated fats to be burned for energy — is not known, but it probably occurs with not more than 3 per cent of energy as PUFA.

Looking instead at HUFA levels in tissue, intake of 1 to 4 per cent of calories as omega-6 fats enables the body to optimise HUFA ratios. However, when omega-6 intake exceeds 4 per cent of energy, tissue levels of omega-6 DGLA and omega-3 EPA are suppressed. DGLA is a long-chain omega-6 fat, but one that moderates the inflammatory effects of AA. Due to this effect, omega-6 consumption above 4 per cent of energy increases AA-to-DGLA and AA-to-EPA ratios with inflammatory effects.[17]

A number of toxicity effects appear with omega-6 intake above 4 per cent of calories. This omega-6 intake has been shown to reduce EPA and DHA levels in pregnant mothers.[18] In piglets, 1.2 per cent omega-6 consumption with adequate omega-3 leads to healthy brain development, but increasing omega-6 intake to 10.7 per cent of calories deprives brains of DHA and compromises neurodevelopment.[19]

. . . .

Four per cent of calories as omega-6 fats is the threshold of health impairment.

. . . .

Further problems appear when omega-6 fat intake reaches 6 per cent of calories. At this intake level, oxidation can't remove the omega-6 fats fast enough, and they start to build up in the body, especially in adipose tissue.

Accumulation of omega-6 fats in adipose tissue is observed in clinical trials. In the Finnish Mental Hospital Study, over four years on a diet rich in soybean oil, participants' omega-6 fats rose from 10.2 per cent of adipose tissue fats to 32.4 per cent.[20] In the Los Angeles Veterans Administration Study, on a diet that was 15 per cent omega-6 by calories, participants' adipose tissue omega-6 levels rose from 10 per cent at the start of the study to 33.7 per cent over a five-year period.[21]

A similar accumulation of omega-6 in adipose tissue has occurred in Americans over the last 50 years, according to data assembled by Stephan Guyenet of the University of Washington. Here's how it looks.[22]

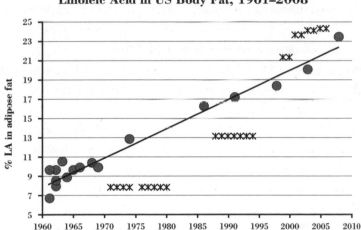

Linoleic Acid in US Body Fat, 1961–2008

The circles mark the percentage of body fat that is linoleic acid (the major omega-6 fat); the crosses mark the fraction of 18- to 29-year-olds who are obese. The obesity epidemic began at the same time, or a few years after, omega-6 fats began accumulating in Americans' bodies.

Americans currently obtain 9 per cent of calories as omega-6 fats, their adipose fats are 23.4 per cent omega-6, and fully a quarter of 18- to 29-year-olds are obese. Back in 1961, omega-6 fats made up 5.8 per cent of the diet, adipose fats were about 9 per cent omega-6, and obesity was rare. A similar pattern has occurred in Australia and New Zealand, where increasing consumption of omega-6 fats has also been associated with increasing rates of obesity.

It appears that when dietary omega-6 intake exceeds 6 per cent of energy, omega-6 fats start to accumulate in adipose tissue, and obesity often follows.

It's a safe bet that 6 per cent of energy as omega-6 fats is far above the peak health range.

Health Effects of Omega-6 Toxicity

Americans are now getting 9 per cent of their energy as omega-6 fats, and Australians and New Zealanders nearly as much. But toxicity begins at 4 per cent of energy; so we ought to be able to see negative effects from this excess.

And we do. As a result of their excessive intake of omega-6 fats, Americans are experiencing elevated rates of liver disease, atherosclerosis, obesity, allergies and asthma, mental illness, bowel disorders, and cancer, not to mention elevated mortality rates. Let's look at some of the evidence.

Liver Disease Caused by High-PUFA Diets

Polyunsaturated fats — both omega-6 and omega-3 — readily produce liver disease when eaten in conjunction with fructose or alcohol, which increase oxidative stress in the liver.

High PUFA intake (say, from soybean oil or corn oil) is a prerequisite for liver disease, while low-PUFA diets (say, with coconut oil or butter) prevent liver disease.

Here is a sampling of studies in which PUFA destroyed and SaFA rescued the health of lab animals' livers:

- Researchers induced fatty liver disease in mice by feeding diets deficient in key nutrients. One diet provided 34 per cent of calories as corn oil, the other as coconut oil. (Corn oil is 57 per cent omega-6 PUFA, while coconut oil is 2 per cent omega-6 PUFA and 92 per cent SaFA.) The mice fed corn oil had severe liver damage, but 'histological scores demonstrated significantly less steatosis, inflammation and necrosis in SaFA-fed mice of all mouse strains'.[23]
- Researchers induced liver disease by feeding mice a combination of alcohol and omega-3-rich fish oil. They then stopped the alcohol and split the mice into two groups, one fed fish oil plus glucose, the other SaFA-rich palm oil plus glucose. Livers of the fish oil group failed to recover, but the palm oil group 'showed near normalization'. The researchers hailed SaFA as 'a novel treatment for liver disease'.[24]

- A study compared a high-carb corn oil diet (62 per cent of calories as carbs, 21 per cent as corn oil, 17 per cent as protein) with low-carb coconut oil or butter diets (17 per cent of calories as carbs, 71 per cent as coconut oil or butter, 12 per cent as protein). Mice eating the coconut oil and butter diets maintained healthy livers despite nutrient deficiencies that normally induce liver disease, while mice on the high-carb corn oil diet developed severe disease.[25]

- Scientists induced liver disease in mice by feeding alcohol plus corn oil. They then substituted a saturated fat–rich mix based on beef tallow and coconut oil for 20 per cent, 45 per cent, and 67 per cent of the corn oil. The more saturated fat, the healthier the liver.[26]

- Mice fed 27.5 per cent of calories as alcohol developed severe liver disease and metabolic syndrome when given a corn oil diet, but no disease at all when given a SaFA-rich cocoa butter diet. (The first line of this paper reads, 'The protective effect of dietary saturated fatty acids against the development of alcoholic liver disease has long been known' — yet somehow this knowledge has eluded many nutritionists.)[27]

The pattern is obvious: give sugar or alcohol in combination with either omega-6 or omega-3 PUFA, and mice develop fatty liver and metabolic syndrome. Give a diet without PUFA, and the liver does fine.

Dyslipidemia and Atherosclerosis
Peroxidation of PUFA creates oxidised LDL, a contributor to elevated serum cholesterol and atherosclerosis.

In studies in 1996 and 1997, volunteers ate, for five weeks each, diets supplemented with four different kinds of fat: a SaFA-rich diet, a MUFA-rich diet, an omega-6-rich diet, and an omega-3-rich diet.[28] The levels of LDL oxidation after each period were as follows.

Levels of Ox-LDL on Various Diets

Diet	TBARs,* 1996 Study	TBARs, 1997 Study
SaFA	1.15	0.89
MUFA	1.15	1.06
Omega-6	1.51	1.56
Omega-3	1.69	1.70

*Thiobarbituric acid reactive substances in LDL,
in nmol of MDA per mg of LDL protein.

In the PUFA-supplemented diets, ox-LDL was increased by at least 30 per cent compared to SaFA- or MUFA-supplemented diets. Overall, the amount of ox-LDL in the body was roughly proportional to the amount of PUFA, and highest on the high-omega-3 diet (since omega-3 fats have a higher peroxidation index than omega-6 fats).

Omega-6 Fats and Obesity

In both rodents and humans, fat mass increases as omega-6 consumption increases.

In one study, rats were divided into three groups receiving diets identical in fat, protein, and carbohydrate calories but differing in the source of the fats: one group was given beef tallow (low in omega-6), another olive oil (moderate in omega-6), and the third safflower oil (very high in omega-6). Relative to the tallow group, the rats in the olive oil group had a 7.5 per cent increase in total body weight, and those in the safflower group had a 12.3 per cent increase.[29]

In another study, 782 men were kept on calorie-controlled diets for five years. They were split into two groups, one consuming animal fats and the other omega-6-rich vegetable oils. The vegetable oil–consuming group had steady gains in body fat and weight compared to the animal fat group; in later years of the study, the vegetable oil group averaged about 5 per cent, or 3.6 kilograms, more weight.[30]

In a third study, four groups of rats were given 52 per cent fat diets with varying amounts of saturated and polyunsaturated fats. The more polyunsaturated fat was consumed, the more rapidly the rats gained weight.[31]

The obesogenic effects of omega-6 fats are strongest on diets high in sugar, but are weak on low-carb diets.[32]

Immune Function, Allergies, and Asthma

Omega-6 fats are generally considered to be inflammatory, and they are. However, excess omega-6 fats actually suppress and distort the immune system.[33] This distorted immune response is doubly bad because:

- The response to extracellular pathogens becomes exaggerated, leading to **allergies.**[34] Young children seem to be especially vulnerable: higher levels of omega-6 fats in mother's milk are associated with **runny nose, asthma, and skin rashes.**[35]
- The response to intracellular viruses and bacteria is weakened. This presumably increases the likelihood of diseases associated with intracellular infections, such as **atherosclerosis, Alzheimer's disease, multiple sclerosis, Lyme disease, Parkinson's disease,** and other **diseases of ageing.**

Omega-6 Fats and Mental Illness

High vegetable oil consumption is associated with depression, mental illness, and high rates of violence. We'll cite papers demonstrating such links later, in our discussion of omega-6 to omega-3 balance, but for now, let's look at an intriguing correlation.

Throughout the industrialised world, omega-6 consumption has increased sharply since 1960 due to increasing use of vegetable oils. Joseph Hibbeln, Levi Nieminin, and William Lands had the idea of comparing omega-6 consumption to rates of violence. They found, across a panel of five countries for which good data were available, two patterns:

- The more omega-6 a country consumed, the higher its homicide rate. The United States, with the highest omega-6 consumption, had the highest homicide rate. Australia, with relatively low omega-6 consumption, had a much lower homicide rate.
- As omega-6 consumption increased between 1960 and 2000, each country — Australia included — saw an increase in its homicide rate.

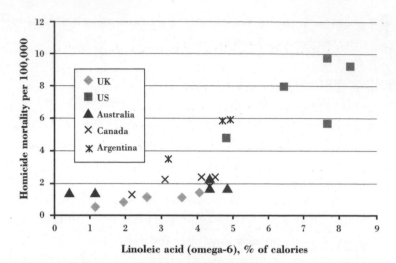

Homicide mortality rates versus consumption of omega-6 linoleic acid,
plotted for 1961, 1970, 1980, 1990, and 2000 in five countries. Within each
country, homicide rates go up as linoleic acid consumption goes up.[36]

Omega-6 Fats and Digestive Health

The incidence of digestive ailments scales with consumption of omega-6
fatty acids. The EPIC study found that those in the highest quartile of consumption of linoleic acid, the omega-6 fat in vegetable oils, have 2.5 times
the risk of ulcerative colitis as those with the lowest consumption.[37]

Omega-6 Fats and Cancer

Omega-6-rich oils promote cancer progression and metastasis. For instance, corn oil, but not saturated fat, stimulates the progression of prostate
cancer.[38]

When mice with implanted tumours were fed a diet high in linoleic
acid, the omega-6 fat in vegetable oils, they experienced a rate of metastasis
four times higher than mice fed oleic acid, a monounsaturated fat.[39]

Mortality Rates

We know of eight clinical intervention trials that directly compared a high-
omega-6 diet with a high-SaFA diet and measured total mortality rates. The
high-omega-6 diet was clearly harmful in three, possibly harmful in two
others, clearly superior in none.

READER REPORTS: healing gut disease

Perhaps this is as good a place as any to share the improvements I experienced after switching from a gut-healing diet that generally can be described as VLC Paleo to PHD. What's even more remarkable than the improvements themselves is that they occurred *within 48 hours* of seriously increasing my safe starch consumption. I couldn't have special ordered it any better.

1. Constipation is gone.
2. Mysterious, persistent rash is gone.
3. Energy and mood are way better.
4. I like what I'm eating now, I am satiated after meals, and my instincts are no longer telling me something's missing. This intangible effect has made perhaps the biggest impact on my day-to-day quality of life.

Also, the final lingering symptoms of my husband's ulcerative colitis resolved after switching to PHD.

Thank you Paul and Shou-Ching! Your PHD came into my life at exactly the right time and produced exactly the changes I needed. So indulge me in a bit of gushing when I tell you I'm utterly grateful for both your product (the book) and service (advice on your site). The one-on-one advice is a very powerful way to connect with your audience. It's as though I can feel the sense of community and healing when I'm on your site. You've got a special thing going, and we appreciate all your efforts.

— Anonymous

- In three — the **Rose Corn Oil Study,**[40] **Anti-Coronary Club Program,**[41] and **Sydney Diet-Heart Study**[42] — the high-PUFA diet seemed clearly harmful, raising death rates 364 per cent, 156 per cent, and 49 per cent, respectively. The Rose Corn Oil trial is particularly interesting: it was the only trial to supply

PUFA in a form — corn oil — that does not contain omega-3 fats, and it had an extraordinarily high death rate in the PUFA group. Omega-3 fats are a partial antidote to omega-6 toxicity!

- In two — the **Minnesota Coronary Survey**[43] and the **Los Angeles Veterans Administration Study**[44] — the high-PUFA diet raised the death rate by less than 10 per cent. The increases were not considered significant. The Los Angeles Veterans Study is interesting: a later retrospective search found 31 cancer deaths among the high-PUFA group and 17 among the controls,[45] even though the number of smokers was much larger in the control diet group.[46]

- The **Oslo Diet-Heart Study** saw 6.5 per cent fewer deaths in its omega-6+fish oil arm, a difference that was not considered significant. Heart attack death rates were lower, but cancer and infectious disease death rates were higher.[47] Given the powerful ability of fish oil to suppress cardiac mortality rates, it seems plausible that the high-PUFA arm would have seen higher death rates than the control if it had not included a large amount of fish oil.

- The **Medical Research Council Study** saw three, or 10 per cent, fewer deaths on its high-PUFA arm but two (8 per cent) more cardiac deaths.[48] These differences were judged to be insignificant, and that judgement is supported by the unexpectedness of this pattern: in other studies, the high-PUFA arm saw a higher overall mortality rate but a reduced cardiac mortality rate.

- The **Finnish Mental Hospital Study**[49] was beset by a crossover design that clouded the results. If dietary omega-6 affects mortality only at the moment it is consumed, the high-PUFA diet lowered the mortality rate by 14 per cent; however, if omega-6 fats affect mortality as long as they remain in the body, the high-PUFA diet increased the mortality rate by at least 28 per cent. (In the hospital that was assigned the high-omega-6 diet first, adipose-tissue omega-6 levels were still elevated four years after residents had switched back to a lower-omega-6 diet. In that hospital, death rates were much higher than in the hospital that used a low-omega-6 diet for the first six years of the study.)

Overall, results of the eight clinical trials indicate a significant increase in mortality rates, especially from cancer, when omega-6 intake reaches 10 per cent of calories.

This is disturbing, because Americans currently average 9 per cent of calories as omega-6 fats!

Takeaway

The optimal intake of omega-6 fats is probably about 2 to 3 per cent of energy, toxicity begins at 4 per cent of energy, and Americans' intake averages 9 per cent of energy.

Most Americans should cut their omega-6 intake by a factor of three, and even reducing it by a factor of nine would still be safe and health-improving!

The Peak Health Range for Omega-3 Fats

It is difficult to identify the omega-3 intake at which toxicity begins, because high omega-3 intake is a partial antidote to omega-6 toxicity. Most people consume far too much omega-6. For them, a high omega-3 intake may be toxic and yet beneficial because it relieves omega-6 toxicity.

Thus, the omega-3 intake that is optimal for Americans on a high-omega-6 diet may be much higher than is optimal for those of us on a lower-omega-6 diet.

We have a bit of evidence for omega-3 toxicity in general and a lot of evidence for the optimal omega-6 to omega-3 ratio. Let's look at those in turn and see what they tell us about our optimal omega-3 intake.

Omega-3 Toxicity

The peroxidative index of omega-3 fats is even higher than that of omega-6, so they can certainly cause mitochondrial damage, DNA mutations, shortened life span, and the other negative effects of lipid peroxidation.

Known toxicity effects of high omega-3 intake include:

- **Liver damage.** When omega-3 fats are eaten in conjunction with alcohol or fructose, they are just as effective as omega-6 fats at causing liver disease.[50]

- **Bleeding and stroke.** High omega-3 intake, especially of EPA and DHA, prolongs bleeding times and may increase the risk of stroke. In Greenland Eskimos with very high intakes of EPA+DHA (6.5 grams per day, equivalent to about 2.25 kilograms of salmon per week), an increased incidence of hemorrhagic stroke has been observed.[51]

- **Early ageing and shortened life span.** We saw that a higher peroxidation index was associated with shortened life span in animals. Animal studies show that high omega-3 intake can shorten life span, probably through increased peroxidation. One study showed that when pregnant rats are given excessive doses of omega-3 fats, their offspring have shortened life span and greater neural degeneration in old age. The authors concluded, 'both over- and under-supplementation with omega-3 FA can harm offspring development'.[52] In another study, feeding mice a high-fish-oil diet shortened their average life span because of peroxidative stress.[53]

Omega-3 toxicity is even greater if the omega-3 fats are allowed to become rancid. In general, fish are refrigerated or frozen immediately after catch and their omega-3 oils remain fresh. However, fish oil capsules are usually stored at room temperature for long periods of time. The fish oil in capsules must therefore often become rancid, since omega-3 fats are so easily oxidised.

It is interesting that fish consumption has an excellent record in clinical trials, but fish-oil capsule supplements do not. In the Diet and Angina Randomized Trial (DART-2), 3114 men with stable angina were followed for three to nine years. There were a control group, a group advised to eat oily fish, and a group taking three fish oil capsules daily. There was a significant increase in sudden cardiac death among the subgroup taking fish oil capsules.[54]

· ·

Do not *take fish oil capsules. Get your omega-3 fats from fish.*

· ·

The Benefits of Omega-6 and Omega-3 Balance

Dr William E. Lands and collaborators did much to elucidate the optimal ratio of omega-6 to omega-3 fats. His work was helpful because it separated the EFA puzzle into two more tractable issues: how tissue abundances affect health, and how dietary intake affects tissue abundances.

In humans and other animals, the most biologically active PUFAs are the HUFAs: principally, the 20-carbon omega-6s **arachidonic acid (AA)** and **dihomo-gamma-linolenic acid (DGLA),** the 20-carbon omega-3 **eicosapentaenoic acid (EPA),** and the 22-carbon omega-3 **docosahexae-noic acid (DHA).** In the body, AA, DGLA, and EPA are precursors of eicosanoids; EPA and DHA are precursors of compounds called resolvins; and DHA is a structural fat in the brain, nerves, and retina.

Nature has turned the fragility of polyunsaturated fats to its advantage by using oxidised PUFA as signalling molecules, called **eicosanoids** and **docosanoids.** When a cell is damaged, enzymes release 20-carbon PUFAs from the cell membrane and turn them into eicosanoids. The eicosanoids trigger inflammation that brings in the immune system to help fight pathogens or remove toxins.

Some of the most popular drugs in the world — aspirin and ibuprofen — work by preventing omega-6 fats from being turned into eicosanoids.

Omega-3 HUFA also are intentionally oxidised by the body into eicosanoids and docosanoids. While the eicosanoids from omega-6 HUFA tend to be inflammatory, the derivatives of omega-3 HUFA are generally anti-inflammatory. They moderate the effect of omega-6 eicosanoids and act as an antidote to some forms of omega-6 toxicity.

Cardiovascular disease risk is strongly influenced by the balance between omega-6 HUFA and omega-3 HUFA in tissue. Dr William E. Lands discovered the relationship shown on the next page.[55]

Heart disease mortality rates rise as the omega-6 fraction rises and the omega-3 fraction decreases, and approach zero when tissue HUFAs are 72 per cent omega-3, 28 per cent omega-6. The total mortality rate is also minimised at about the same tissue ratio.[56]

The tissue percentages of most Americans (see 'USA' at the upper right of the graph) are less than 25 per cent omega-3 HUFA, more than 75 per cent omega-6 HUFA. The omega-6 to omega-3 tissue HUFA ratio is about ninefold higher than the optimum: it should be three to one in favour of

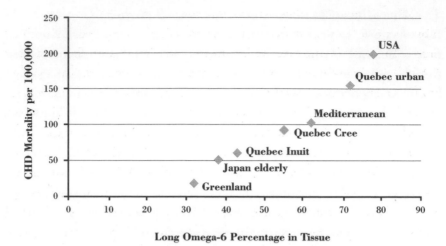

The horizontal axis is the percentage of long-chain (20-carbon or longer)
PUFA in tissue that are omega-6, not omega-3. The greater the omega-6
fraction, the higher the cardiovascular mortality rate.

omega-3 but instead is 3 to 1 in favour of omega-6. This imbalance alone more
than triples the United States' cardiovascular mortality rate relative to Japan's.

Achieving balance between omega-6 and omega-3 HUFA has benefits
for other parts of the body, too:

- Reducing the omega-6 to omega-3 ratio improves bone mineral
  density.[57]
- Reducing the omega-6 to omega-3 ratio relieves depression.[58]
- Reducing the omega-6 to omega-3 ratio decreases anger and
  anxiety, reduces aggression, and reduces suicidal behaviours
  and self-harm.[59]
- A low omega-6 to omega-3 ratio improves recovery from sepsis
  and operations and shortens stay in intensive care units.[60]

More evidence of the benefits of omega-6 and omega-3 balance comes
from a fascinating experiment. A gene from nematodes that converts omega-6
fats to omega-3 fats was inserted into the genome of mice. Regardless of diet,
these transgenic mice have equal amounts of omega-6 and omega-3 fats
in their membranes. They develop stronger vertebrae[61] and are protected
against nerve injury,[62] Alzheimer's disease,[63] allergies,[64] diabetes,[65] macular
degeneration,[66] bowel disease,[67] and cancer.[68]

Clinical trials also support a low omega-6 to omega-3 ratio. Among the most successful clinical trials at reducing mortality was the Lyon Diet Heart Study. This study compared the American Heart Association Step One diet (a high-carb, high-omega-6 diet) with a Mediterranean diet that was low (less than 7 grams per day, about 3 per cent of energy) in omega-6 and high in omega-3 due to a supplement providing 2 grams per day of ALA. The result: a striking reduction in all-cause mortality rates, heart attacks, and cancer.

After a mean follow-up of 27 months, the number of cardiac deaths was 16 on the AHA diet, three on the Lyon diet; the number of all-cause deaths was 20 on the AHA diet, eight on the Lyon diet.[69] At four years follow-up, there had been 19 cardiac deaths on the AHA diet, six on the Lyon diet; 24 total deaths on the AHA diet, 14 on the Lyon diet; 17 cancer cases and four cancer deaths on the AHA diet, seven cancer cases and three cancer deaths on the Lyon diet.[70]

Another clinical trial that tested increased dietary omega-3 was the Diet and Reinfarction Trial (DART), which enrolled 2033 British men who had previously suffered a heart attack. In this trial, a fish-eating group tripled their weekly omega-3 intake from 0.6 to 2.4 grams of EPA. This group saw a significant reduction in both heart attacks and all-cause deaths: 9.3 per cent of the fish-eating group died, 12.8 per cent of the control group.[71]

Dietary Intakes for Omega-6 and Omega-3 Balance

Different cultures around the world have widely different omega-6 and omega-3 intakes. This has allowed scientists to develop a formula relating tissue abundances of long-chain PUFAs to dietary intake of the various PUFAs.[72] An Excel calculator is available online.[73]

The plant-derived PUFAs LA and ALA have little direct use in the body; but they serve as a reservoir from which longer-chain PUFAs can be manufactured. Typically, only a fraction of these shorter PUFAs are converted to the longer-chain PUFAs that control mortality risk.

In practice, for most people, three fatty acids determine tissue abundances of the long-chain PUFAs:

- The 18-carbon omega-6 **linoleic acid (LA)** is the dominant omega-6 fat in most diets; internationally, LA generally makes up more than 90 per cent of dietary omega-6 fats, ranging from about 90 per cent in Filipino diets to about 98 per cent of the omega-6 in American diets. Many of the long-chain omega-6 fats (such as AA and DGLA) in tissue are derived from LA, not obtained directly from diet. The main dietary sources of LA are vegetable oils and baked or fried foods cooked with vegetable oils.

- Although the 18-carbon omega-3 alpha-linolenic acid (ALA) is a larger component of diet, tissue long-chain omega-3 levels depend mainly on dietary intake of the long-chain omega-3s **EPA, DPA,** and **DHA.** This is partly because LA inhibits the conversion of ALA into long-chain omega-3s, so that at the high vegetable oil intakes of most Americans, the conversion rate of ALA into EPA is small.

Thus, two foods largely control the tissue omega-6 to omega-3 ratio: vegetable oils (supplying omega-6 LA) and cold-water fish (supplying long-chain omega-3s). We can calculate the key tissue abundance ratio from just two inputs — LA intake as a fraction of total energy and long-chain omega-3 intake as a fraction of total energy. A graph of the results of this calculation is available online at the U.S. National Institutes of Health EFA Education site.[74]

The table below gives the salmon intake required at different LA intakes to achieve the optimal 28 per cent long-chain omega-6, 72 per cent long-chain omega-3 tissue ratio.

LA g/day (% of energy)	EPA+DPA+DHA g/day (% of energy)	Salmon (450 g/week)
4.8 (2%)	1.8 (0.74%)	1.2
7.2 (3%)	2.6 (1.1%)	1.7
9.6 (4%)	3.5 (1.4%)	2.3

The conversion between grams and percentage of calories is based on a diet of 2200 calories per day. The salmon estimate assumes 10.7 grams of EPA+DPA+DHA per 450 grams of salmon, which is typical of farm-raised Atlantic salmon.

These omega-6 intakes of 2 to 4 per cent of energy are within our peak health range.

The Japanese consume about 1.5 grams of long-chain omega-3s per day, equivalent to about 450 grams of salmon per week. Clear evidence of omega-3 toxicity begins at about 3 grams of long-chain omega-3s per day, meaning that it's important to eat less than 900 grams of salmon per week.

So this leaves a narrow window of omega-6 and omega-3 intakes that can achieve balance while avoiding toxicity. We must ruthlessly minimise our omega-6 intake while eating as the Japanese do — about 450 grams of oily marine fish per week.

This would require big changes to the diets of those in countries such as the United States, Canada, Australia, and New Zealand:

- Australians eat less than 0.25 gram per day of long-chain omega-3s. Eating 450 grams of salmon per week would **increase the average Australian's EPA plus DHA intake fivefold.**
- Americans now consume about 36 grams per day of LA, 8.9 per cent of calories.[75] This is up from about 12 grams per day in 1909.[76] Getting LA intake down to 7 grams per day (3 per cent of energy on 2000 calories per day) would require **a fivefold reduction in omega-6 consumption.**

Such big changes can be achieved, but only with total elimination of vegetable seed oils and foods prepared with them (including most commercial breads, doughnuts, cookies, crackers, and chips) and the inclusion of cold-water fish as a once-a-week feature of the diet.

Optimal Meats and Oils

We've found that for optimal health we want to minimise omega-6 fats, keeping them below 4 per cent of energy and preferably near 2 per cent of energy, while eating about 450 grams of salmon (or similar fish, such as sardines) per week to achieve omega-6 and omega-3 balance.

On the following page there is a table of the omega-6 and omega-3 content of various animal foods.

Table: macronutrient profile of meats, seafood, and eggs

Food	Calories per 450 g	Fat/Protein Content, Calories	Omega-6 as Per Cent of Fat	Omega-3 as Per Cent of Fat
Ribeye steak	1202	59%/41%	3%	1%
Ground beef (85%)	1164	55%/45%	2%	0%
Prime rib	1321	64%/36%	3%	1%
Lamb, leg	1152	71%/29%	3%	1%
Goat, wild (lean)	649	20%/80%	4%	1%
Chicken leg	866	41%/59%	19%	2%
Chicken breast, meat and skin	837	38%/62%	18%	1%
Chicken breast, skinless	749	21%/79%	17%	2%
Chicken liver	781	36%/64%	1%	0%
Duck, roasted	1531	77%/23%	12%	1%
Pork, country ribs	1490	71%/29%	7%	0%
Ham	807	47%/53%	13%	3%
Bacon	2420	70%/30%	10%	0%
Salmon, Atlantic (farmed)	936	56%/44%	5%	18%
Salmon, Atlantic (wild)	825	42%/58%	3%	32%
Herring	921	53%/47%	1%	19%
Cod	477	8%/92%	1%	21%
Tilapia	581	19%/81%	11%	9%
Shrimp	449	10%/90%	2%	33%
Mussels	780	28%/72%	1%	19%
Eggs	704	65%/35%	11%	1%

The essential points to take from the table are:

1. The best sources of omega-3 fats are **marine fish** and **shellfish:** salmon, herring, sardines, mussels, clams, and shrimp. Other animal foods have few omega-3 fats.
2. To minimise omega-6 consumption, the best foods are **fish, shell-fish,** and **ruminant meats — beef, lamb,** and **goat.** Ruminant

meats generally provide 3 per cent of fats and less than 2 per cent of calories, as omega-6 fats. Fish and shellfish generally have minimal omega-6 — below 1 per cent of calories.

3. Many popular meats — chicken, pork, eggs, duck, and tilapia, which is a farmed fish — have omega-6 levels between 10 and 20 per cent of fats. The exception: some organ meats are low in omega-6, such as **chicken liver.**

We recommend making fish, shellfish, and ruminant meats your principal meats, eaten five days of the week. Eat chicken and pork only occasionally for variety.

What about oils? Here are the omega-6 and omega-3 contents of some animal fats.

Fat	SaFA, %	MUFA, %	Omega-6, %	Omega-3, %
Salmon (wild) oil	19.9%	29.0%	1.5%	35.3%
Tallow (beef)	49.8%	41.8%	3.1%	0.6%
Butter	63.6%	25.9%	3.4%	0.4%
Salmon (farmed) fat	22.6%	28.2%	7.3%	18.7%
Lard (pork)*	39.2%	45.1%	10.2%	1.0%
Duck fat	33.2%	49.3%	12.0%	1.0%
Egg yolks	37.5%	46.0%	15.5%	1.0%
Chicken fat	29.8%	44.7%	19.5%	1.0%

* Warning: lard from confined grain-fed pigs can range up to 33 per cent omega-6.

And here are some healthful plant oils.

Oil	SaFA, %	MUFA, %	Omega-6, %	Omega-3, %
Palm kernel oil	81.7%	11.4%	1.6%	0.0%
Coconut oil	86.7%	5.8%	1.8%	0.0%
Cocoa butter	59.6%	32.9%	2.8%	0.1%
Palm oil	49.1%	37.0%	9.1%	0.2%
Olive oil	13.8%	73.1%	9.8%	0.8%

(continued on next page)

Oil	SaFA, %	MUFA,%	Omega-6, %	Omega-3, %
Avocado oil	11.6%	70.6%	12.5%	1.0%
Cashew butter	20.3%	59.5%	16.5%	0.3%
Almond butter	9.5%	64.8%	20.1%	0.7%

Oils used in cooking or sauces and dressings should be low in both omega-6 and omega-3 fats. Cooking exposes polyunsaturated fats to high temperatures that can denature them; shelf storage may also lead to rancidity.

The best fats and oils to use in cooking and for sauces and salad dressings are **beef tallow, clarified butter** or **ghee, coconut oil** or **coconut milk, palm kernel oil, cocoa butter,** and **macadamia nut butter.** Duck fat, olive oil, and avocado oil are also healthful but fall into a second tier of healthfulness, rather like duck, chicken, and pork among meats.

Here are some oils that should be eliminated from your diet.

Oil	SaFU, %	MUFA, %	Omega-6, %	Omega-3, %
Canola oil	7.4%	63.3%	18.6%	9.1%
Peanut oil	16.9%	46.2%	32.0%	0.0%
Soybean oil	15.6%	22.8%	50.4%	6.8%
Corn oil	12.9%	27.6%	53.5%	1.2%
Wheat germ oil	18.8%	15.1%	54.8%	6.9%
Safflower oil	6.2%	14.4%	74.6%	0.0%

Though canola oil has one redeeming feature — a good balance between omega-6 and omega-3 — it has two disqualifying traits: 27.7 per cent of its fats are PUFA, which is too much; and it may contain toxins, as we'll discuss in Part III.

In short:

- Minimise your dietary omega-6 intake by eliminating omega-6-rich vegetable oils from your diet; relying on low-omega-6 oils such as butter, beef tallow, and coconut oil; and eating low-omega-6 animal foods such as fish, shellfish, beef, and lamb.
- Eat at least 225 grams, and up to 450 grams, per week of salmon or other fatty fish for omega-3 fats.

12
The Safe Fats: SaFA and MUFA

- *Saturated and monounsaturated fats are safe to consume, even in large quantities.*
- *They are the most adjustable macronutrient of our diet: the quantity eaten can be adjusted up or down to satisfy appetite.*
- *On calorie-restricted weight-loss diets, these are the macronutrients to cut.*

The macronutrients we've considered so far all become toxic above a threshold: protein above 600 calories per day; carbs (if there is any impairment of disposal pathways) above 600 calories per day, plus up to 500 calories per hour of athletic training; PUFA above 100 calories per day.

We've considered every macronutrient except SaFA and MUFA — and we have only about 1300 calories per day before toxicity effects begin.

What about athletes who consume very large amounts of calories, for example, 5000 calories per day? Can they consume so many calories without experiencing macronutrient toxicity?

Yes: SaFA and MUFA are non-toxic; they are beneficial, for that matter, even when eaten in very large amounts. The body can accommodate longer (14-carbon or more) SaFA and MUFA in large quantities because:

- They are the core structural fats of the human body, making up 75 to 80 per cent of the fatty acids in most cells.

Notes for this chapter may be found at www.perfecthealthdiet.com/notes/#Ch12.

- They are the primary energy source for most of the body and a more healthful form of energy than glucose.

They also have no known toxicity, even at very high doses, as long as metabolic damage or high insulin does not prevent fats from being utilised or stored in their safe triglyceride and phospholipid forms. This makes saturated and monounsaturated fats a benign source of calories.

SCIENCE OF THE PHD
Lipotoxicity of Free Fatty Acids

Although the triglyceride and phospholipid forms of fats are entirely safe, another chemical form — free fatty acids — is potentially dangerous. Free fatty acids do have some chemical reactivity — they can bond to other molecules, a process called 'esterification'. (Free fatty acids are also called 'nonesterified fatty acids', or NEFA.) This can prevent those other molecules from performing their proper functions.

In healthy people, this does not lead to problems: free fatty acids are burned in mitochondria soon after their release (or 'lipolysis') from phospholipids or triglycerides, and free fatty acid levels are low.

However, in people with metabolic syndrome and diabetes, free fatty acid levels can become elevated even as mitochondria are blocked from burning fats by, for instance, high insulin levels. This excess of free fatty acids in cells can lead to 'lipotoxicity'. For instance, in a study of lipotoxicity and sudden cardiac death, only patients with metabolic syndrome died:

> Increases in blood pressure and in levels of plasma glucose, insulin, and triglycerides are features of the metabolic syndrome (syndrome X). Besides an increase in NEFA, all of these variables were increased at inclusion in subjects who died suddenly during follow-up.[1]

We thus have a seemingly parallel situation with fats and carbs: in conditions of energy excess, either can be dangerous. An excess of carbs

---

leads to hyperglycemic toxicity; an excess of free fatty acids leads to lipotoxicity.

However, there are crucial differences that make intake of dietary fats safer than dietary carbs in metabolic syndrome. First, the body's ability to store glucose as glycogen is severely limited, while the body's storage capacity for fats is virtually unlimited. Second, dietary carbs are allowed to circulate in their toxic form (glucose), whereas dietary fats are not released into circulation in the toxic form (free fatty acids), but rather are packaged by the intestine in non-toxic forms (triglycerides and phospholipids in particles called chylomicrons) and transported directly into storage.

The upshot is that if one has metabolic syndrome, it's safer to eat an excess of dietary fats than dietary carbs. Best of all, however, is to *cure* metabolic syndrome, which is best achieved by avoiding the various toxicities of excess fructose and polyunsaturated fats. High-SaFA and high-MUFA diets, by removing food toxins, are a crucial step in the restoration of healthy metabolic control and the elimination of lipotoxicity.

Benignity of SaFA and MUFA

Since they are more chemically stable and not easily oxidised, SaFA and MUFA are essentially non-toxic. The primary places in the body they are chemically modified are:

- In the liver primarily, SaFA and MUFA can be elongated and desaturated to transform particular fatty acids that are present in relative excess — typically, 16-carbon SaFAs created from carbs or PUFA — into SaFA or MUFA that are relatively deficient.
- In mitochondria throughout the body, SaFA and MUFA are burned for calories, a process that steadily shortens them two carbons at a time until nothing is left but carbon dioxide and water.

Each of these transformations is benign and creates no toxic products.

We mentioned earlier that SaFA and MUFA are invulnerable to peroxidation, unlike PUFA, which are readily peroxidised.

Another factor ensuring the safety of SaFA and MUFA is our ability to store them in quantity. The body has large reservoirs for the storage of excess SaFA and MUFA. As structural elements of cells, these fatty acids constitute almost half the lean mass of the body. Several kilograms of SaFA and MUFA, containing tens of thousands of calories, are stored in skeletal muscle alone. Adipose cells store further amounts.

These reservoirs are evolutionarily valuable, because, as the preferred fuel of mitochondria, SaFA and MUFA are desirable things to have in storage. Note that a lean person has reservoirs of 15 kilograms (135,000 calories) of SaFA and MUFA, but glycogen stores are only about 70 to 100 grams in the liver and 300 to 500 grams in skeletal muscle — about 2000 calories total, or less than a day's energy. As a reserve for high-intensity exertion and management of blood glucose levels, this glycogen is not intended to be used for ordinary energy needs. During food scarcity, *it cannot be,* or a person would starve in a few days.

Clearly, SaFA and MUFA, not carbs, are what nature wants us to use as our primary energy source in times of food scarcity — and, for that matter, in times of food abundance. If glucose were a superior energy source, we would have evolved ways to store it in quantity, the way plants store starch.

If the body has the ability to store SaFA and MUFA equaling 60 days or more of total energy needs, the body can safely handle even a large but transient dietary excess of these fats.

Benefits of High SaFA and MUFA Consumption

In addition to their lack of toxicity, SaFA and MUFA in high amounts deliver several benefits:

1. **Improvements in lipid profiles,** diminishing the risk of heart disease.
2. **Increases in muscle mass.** Muscle is composed of both fat and protein. One way to store fat, without making individual cells

excessively fatty, is to increase the number of cells. Muscle is, along with adipose tissue, the primary body component that grows in order to store excess fat.

Clinical trials further support the idea that SaFA and MUFA are the safest and most beneficial source of marginal calories.

Improved Lipid Profiles

Saturated fat consumption improves lipid profiles in two ways:

- It increases levels of protective HDL cholesterol.
- It makes LDL particles larger and more buoyant, protecting them from glycation and oxidation. This is Dr Ronald Krauss's 'pattern A', the healthful pattern of LDL cholesterol-carrying particles.

As a result of its improvements to LDL particle size, saturated fat reduces the level of atherogenic oxidised-LDL.

Monounsaturated fat is also superior to carbohydrates and PUFA in its effect on lipid profiles. MUFA do not increase levels of small, dense LDL and ox-LDL, as carbohydrates and PUFA do.[2]

SaFA and MUFA also improve another blood lipid marker, triglyceride levels. Triglyceride levels are largely determined by carbohydrate consumption and insulin levels; insulin inhibits the removal of triglycerides from the blood. On the Perfect Health Diet, fasting triglyceride levels are typically around 50 to 60 milligrams per decilitre — the healthiest levels.

Benefits of SaFA and MUFA: increased muscle mass

Many people believe that excess calories are stored in adipose tissue and that obesity is the result of summer storage of calories in preparation for a harsh winter. We disagree.

In animals that are seasonally obese, summer builds both muscle and fat. We believe that in humans, who lack a seasonal tendency to store fat and have a greater need for glucose (which during fasting is derived from protein), muscle is the primary summer energy storage organ. Summer is not meant to make people fat; it is meant to make them strong. Muscle builds up when food is abundant and is scavenged when food is scarce. Muscle, by calories, is majority fat and less than half protein — after conversion of some protein to glucose, not far from the ratios of breast milk. A typical adult male contains 30 kilograms of skeletal muscle, or about 200,000 calories — enough to maintain life for 60 to 70 days without food.

By contrast, adipose tissue, which stores little protein, is an unbalanced nutrient reserve. Stored adipose fat would not extend the life of a starving man for long. Nor would abdominal flab be as useful as muscle in helping a hungry Paleolithic hunter obtain food. No, the natural storage reservoir of excess calories is muscle.

The way to build muscle is to supply an excess of macronutrients in the proportions lean tissue needs — with a majority fat diet. Bodybuilders and weightlifters have long known of the benefits of fat-rich diets for muscle gain:[3]

- George Hackenschmidt, the 'Russian Lion', drank 11 pints of milk per day. Milk is about 50 per cent fat by calories, 90 per cent SaFA and MUFA.
- Vince Gironda, the 'Iron Guru', stated that nutrition was 85 to 90 per cent of bodybuilding and advocated eating 36 eggs per day. Eggs are 68 per cent fat by calories, 83 per cent SaFA and MUFA. Gironda sometimes ate ⅓ cup of protein powder with a dozen eggs and 340 grams of raw cream; the mix had about 740 protein calories and 1440 fat calories, for 66 per cent fat.
- Casey Viator, who became Mr America as a teenager, consumed two dozen eggs and 7.57 litres of raw milk per day.
- Arnold Schwarzenegger recommended consuming between 60 and 100 grams of carbohydrate per day — 240 to 400 calories — which necessarily requires obtaining the bulk of calories from fat.[4]

In short, the optimal macronutrient proportions for building muscle are to eat carbs at the natural carb intake — about 30 per cent of calories — and protein and fat in the proportions found in the body as a whole — thus, splitting the remaining calories 74 per cent as fat and 26 per cent as protein. That

How High-Fat Diets Produce Muscle Gain

A few scientific studies indicate how high SaFA and MUFA intake causes muscle gain.

- Testosterone promotes muscle growth,[5] and in men testosterone levels are proportional to dietary fat intake.[6]
- Higher-fat diets inhibit muscle breakdown, preserving muscle.[7]
- Growth hormone is the main muscle-promoting hormone and is released during fasting.[8] Fasting closely resembles the adoption of a 'carnivore strategy' diet of 74 per cent fat, 26 per cent protein, 0 per cent carbs. Eating a low-carb, high-fat diet, which reproduces the fasting pattern of gene expression, increases growth hormone release during the overnight fast. A moderate-carb majority-fat dietary pattern reduces hunger, causing people to spend more time in negative caloric balance and thereby promoting growth hormone release.

Growth hormone is increased not only by a high-SaFA-and-MUFA diet, but also by consumption of shorter-chain (10- and 12-carbon) saturated fats.[9]

works out to a 30 per cent carbs, 18 per cent protein, 52 per cent fat diet. But the fat needs to be low in PUFA and thus high in SaFA and MUFA.

By supplying all the ingredients for building lean tissue in exactly the right proportions, these macronutrient ratios make it easy for the body to add muscle. But these percentages — 30 per cent carbs, 18 per cent protein, and 52 per cent fat — are the PHD recommendations. (They're also the proportions found in milk — one reason bodybuilders have always loved milk. Eggs are a good combination with milk because their choline helps the body handle a high intake of fat.)

Evidence from Clinical Trials and Prospective Studies

Ever since Ancel Keys accused saturated fat of causing heart disease, it's been considered suspect. It's taken decades and numerous clinical trials for medical researchers to realise that the concern about SaFA was misplaced.

We've already reviewed randomised intervention trials comparing SaFA with PUFA. In our analysis, SaFA came out clearly more healthful than PUFA in three trials, probably more healthful in three, and as healthful as PUFA in the other two.

A recent meta-analysis of epidemiological and prospective cohort studies concluded that:

> [T]here is no significant evidence for concluding that dietary saturated fat is associated with an increased risk of CHD or CVD.[10]

Another review concluded that dietary saturated fats are clearly superior to carbohydrates.[11] If our belief that SaFA and MUFA are benign and other macronutrients are toxic at common intake levels is right, eating more SaFA and MUFA should improve health by displacing toxins from the diet.

Recent studies are verifying this. A Japanese study followed 58,453 Japanese adults, aged 40 to 79 at the start of the study, for 14.1 years.[12] Higher saturated fat intake was associated with:

- A 31 per cent reduction in mortality from stroke
- An 18 per cent reduction in mortality from cardiovascular disease

In the United States, the Framingham Study found that the more saturated and monounsaturated fat people ate, the fewer strokes they had.[13] (Polyunsaturated fat had no such benefit.) Another study found that higher saturated fat consumption was associated with slower progression of heart disease and clearer coronary arteries; lower saturated fat consumption, with narrowing of arteries and rapid disease progression.[14]

Restriction of SaFA and MUFA for Weight Loss

The Perfect Health Diet premise is that we should eat to precisely satisfy our nutrient needs. **This is true even on calorie-restricted weight-loss diets.**

Because carbs are not stored in the body, the optimal carb intake *does not change* when one is restricting calories. So dieters should continue to eat the same number of carbs — about 600 calories per day — even while restricting total calories.

Similarly, protein intake should not change on a weight-loss diet. Muscle is the body's primary storage reservoir for protein, and it is not desirable to lose muscle. So dieters should consume the same number of protein calories — about 300 per day — while restricting total calories.

Fat, however, is different. The body has a large internal store of fat, and any calorie deficit will be met by releasing fats from adipose tissue. So fat intake, strictly speaking, is not nutritionally necessary for an overweight person.

However, there are many fat-associated nutrients, such as choline and vitamin A, that it is necessary to obtain from food. Also, it's probably a good idea to continue eating omega-3 fats while dieting. These considerations imply that a healthful weight-loss diet should not be extremely low in fat.

That leads us to this conclusion: the ideal weight-loss diet should not restrict daily calorie intake below about 1300 calories. A lower calorie intake would generate nutrient deficiencies of one kind or another. Even at 1300 calories, the diet must be carefully designed to achieve adequate nutrition. The proper macronutrient mix is:

- About 500 carbohydrate calories
- About 300 protein calories
- About 500 fat calories — as low in omega-6 fats and as high in fat-associated micronutrients as possible

Restricting fat intake for weight loss is just the mirror image of the situation for athletes, who have increased caloric needs. When endurance athletes burn lots of calories in training, they should increase SaFA and MUFA intake (and some carbs) to provide benign fats for energy. SaFA and MUFA are the adjustable macronutrients of the diet.

Takeaway

Saturated and monounsaturated fats, in their dietary and tissue storage forms as triglycerides or phospholipids, are chemically stable compounds with no toxicity. They are the body's major storage form of energy and therefore the macronutrients we can most easily do without during periods of calorie restriction. They are therefore the most innocuous macronutrients — the safest to eat in large quantities to support high activity levels and the safest to restrict during weight loss.

13
Medium-Chain Fats and Therapeutic Ketogenic Diets

. . . .

- *Three to 6 teaspoons of coconut oil per day may be beneficial for everyone.*
- *A ketogenic diet is therapeutic for some conditions, especially neurological disorders.*

. . . .

Short-chain (less than 6-carbon) and medium-chain (6- to 12-carbon) fatty acids make up about 58 per cent of coconut oil, 54 per cent of palm kernel oil (not palm oil), and 14 per cent of butter.

Most people eat few of these fats. The best plant sources were never part of the Western diet, and butter has been displaced by vegetable oils.

For Everyone: 6 teaspoons a day?

Human breast milk provides about 10 per cent of fat calories (6.5 per cent of total calories) as short- and medium-chain fats. If this is optimal for adults, most Australians and New Zealanders would be starved for these fats. But the deficiency could be easily made up: 6 teaspoons of coconut oil provides about 140 calories of medium-chain fats — about 6 per cent of total calories.

Is the composition of breast milk a good indicator of how much coconut oil we should be eating?

Notes for this chapter may be found at www.perfecthealthdiet.com/notes/#Ch13.

Functions of the Short- and Medium-Chain Fats

These fats are rarely incorporated into cell membranes. They are specially treated by the digestive system: rather than being released into the blood as are most fats, these fats are shunted to the liver via the portal vein. In the liver, short-chain fats are disposed of by oxidation.

Short- and medium-chain fats are the most 'ketogenic' of all fats, meaning they are the most likely to be turned into ketone bodies and released into the blood.[1] This is why these fats provide a large share of the calories in therapeutic ketogenic diets. Ketosis can be maintained with a higher level of carbohydrate consumption if short-chain fats are consumed.[2]

Due to the neuroprotective nature of ketones, ketogenic diets are therapeutic for neurological disorders. Even people without neurological disorders may benefit from occasional ketosis to improve neurological function and, potentially, delay neurological ageing.

In addition to their ability to induce production of ketones, short- and medium-chain fats have other benefits:

- They are antimicrobial: they kill or inhibit parasites, bacteria, viruses, and fungi.
- They stimulate some of the same pathways as niacin, leading to increased HDL and improved blood lipids.
- They appear to promote weight loss.

Now for a closer look at these benefits.

Protection of the Gut and Liver Against Pathogens

Medium-chain fatty acids and their monoglycerides (such as monolaurin, the monoglyceride of 12-carbon lauric acid, and monocaprin, the monoglyceride of 10-carbon capric acid) have antimicrobial actions against:

- yeast and fungi[3]
- parasites such as giardia[4]
- bacteria including Salmonella,[5] Propionibacterium (a cause of acne),[6] E. coli and Bacillus subtilis,[7] Chlamydia,[8] and Heliobacter pylori[9]
- enveloped viruses including HIV, herpes, and cytomegalovirus[10]

Medium-chain fatty acids seem to be benign toward probiotic bacteria but suppressive of pathogens.

Dietary medium-chain fatty acids are generally absorbed in the intestine and shunted to the liver, although some lauric acid enters the body.[11] As such, they are likely to give most protection to the gut and liver. Still, protection of the gut and liver is important because:

- The gut is where most pathogenic bacteria enter the body, and biofilms in the gut may provide a reservoir that shelters pathogenic bacteria from the immune system and maintains chronic infections.
- Liver infections (or gut infections that spread bacterial toxins to the liver) may be a primary cause of metabolic disorders.

Indeed, as far as we know, the entire benefit of dietary fibre comes through its conversion to short-chain fats by probiotic gut bacteria. It is the short-chain fats, not the fibre per se, that are beneficial.

Better Lipid Profiles and Reduced Heart Disease

Some doctors reject the idea that medium-chain fats are cardioprotective. For example, Dr Walter Willett, in the September 2006 *Harvard Heart Letter*, said that 'coconut and coconut oil can't be considered heart-healthy foods' because 'coconut oil substantially elevates LDL (bad) cholesterol' even though 'coconut oil has a powerful HDL-boosting effect'.[12]

With finer measurement of blood lipids using new techniques, however, it has been established that it is not LDL cholesterol that is dangerous, but 'small, dense LDL' — LDL particles with insufficient fats and cholesterol around their lipoprotein. Small, dense LDL is vulnerable to protein glycation and conversion to oxidised LDL, which causes atherosclerotic plaque formation.[13] Having large, buoyant LDL particles with lots of fat and cholesterol protecting each lipoprotein is actually healthful.[14]

Tests for whether LDL is in the small, dense or large, buoyant form are expensive. However, a good proxy is the triglyceride-to-HDL ratio. When this is high, LDL particles are mostly in the small, dense form; when it is low, LDL particles are in the healthful, large, buoyant form.[15]

What do medium-chain fats do? They reduce triglyceride levels[16] and they raise HDL levels — often doubling them to 100 milligrams per decilitre or higher.[17] Their effect on lipids — higher HDL levels, lower triglyceride levels, and very likely lower small, dense LDL and lower Lp(a) levels — is unambiguously positive.

The heart's hydraulic efficiency is 28 per cent higher on ketones than glucose, suggesting that short-chain fats may be therapeutic for heart disease.[18]

Epidemiological data supports the benefits of coconut oil:

- Among countries with reliable data, Sri Lanka has the highest intake of coconut oil and the lowest rate of ischemic heart disease.[19]
- Stroke and heart disease appear to be entirely absent among the islanders of Kitava, who obtain almost 20 per cent of calories from coconut oil.[20]
- Tokelau Islanders, who obtain 50 per cent of calories from coconut oil, are similarly free of stroke and heart disease.[21]

SCIENCE OF THE PHD
Coconut Oil Is Better than Niacin for Cardioprotection

Recently scientists have been investigating the mechanisms by which dietary short-chain fats raise HDL levels and lower triglyceride levels. It turns out that short-chain fats stimulate some of the same pathways as niacin, another compound that raises HDL levels and lowers triglyceride levels. For instance, niacin and ketone bodies both stimulate the receptor GPR109A and through this receptor increase levels of adiponectin, a beneficial hormone.[22]

Niacin is much recommended by doctors, even though its conversion to niacinamide in the body can lead to flushing and liver toxicity. Coconut oil achieves the benefits of niacin with no flushing and no liver toxicity.

Weight Loss

Short- and medium-chain fats seem to strongly promote weight loss. In one study, eight weeks of taking the equivalent of 3 teaspoons per day of coconut oil caused a significant decrease in body weight, waist size, and blood triglyceride levels.[23] In another, obese women who were given 6 teaspoons of coconut oil per day slimmed their waist and increased their HDL levels without an increase in LDL levels, while a comparison group receiving soybean oil did not slim their waist and had lower HDL levels with higher LDL and total cholesterol levels.[24]

Polynesian Islanders who eat a lot of coconut have always been noted for 'their extreme leanness'.[25]

Short- and Medium-Chain Fats Are Safe

At the doses achievable in human diets, short- and medium-chain fats seem to be entirely safe.

There are no reports of toxicity from short- and medium-chain fats in human diets, even when they constitute the bulk of the diet.

- Ketogenic diets providing 60 per cent of calories as medium-chain fats have been safely followed for years by epilepsy and brain cancer patients.[26] Problems on ketogenic diets arise not from the fats, but from nutrient deficiencies — notably selenium[27] and vitamin C[28] deficiencies.
- Coconut oil delivered intravenously to people who cannot eat — parenteral nutrition — is comparable in safety to olive oil and fish oil, and safer than soybean or safflower oil.[29]

Ruminants and other vegetarian mammals typically obtain 60 to 70 per cent of calories from short-chain fats — another argument that short-chain fats are safe.

Takeaway

Short- and medium-chain fats may improve gut health, protect against infections, improve neurological function and reduce cardiovascular disease risk. They have no known negative effects.

It seems prudent to follow nature's recommendation and mimic the share of short- and medium-chain fats found in mother's milk — about 6.5 per cent of total calories. This can be achieved by eating up to 6 teaspoons of coconut oil or 18 teaspoons of coconut milk per day, perhaps as a sauce or soup flavouring or cooking oil.

Therapeutic Ketogenic Diets

Ketones are special: they are manufactured from fats and can be burned for energy like fats, yet don't require transport through the blood and cells as fats do. Instead, they are water-soluble small molecules that diffuse across cell membranes. They reach mitochondria and are metabolised for energy without any active transport process. Moreover, ketones need less oxygen to produce energy.

This means that even when a heart attack or stroke deprives the heart or brain of blood — and the glucose, fat, and oxygen it carries — ketones may still reach the blood-deprived tissues and nourish them. Ketones have shown promise as therapies for stroke and heart attack.[30]

READER REPORTS: traumatic brain injury

Thank you for the gift of better brain function you have given me! A few months ago I switched to a ketogenic diet, and now a completely Paleo diet based on your Perfect Health Diet. The differences I've experienced are amazing. The more ketogenic my diet, the better my brain capacity, cognitive energy, energy stability, endurance, and the better I feel.

— Patrick Jones, www.mindyourheadcoop.org

Because of their ability to diffuse into the brain, ketones are an alternative fuel for neurons. This makes them of special interest for neurological disorders, especially cases of genetic impairment of glucose metabolism.

Neurodegeneration with brain iron accumulation (NBIA) is a genetic disease that kills children in their teens and generates extreme pain from dystonia (muscle spasms) for years before that. The ketogenic version of the

Perfect Health Diet has eliminated pain and improved function for several children with NBIA.

READER REPORTS: ketogenic dieting for NBIA

My son, who is 6, has been on the [ketogenic version of PHD] and his hands have relaxed enough for him to regain his pointing ability (which had been lost). He is in no pain. This is pretty much a miracle given the extremely aggressive and progressive nature of this illness. Mathias has no botox, nor does Zach. Both are without pain . . .

Zach, who is 13 years old, is much further progressed in the disease. Zach has been on the diet since late October, 2010. The diet worked fantastically for him. He gained over 30 pounds [13.6 kilograms], which is an incredible feat when considering that our kids can burn in the range of 5000 to 7000 calories a day due to dystonia. At 13 years old, he now weighs 70 pounds [31.8 kilograms].

Zach has begun holding up his head even though his neck has been hyper extended backwards since he was 9, he has begun pointing with his finger again instead of the palm of his hand, he is moving his right arm again, and he is now able to go from a lying position to a sitting position on his own by hanging on to something or someone. He has not done this since he was 9 years old. Recently, Zach began to use his left arm again after years of not using it.

Both boys have begun smiling and laughing all the time. Zach has gotten off all pain medicine and only has a small amount of 3 [antispasmodic] medicines left.

Thank you for all your help. You cannot imagine how much it means to us.

— Mathias Flyvholm

Ketogenic Diets for Neurological Disorders

Ketogenic diets have long been in clinical use for the treatment of epilepsy. The ancient Greeks used fasting and calorie-restricted diets to treat epilepsy.

The Greek physician Erasistratus declared, 'One inclining to epilepsy should be made to fast without mercy and be put on short rations,' and Galen recommended an 'attenuating diet'.[31] A fasting-based approach to epilepsy treatment was revived in the 1910s by the American osteopath Hugh Conklin of Battle Creek, Michigan, who recommended an 18- to- 25-day 'water diet'.

By 1921, the three ketone bodies — beta-hydroxybutyrate, acetoacetate, and acetone — had been identified and shown to be produced in the liver during starvation or on low-carb, high-fat diets. Research soon revealed that it was the presence of ketones that made fasting effective against epilepsy. In 1921, Russel Wilder of the Mayo Clinic conducted the first trial of a low-carb, high-fat 'ketogenic diet' in epilepsy patients.

In the pharmaceutical drug era, interest in therapeutic ketogenic diets waned, but revived in the 1990s after the NBC *Dateline* television show reported the recovery of two-year-old Charlie Abrahams, the son of Hollywood producer Jim Abrahams, from epilepsy using a ketogenic diet after all pharmaceutical therapies had failed. They are now a standard tool in clinical practice.

Ketogenic diets are likely beneficial for many other neurological disorders besides epilepsy. For instance, there is evidence of benefits in Alzheimer's and Parkinson's.[32] But ketogenic diets may be beneficial for nearly all neurological disorders; they just haven't been tried.

Let's explore some of the benefits of ketones for the brain and nerves.

- Ketogenic diets protect neurons from glucose deprivation and excitotoxicity,[33] from other types of injury,[34] improve recovery from spinal injury,[35] and prevent brain damage after heart attacks.[36]
- Ketogenic diets are therapeutic for epilepsy,[37] Parkinson's disease,[38] Alzheimer's,[39] ALS,[40] and infantile spasms (West syndrome).[41]
- Ketogenic diets improve the behaviour of children with autism,[42] are antidepressant,[43] and may stabilise mood in bipolar disorder.[44] A ketogenic diet cured one case of schizophrenia.[45]

We believe that *everyone* with a mental or neurological disorder should experiment with a healthful low-carb ketogenic diet to see if it helps.

Perfect Health Diet readers have cured or greatly improved a number of neurological disorders using the ketogenic variant of our diet, including migraines, depression, anxiety, obsessive-compulsive disorder, and borderline personality disorder.

READER REPORTS:
curing migraines and anxiety with ketogenic PHD

I started getting migraine headaches in my late 30s (I am now 52). In the beginning I thought I had the stomach flu, because in addition to the headache I would always throw up or have dry heaves. The worst headaches would keep me immobilized in bed for up to two days. My brother-in-law, a neurologist, convinced me they were migraines. I finally consulted a doctor, who put me on midrin, which did not help, and a few months later I started on imitrex, which did help, at least at first. Eventually, my headache pattern evolved, and I had at least a mild headache every day, punctuated by the occasional doozy. Apparently, this is a pretty common progression, especially with women my age. I always suspected there was something wrong with my lifestyle or diet, and over the years I have tried numerous experiments, but nothing ever worked.

In January 2011, in my blog travels, I stumbled on your site. I ordered the book and was intrigued by your and Shou-Ching's ideas about disease and chronic conditions. I was already familiar with the idea of a ketogenic diet for epilepsy, so I was immediately interested in trying a more ketogenic diet for myself. I ordered all your basic supplements, and immediately upped my kelp to two capsules. I had been using coconut oil for curries, so I started using it habitually. Started eating 200 calories of starches that you recommended — this was a little scary, after studiously avoiding them for four years! I was afraid they might keep me awake at night, but I am sleeping like a log. Started fasting 16/8, which was easy once you absolved me for having cream in my morning coffee! Within a week of starting this regimen my

(*continued on next page*)

chronic headache started to disappear! Some days I would only have a headache for part of the day, and occasionally I would have no headache at all! I read somewhere on your site that NAC is good on a ketogenic diet, so I ordered it too. I had never heard of this supplement before. It seems to have made a further positive difference. I have started taking it twice a day. Once before bed, and once in the late afternoon, when the headache sometimes starts coming back. Since I added NAC, I have been nearly headache free.

My Raynaud's, which I've had all my life, has improved, as measured by the fact I sometimes forget to turn the heat up in the morning, and cold extremities don't always alert me to my forgetfulness!

Another amazing development concerns anxiety. Over the years I have become somewhat anxious when I drive on highways. I grip the steering wheel tightly, sit forward in the seat, and am generally hyper vigilant. I always chided myself for my lack of nerves, but that didn't help. As mentioned above, this was magnified by the Topomax. I never had this issue when I was younger; indeed I used to fly helicopters in the army. Two weeks ago I drove up to New Jersey to pick up my daughter, a 3.5 hour trip from where I live in Northern Virginia. I stopped two hours into the trip to make a pit stop, and I suddenly realized I was totally relaxed, and had been for the entire trip! The PHD is strong brain medicine indeed! Thanks for all your research, insights, and ideas. I think the Perfect Health Diet is going to be a game changer for many people. Hopefully it is the start of a sea change at how we approach the chronic maladies of our times.

— Kate

READER REPORTS: another migraine cure

I have particularly severe, chronic, complicated, and often silent migraines. I have had these since childhood all day every day. Because they were often silent (no pain) they would manifest in various other ways, thus leading to misdiagnoses of mood disorders and schizophrenia for many years. At one point I was also misdiagnosed with epilepsy as well. After one particularly smart neurologist saw and tested me, I was placed on blood pressure medications for migraines. This worked. The problem is that my body constantly fights to readjust to the medications. After a few months at one dose, it seems I start to get migraines again. So it would go up and the same thing would repeat again. I was looking for a different solution and I stumbled across this article.

I've been on the keto diet for nearly a month and it is the best thing that has happened to me. I'm migraine free and medication free. My mood is incredibly stable, I fall asleep quickly and stay asleep all night, I have lots of energy, I can concentrate for hours on end, etc. I've lost weight also, a much loved side effect. Thank you for writing this!

— Karin

Ketogenic Diets for Cancer

In addition to neurological disorders, cancer, heart disease, and chronic bacterial infections might benefit from (intermittent or routine) consumption of a ketogenic diet. Let's take a quick look at cancer.

It's been proposed that ketogenic diets may be beneficial against cancer, because cancer cells are highly dependent on glucose metabolism and, in test tubes, frequently die if they are obliged to use ketones or fats for energy.[46] Consumption of short-chain fats for ketone generation, along with carb restriction, can lower blood glucose levels while still nourishing neurons with ketones. A ketogenic diet recently tested in cancer therapy consisted of 60 per cent medium-chain fats, 10 per cent longer-chain fats, 10 per cent carbs, and 20 per cent protein.[47]

So far, at least, positive results have only been reported for ketogenic diets in brain cancer.[48] There are case reports of ketogenic diets reducing tumour activity and halting brain cancer progression.[49]

However, studies of ketogenic diets in other cancers have been disappointing. Here are the results of a pilot trial in which 16 patients with advanced metastatic cancer were put on ketogenic diets:

One patient did not tolerate the diet and dropped out within 3 days. Among those who tolerated the diet, two patients died early, one stopped after 2 weeks due to personal reasons, one felt unable to stick to the diet after 4 weeks, one stopped after 6 and two stopped after 7 and 8 weeks due to progress of the disease, one had to discontinue after 6 weeks to resume chemotherapy and five completed the 3-month intervention period.[50]

A possible reason why ketogenic diets may work well in brain cancers but not other cancers is that tumours in the body may evade the metabolic restrictions of a ketogenic diet by manipulating neighbouring normal cells into providing them with lactic acid, which the cancer cells can metabolise.[51]

However, ketogenic diets may still be a valuable adjunct to chemotherapy. Fasting prior to chemotherapy reduces toxicity to normal cells but increases toxicity to cancer cells.[52] Fasting is ketogenic, and a ketogenic diet might have the same effect during chemotherapy.

READER REPORTS: multiple sclerosis

I am a non-menstruating woman who has MS . . .

I do practice ketogenic dieting (thanks to you!) and I definitely feel the benefit. I do the coconut oil but I am prone to fungal infections so I am careful not to take too much. I once lived in an apartment for over 2 years working out of my home and when it was time to move out noticed mold on the ceiling and after further investigation discovered that the heating ducts were filled with it. I'm pretty sure this is where my health problems began.

I have had no new lesions and looking at me you would not know that I have MS.

— Sara H., Louisville, KY

Ketogenic Diets for Bowel Disorders
Bowel diseases, too, often benefit from lower-carb dieting. Usually, bowel diseases are due to infections, and gut pathogens are generally dependent

on carbohydrates for energy. Thus, low-carbohydrate dieting can help starve the pathogens.

In any low-carb diet, generation of ketones improves the safety of the diet, by providing neurons with an alternative fuel to glucose.

Infections of the small intestine, which typically cause SIBO, Crohn's disease, and acid reflux/GERD, will typically benefit from avoidance of fructose and other simple sugars. Since food passes through the small intestine fairly quickly, simple sugars are the most available to small intestinal pathogens. Glucose is the least dangerous sugar, since it is well absorbed by the human cells of the small intestine.

Infections of the large intestine, which cause irritable bowel syndrome, ulcerative colitis, and other colonic disorders, are typically fed by starches, fibre, and indigestible sugars (the fermentable oligo-, di-, and monosaccharides and polyols, or 'FODMAPs'). Simple sugars, such as dextrose, rice syrup, and honey, may be the best carb sources in these conditions. The Specific Carbohydrate Diet specifies foods that, experience has shown, are most likely to be tolerated in these conditions.

If the gut infections are bacterial, low-carb ketogenic dieting often aids in recovery. Joan's story of recovery from Crohn's illustrates the process.

- -

READER REPORTS:
low-carbohydrate dieting for bowel disease

Quick background: Crohn's for 16.5 years. Steroids for most of that time as other Crohn's meds ineffective. Got off steroids in Oct 2011 after 14 months on an almost zero carb diet. Glucose deficiency symptoms led me to your site. Added in safe starches in November and started to implement PHD with recommended supplements. Did a home fecal transplant in December.

All these things improved my general sense of wellbeing and energy levels but the Crohn's was still a problem.

During this time, since coming off steroids, I was able to observe the nature of the Crohn's without the confusion of medications. My

(continued on next page)

observations convinced me that it was an infection and research indicates *mycobacterium avium paratuberculosis* (MAP) is the most likely pathogen. High *E. coli* counts in my stool test seem to confirm this.

So, re-reading your assertion that intra-cellular bacteria can only feed on glucose not ketones, I realised that the exacerbation of the Crohn's was due to coming off the ketogenic zero carb diet and adding in too many starches (300–400 cals). For the last month I've dropped back to 200 cals, kept to a daily 6 to 7 hour feeding window, and added in BCAAs and MCT oil (I was already taking coconut oil). My Crohn's symptoms have improved steadily. I have very little tummy pain now.

I'm convinced a ketogenic, low-fibre form of PHD is the best way to manage my Crohn's.

— JC

How Not to Implement a Ketogenic Diet

Ketogenic diets used in clinical practice have often been terribly unhealthy. Doctors mistakenly assumed that since ketones are produced in starvation, starvation must be the best way to make a diet ketogenic. So they designed ketogenic diets to be starvation diets, deficient in glucose and protein.

Glucose and protein starvation cause a host of problems, especially in children. One study followed 28 children on the ketogenic diet for epilepsy for six years and tracked their health problems:[53]

- **Weak bones.** Six children had skeletal fractures; four had multiple fractures at separate times and locations.
- **Stunted growth.** By the sixth year, 23 of the 28 children were in the bottom tenth of their age group by height.
- **Kidney stones.** Kidney stones occurred in seven children.
- **Dyslipidemia.** Total cholesterol was elevated to as much as 383 milligrams per decilitre.

Compounding the problem of glucose and protein deficiencies, these clinical ketogenic diets were formulated not with food, but with purified nutrients. Worse, high-omega-6 seed oils were the source of fat!

The 28 children who had all those problems were eating a mix of pharmaceutical products: Ross Carbohydrate Free, which consists of soy protein isolate, high-oleic safflower oil, soy oil, and coconut oil, plus vitamins and minerals; Mead Johnson Microlipid, a safflower oil emulsion; and Ross Polycose, hydrolysed cornstarch. Another commonly prescribed formula is Ketocal, which consists of hydrogenated soybean oil, dry whole milk, refined soybean oil, soy lecithin, and corn syrup solids. One of our commenters, Jake, summed up the formulas: 'You might as well hold a gun to the head of the child and pull the trigger.'

A Better Way: MCT oil, carbohydrates, and protein

Fortunately, clinicians have gradually realised that starvation is both dangerous and unnecessary.

The better way is to meet carbohydrate and protein needs and to generate ketones not by starvation but by eating large amounts of medium-chain fats. These fats flood the liver, where they are disposed of by conversion to ketones, regardless of how many carbs are in the diet.

In epilepsy and probably all other diseases, it's better to include carb calories in a ketogenic diet. A study using a blinded crossover design switched 20 epileptic children between (1) a zero-carb ketogenic diet and (2) the same diet with 240 glucose calories. On both diets, ketones were produced. The glucose group had fewer seizures.[54]

To prevent a protein deficiency, it's desirable for carbohydrate plus protein intake to equal at least 600 calories.

Finally, on ketogenic diets it's desirable to supplement branched-chain amino acids. The most important branched-chain amino acid, leucine, is itself ketogenic; it also supports muscle synthesis and protects protein stores. A 2009 study among epileptics found that adding branched-chain amino acids to the classic ketogenic diet reduced seizures and did not reduce ketone production.[55]

How to Implement a Ketogenic Diet
Here is a strategy for implementing a ketogenic diet.

- Consume *at least* 200 carb calories per day from fibre-rich safe starches such as taro and white potato. But *eliminate fructose sources* from the diet; fructose metabolism depletes the liver of ATP and reduces its production of ketones.
- Consume sufficient protein to reach a minimum of 600 calories of carbs plus protein per day. Supplement with 5 grams per day of branched-chain amino acids.
- Consume copious amounts of short-chain fats. Somewhere between 500 calories (12 teaspoons) and 1500 calories (36 teaspoons) of MCT oil per day may be optimal.
- Engage in intermittent fasting. During a 16-hour daily fast, take MCT oil but no other food except water and electrolytes. Eat during an eight-hour daily window.
- Supplement with various nutrients including vitamin C and glutathione or its precursor N-acetylcysteine, plus vitamins involved in gluconeogenesis such as biotin.
- Finally: apart from the MCT oil and branched-chain amino acids, eat food. Do not drink purified-nutrient shakes!

This strategy should minimise the risks while still generating abundant ketones to nourish the brain and nerves.

14
Fibre

- *Fibre is beneficial in the amounts found naturally in PHD plant foods.*
- *There is no need to seek out extra fibre.*

Within the human body, bacteria outnumber human cells by ten to one.[1] (Bacteria are small and add only a few kilograms to our weight — luckily, or they would be hard to carry around!) These bacteria can be either friendly or harmful:

- **Cooperative, 'probiotic' bacteria** aid digestion, release nutrients, and guard the gut against more dangerous pathogens.
- **Uncooperative, 'pathogenic' bacteria** steal food and nutrients, release toxins, and invade the body to cause infectious diseases.

A healthy person has about 1000 bacterial species in the gut; people with bowel disease typically have fewer, about 750 species, because pathogenic bacteria drive out some probiotic species.[2] The quality of one's gut bacteria plays a powerful role in one's health.

Dietary fibre — plant matter that is indigestible to humans, but digestible by gut bacteria — helps to determine the nature of one's gut bacteria. The amount of fibre determines how many bacteria live in the gut, and the type of fibre determines which species flourish.

Notes for this chapter may be found at www.perfecthealthdiet.com/notes/#Ch14.

SCIENCE OF THE PHD
Ways to Change Your Gut Bacteria

Probiotic supplements provide species of bacteria that flourish in infants who suckle breast milk; they are healthful species but make up only a small part of the adult gut microbiome. Such supplements are great for overcoming food poisoning but rarely supply the species a chronically unhealthy gut needs.

Fermented foods provide a much wider array of bacterial species. The best way to ferment: place fresh organic vegetables in a salty brine with no exposure to oxygen, and keep the container sealed for several weeks until the brine is sour with acid. The acidic, salty, oxygen-free environment is similar to that in the human gut and will create a healthy mix of bacterial species.

Fecal transplants — moving the stool of a healthy person into the colon of a sick person — are the most effective probiotic. They provide all of the thousand or so bacterial species in the donor's colon. Fecal transplants have been startlingly effective at curing some bowel diseases and may be a therapy of the future for conditions such as obesity.[3]

Harmful Fibre

Some fibre, such as that in cereal grains, seems to be harmful. Grain fibre has two major problems. It contains toxic proteins such as gluten, which we will discuss in Part III; and it contains roughage that can injure the intestinal wall.

Conventional medical opinion recommends whole-grain fibre despite these issues. Dr Paul L. McNeil explains:

When you eat high-fibre foods, they bang up against the cells lining the gastrointestinal tract, rupturing their outer covering. What we are saying is this banging and tearing increases the level of lubricating mucus. It's a good thing.

It's a bit of a paradox, but what we are saying is an injury at the cell level can promote health of the GI tract as a whole.[4]

This is one of those clever ideas that, as George Orwell said, 'only an intellectual could believe'.

Whole-grain fibre has been tested in a clinical trial — the Diet and Reinfarction Trial (DART), published in 1989. This study included 2033 British men who had previously suffered a heart attack and compared a high-fibre group with a control group. The high-fibre group ate whole grains and doubled their grain fibre intake from 9 to 17 grams per day.

The result? The number of deaths in the high-fibre group was 22 per cent higher over the two-year study — 9.9 per cent of the control group died versus 12.1 per cent of the high-fibre group.[5]

The Benefits of Butyrate

The gut is an anaerobic environment, meaning it lacks oxygen. That prevents bacteria from metabolising fats, forcing them to rely on carbohydrates, which carry their own oxygen. As a byproduct of carbohydrate fermentation, bacteria generate short-chain fats such as propionate, butyrate, and acetate. Since they cannot exploit these fats themselves, they are released to the body. Short-chain fats from gut bacteria are the primary energy source for certain intestinal cells called colonocytes[6] and may meet up to 7 per cent of the whole body's caloric needs.[7]

The most important of these short-chain fats is butyrate, a 4-carbon saturated fat. Butyrate improves health in a remarkable number of ways. It:

- **Prevents obesity.** Butyrate improves insulin sensitivity and prevents rats from becoming obese.[8] Perhaps what obese people need most is more butyrate.
- **Heals the intestine.** Butyrate supplements or enemas have been used to treat Crohn's disease and ulcerative colitis.[9]
- **Improves gut barrier integrity.** Butyrate decreases intestinal permeability, preventing entry of toxins and pathogens to the body.[10]

- **Relieves constipation.** A rye fibre that increased butyrate production by 63 per cent compared to wheat bran increased weekly defecations 1.4-fold, softened feces, and eased defecation.[11]
- **Prevents colon cancer.** Butyrate induces differentiation of cancer cells into normal types[12] and prevents cancer-causing mutations.[13] Its protection against colon cancer is enhanced by fish oil (DHA).[14]
- **Delays neurodegeneration.** Much like its cousins, the ketone bodies, butyrate improves nerve function and survival in mouse models of several neurological disorders, including Huntington's disease.[15]
- **Improves cardiovascular markers.** Butyrate supplementation in rats lowers blood cholesterol, triglyceride, and fasting insulin levels.
- **Reduces the ill effects of diabetes.** Butyrate stabilises blood glucose levels in diabetic rats.[16]
- **Reduces inflammation.** Butyrate downregulates inflammatory cytokines and calms the immune system.[17]
- **Fosters tissue healing.** Injection of butyrate along with hyaluronan and vitamin A into the hearts of rats that had suffered a heart attack 'afforded substantial cardiovascular repair and recovery'.[18]

Given all these benefits, one wonders why butyrate is not commonly available as a dietary supplement. It should be noted that butyrate makes up 3 to 5 per cent of butter: yet more proof that nature has included in mother's milk the most nutritious ingredients.

Healthful Fibre

Although the fibre in cereal bran is harmful, two kinds of fibre seem to be highly beneficial: *resistant starch* and *pectin*. These also happen to be the types that generate the most butyrate.[19]

'Resistant starch' is starch that is indigestible to human digestive enzymes. Potatoes naturally come with high levels of resistant starch. But all starchy foods can form resistant starch after cooking and cooling. Cooking gelatinises starch into a form that is readily digested by human amylase; but if it is allowed to cool, some of this gelatinised starch re-forms into resistant starch.

Starch-rich diets are associated with very low rates of colon cancer, even if they contain very little natural fibre.[20] The likely reason is that butyrate from resistant starch formed after cooking protects against colon cancer.

Pectin, gums, and mucilage — commonly called water-soluble fibre or viscous fibre — are common in fruit and vegetables such as apples and tomatoes. They appear to protect against atherosclerosis.[21] Berries may be an especially good source of pectin, because they often contain antimicrobial agents that improve the gut flora. For example, blueberries reduce the population of pathogenic bacteria while feeding probiotic bacteria. Blueberry husks taken with probiotics generate a rise in circulating butyrate in the blood, and blueberry fibre is more beneficial than rye or oat bran.[22]

Cellulose is probably another useful form of fibre. Cellulose-rich foods include the squashes (pumpkin, zucchini, acorn squash, butternut squash) and stalk vegetables such as celery or bok choy.

There Is a 'Goldilocks' Amount of Fibre

Biology indicates that our bodies function optimally with a 'Goldilocks' amount of fibre — neither too much nor too little.

Fibre is food for gut bacteria, and consumption of more fibre means the creation of more gut bacteria.

There are some downsides to having more gut bacteria, however. In addition to generating beneficial short-chain fatty acids, they generate endotoxins — lipopolysaccharides that excite an immune response.

The Human Body Regulates Bacterial Populations and Endotoxin Levels

Endotoxins are fat-soluble and are carried into the body with dietary fats. The immune system monitors endotoxin levels and tries to keep them — and the bacterial population that produces them — at an appropriate level.

- When endotoxin levels are high, the immune system attacks gut bacteria with antimicrobial peptides to reduce their population.
- When endotoxin levels are low, the immune system relaxes to let gut bacteria proliferate.

It turns out the reason antibiotics often lead to pathogenic infections is that, by killing off probiotic bacteria, antibiotics reduce endotoxin levels and cause immune cells to let down their guard. This makes it easier for pathogens to invade the body.[23]

If the immune system is targeting a certain level of gut bacteria, too much fibre will not lead to more gut bacteria; it will lead to more bacterial 'births' as they feed on the fibre, but also more 'deaths' as the immune system works to keep the bacterial population down. This means that with high fibre intake, the gut will be exposed to more bacterial endotoxins and also to inflammation generated by immune activity.

Gut Bacteria Need a Balanced Diet Too

A few lines of evidence suggest that low or moderate fibre intake may create a more healthful, friendly gut flora.

Bacteria not only need carbohydrates for food, they need other nutrients too: phospholipids for their membranes, amino acids for their proteins, minerals for their enzymes. And well-nourished gut bacteria may be more likely to cooperate probiotically with their host.

This may be a reason that tree nuts are healthful. Almond fats, for instance, have been shown to help probiotic bacteria flourish. The benefits of almonds are lost when the fat content is removed.[24]

If gut bacteria need fats, and if providing fats makes the gut healthier, high-carb, low-fat diets may sabotage the gut by creating a scarcity of nourishing fats for gut bacteria. A low-carb, high-fat diet will create a smaller but healthier — and friendlier — population of gut bacteria.

Maybe the Best Fibre Doesn't Come from Food

Recent work has shown that probiotic strains that flourish in infants, such as *B. bifidum,* are able to digest human mucus.[25] This raises the intriguing possibility that we may not need fibre at all to maintain probiotic gut flora.

Mucin, the main component of mucus, is a glycoprotein, composed of a protein bonded to sugars. It may be that gut mucus, like human breast milk, is designed to feed friendly species of bacteria, enabling them to outcompete pathogenic strains in the mucus layer that is adjacent to human cells. Biofilms of probiotic bacteria heavily colonise the intestinal mucus layer.[26]

Increasing dietary fibre would make gut mucus a smaller share of the 'diet' of gut bacteria. Since dietary fibre is equally nourishing to pathogens as well as probiotic bacteria, too much fibre might make it easier for pathogens to survive in the gut.

Takeaway

The effects of antibiotics show that there are substantial health risks to having too few gut bacteria. However, there are risks to having too many gut bacteria also. There must be an optimal level of dietary fibre — neither too much nor too little.

The Optimal Amount of Fibre

Human breast milk provides 3 per cent of energy as oligosaccharides, the milk equivalent of fibre.

If this is the optimal human fibre intake, the Australian diet is fibre-deficient. Most Australians eat between 18 and 25 grams of fibre a day, providing about 1 per cent of energy.[27] However, it seems unlikely that the oligosaccharide fraction of milk is an indicator of adult fibre needs. Most plant foods have about 8 to 10 grams of fibre per 450 grams, and Australians currently eat about a kilogram of plant food per day. To reach 3 per cent of energy from fibre, they would have to eat more than 3 kilograms of plant food per day. That's a lot!

We incline to the view that 1 per cent of energy as fibre is probably just about perfect, assuming it is the healthiest fibre — resistant starch from starchy plants and pectin from fruits and vegetables. Supporting evidence for this view comes from studies of American fibre intake.

If 1 per cent of energy is optimal, small changes in fibre consumption would have no discernible effect on Americans' health. The reason is simple: at any optimum, small changes have no effect, for the same reason that when a road crests a hill, its slope is level. Only away from the peak will the road be climbing or descending.

Indeed, clinical trials provide few signs that health can be improved by increases or decreases in fibre consumption. The 49,000 women Dietary Modification Trial of the Women's Health Initiative found that increasing dietary fibre had no effect on risk of colon cancer, breast cancer, or heart disease, and no effect on weight loss.[28]

Although clinical trials show, at most, modest benefits to higher fibre consumption, association studies do find an association between higher fibre consumption and good health. For instance, in the NIH-AARP study, the highest fibre intake was associated with a 22 per cent lower chance of death.[29] However, this association may be only that — an association. Higher-income, better-educated, healthier people tend to eat whole grains, whereas poorer and less healthy people tend to eat refined grains and sugars, so people who are less likely to die eat more fibre.

Takeaway: stick to moderate amounts of Paleo fibre

Research into gut bacteria, fibre, and their influence upon health is still in early stages. Any specific prescription might be overturned by future research.

However, a few tentative conclusions seem warranted:

- Foods that have been in the human diet for hundreds of thousands of years — fruits, vegetables, and starchy tubers — are the most healthful sources of fibre. Neolithic foods, such as cereal grains, tend to supply harmful fibre. We can't guarantee that science won't in time identify harmful effects of fibre from some Paleo foods or some benefits of fibre from Neolithic plants. But for now, it appears that the Paleo principle holds: eat what our Paleolithic ancestors ate, and avoid the rest.
- **In people with healthy guts** that keep bacteria and their toxins from entering the body, **fibre from food is generally healthful.** However, there's no need to go out of one's way to get additional fibre. Supplemental fibre may be ill-advised.
- **Too much fibre has the potential to do harm.** In people with leaky guts and those eating diets high in polyunsaturated fats or alcohol, too much fibre can promote 'endotoxemia', a poisoning of the body with endotoxins generated in the gut. People

with bowel disorders may benefit from obtaining short-chain fats such as butyrate from coconut oil and butter, and limiting fibre to keep down endotoxin production.

The Perfect Health Diet, which includes roughly 450 grams of safe starches and 450 to 900 grams of fruits and vegetables daily, probably provides the optimal fibre for gut health.

15
Alcohol

· ·

- *Moderate drinking is healthful — but make it safer by eating a diet rich in saturated fats and nutrients such as choline.*

· ·

Many studies have shown that moderate alcohol consumption — one to three alcoholic beverages per day — is associated with good health.

A recent study followed 1824 adults, initially between ages 55 and 65, for 20 years. Their conclusion: 'abstainers and heavy drinkers . . . show increased mortality risks of 51 and 45%, respectively, compared to moderate drinkers'.[1] A host of prior studies showed similar results.[2]

One might be forgiven for coming to the conclusion that we should all engage in moderate drinking! However, there are confounding factors. Abstainers are less educated, less intelligent, more likely to smoke, less likely to exercise, and less likely to eat vegetables than moderate drinkers are.[3] Many abstainers are former heavy drinkers who are avoiding alcohol, and 'former drinkers are consistently more likely to be heavier smokers, depressed, unemployed . . . to have used marijuana . . . [to be] in poorer health, not religious, and unmarried'.[4]

Some studies find that the benefits of moderate alcohol consumption disappear when these confounders are taken into effect.[5] Others find that moderate alcohol consumption is still superior to abstention.[6] Specific diseases, such as diabetes, may benefit from moderate alcohol consumption.[7]

The upshot is that moderate drinking is probably a healthful behaviour,

Notes for this chapter may be found at www.perfecthealthdiet.com/notes/#Ch15.

so if one or two glasses of alcohol a day bring you pleasure, there's no health reason not to indulge.

There are some actions you can take to further guarantee that your alcohol consumption is safe.

Don't Mix Alcohol and Polyunsaturated Fats

We've previously mentioned that alcoholic liver disease results from mixing alcohol with polyunsaturated fats. Dietary saturated fats protect the liver from alcohol.[8] So does choline.

Unfortunate interactions between alcohol and polyunsaturated fats seem to be behind many of the alcohol-associated health problems.

Alcohol can induce a gut dysbiosis and trigger endotoxemia — a large influx of endotoxins from gut bacteria into the body.[9] Endotoxemia is greatly aggravated when the diet has a lot of polyunsaturated fat, for instance from corn oil and industrial lard.[10] Diets low in polyunsaturated fat minimise endotoxemia.

Metabolism of alcohol generates certain toxins: acetaldehyde, for instance. These toxins tend to oxidise polyunsaturated fat and can deplete the liver and other tissues of arachidonic acid and DHA.[11] A variety of nutrients, such as methionine, choline, glutathione, N-acetylcysteine, vitamin C, pantethine, and thiamin, help eliminate these toxins.[12]

Here are our tips for safe alcohol consumption:

- **Include salmon or sardines in your diet for omega-3 fats,** but avoid consuming alcohol on days when you consume salmon or sardines. The combination can damage your gut. The best foods to combine with alcohol? Beef, lamb, or nonoily fish.
- **Be well nourished.** Eat liver and egg yolks for choline, and get extra antioxidants, especially vitamin C, to support glutathione regeneration and protect against lipid oxidation.
- **Be wary of gut problems.** If you experience symptoms of digestive tract dysfunction, such as acid reflux, consider avoiding alcohol until your gut is healthy.

With these steps there should be little to fear from moderate alcohol consumption.

16

The Best Foods for Energy

. . . .

- *The best meats: fish, shellfish, beef, and lamb.*
- *The best oils: butter, coconut milk, beef tallow.*
- *The best plants: white potatoes, taro, sweet potatoes.*

. . . .

We've covered a lot of ground. You may be asking yourself: what should I eat?

The Perfect Health Diet prescription is:

- About 600 carbohydrate calories per day from about 450 grams of 'safe starches' such as sweet potatoes, yams, taro, white rice, sago, tapioca, and potatoes and 450 grams of fruits, berries, and sugary vegetables such as beets and carrots.
- About 300 protein calories per day from 340 grams of meat, fish, and eggs.
- Some factors influencing carb and protein intake:
    - Athletes should eat extra carbs as needed to accommodate their training; they may also benefit from extra protein.
    - Eating slightly lower amounts of protein may extend longevity.
- Omega-6 fatty acids should be limited to less than 4 per cent of calories. To get down to this level, do not eat any vegetable seed oils; do eat low-omega-6 oils such as butter and coconut oil and low-omega-6 meats such as beef, lamb, fish, and shellfish.

Notes for this chapter may be found at www.perfecthealthdiet.com/notes/#Ch16.

- Long-chain omega-3 fats from cold-water fish such as salmon, sardines, and anchovies should be eaten to balance tissue omega-6s. Up to 450 grams of oily fish per week is likely to be healthful.
- Saturated and monounsaturated fats are the safest calorie source — indeed, the only calorie source that is non-toxic in very high doses — and should provide the bulk of calories. Fish, shellfish, beef, lamb, and dairy fats such as butter and cream are the best animal sources; coconut milk and coconut oil are great plant sources.
- Six teaspoons of coconut oil (18 teaspoons of coconut milk) per day will provide short-chain fats to protect the health of the gut, liver, nerves, brain, and cardiovascular system.
- More short-chain fats are generated in the gut by eating fibre. Fibre should be obtained from 'Paleo' foods: the safe starches, fruits and berries, and vegetables to taste. These are the fibre sources that generate the healthiest portfolio of gut bacteria and the most abundant colonic production of beneficial short-chain fats.

Grading the Best Foods for Energy

Here are our grades for macronutrient-bearing foods.

The Best Animal Food Energy Sources

Grade	Source
A	Fish, shellfish
A	Ruminant meats: beef, lamb, goat
A–	Wild birds or game animals
B+	Organic eggs; farm-raised duck or goose
B	Pork muscle meats and bellies or bacon; full-fat dairy products; organic heritage chickens
C	Industrially raised chickens and their eggs
D	Pork liver, blood, intestines, or processed pork meats such as sausage or hot dogs

We recommend eating grade A/A– animal foods five days or more per week; grade B animal foods for variety; grade C or D animal foods rarely or never.

For variety of flavour and better nutrition, occasionally eat organ meats as well as muscle meats. From cattle, don't just eat steak. Beef tongue, heart, kidney, liver, tripe, and soups made from beef bone and joint tissue are all extremely healthful foods.

Eggs are an unusual food: they don't get top marks (B+ for organic, C for industrial eggs), but we highly recommend them as a source of micronutrition, as we'll see in Part IV. It's good to eat three egg yolks daily, but don't rely on them as your sole animal food.

Some of the pork sold in supermarkets, especially the livers, blood, and intestines, harbours pathogens that can infect humans. Thorough cooking will destroy microbes, but for caution's sake we recommend avoiding those parts of pigs and processed foods made from them.

The Best Plant Food Energy Sources

Grade	Source
A	Safe starches: potatoes, white rice, taro, tapioca, sago, sweet potatoes, yams, winter squash
A	Healthful sugary plants: beets, carrots, onions, fruits, berries
A–	Low omega-6 nuts: macadamia, coconut
B+	Moderate-omega-6 nuts; avocados
B	Buckwheat; yucca/manioc/cassava
C	High-omega-6 nuts and seeds
D	Beans; rye, oats; quinoa
F	Wheat, corn, and other grains; peanuts

Grade A/A– foods should be the staple plants of your diet, eaten at least five days per week. Grade B plant foods can be eaten occasionally for variety, grade C foods eaten rarely, and grade D and F foods should be avoided.

Grade A/A– plant foods consist mainly of the safe starches, which contain essentially no fructose, and of healthful sugary plants, which contain some fructose. If roughly equal weights of safe starches and healthful sugary plants are eaten, and no added sugars, fructose intake will be about 15 per cent of carb calories, which is a good level.

Grade A/A– foods are distinguished from Grade B/C foods by their omega-6 content and their potential to contain possible natural toxins.

Grade D and F foods are generally rich in natural toxins and we consider them unsafe, though some (Grade F) are worse than others (Grade D).

Note that this table leaves out vegetables, which are low in calories. Eat vegetables to taste — they are nourishing and add flavour to meals — but don't consider them a calorie source.

The Best Fats and Oils

Grade	Fat or Oil
A	High-medium-chain, low-omega-6 oils: coconut milk or oil, palm kernel oil
A	Low-omega-6 animal fats: beef tallow, mutton fat, butter
A	Low-omega-6 plant oils: palm oil, macadamia nut oil
B	Moderate-omega-6 plant oils: olive oil, avocado oil, palm oil
B	Moderate-omega-6 tree nut butters: almond butter, cashew butter, pistachio butter
B	Moderate-omega-6 animal fats: duck fat, lard from naturally raised pigs
C	Higher-omega-6 animal fats: pork lard, chicken schmaltz
C	Higher-omega-6 tree nut oils: walnut oil
F	High-omega-6 seed oils: soybean oil, canola oil, safflower oil, corn oil, peanut butter

Once again, we recommend making grade A fats and oils your mainstays for both cooking and flavouring. Grade B fats and oils are healthful and add variety. Pork and chicken fats are a special case: generally, fat from naturally raised and fed animals is healthful, but fat from industrially raised, grain-fed animals is unhealthful and should be avoided. The higher-omega-6 seed oils should be avoided. Walnuts are useful for flavour but shouldn't be a substantial calorie source.

17

Nutrient Hunger: a key to weight loss

- *A nourishing, balanced diet that provides all nutrients in the right proportions is the key to eliminating hunger and minimising appetite.*
- *Eliminating hunger at minimal caloric intake is a key to weight loss.*
- *The Perfect Health Diet is highly effective for long-term weight loss because it does precisely that. Other diets may produce faster early weight loss but will eventually induce malnourishment and a rebound weight regain.*

We began Part II with Michael Pollan's recipe for healthful eating: 'Eat food. Not too much. Mostly plants.'[1] We've already explained why we agree with the first and the last:

- **'Eat food'** means eating *plants and animals*. We're meant to live on other living things, just as our ancestors did in the Paleolithic. Eating real food nourishes us and avoids toxic pretend-foods developed in chemistry laboratories.
- **'Mostly plants'** is good advice because our natural diet has more carbs than protein — around 600 carb calories and 300 protein calories — and *healthful plant foods have about the same*

Notes for this chapter may be found at www.perfecthealthdiet.com/notes/#Ch17.

number of carb calories per 450 grams as healthful animal foods have protein. Our safe starches and other recommended plant foods range from 200 to 600 carb calories per 450 grams, while animal foods consistently have about 400 protein calories per 450 grams. To balance carb and protein intake, our diet should be two-thirds plant foods by weight — and that is without even counting low-calorie vegetables.

But Pollan's middle rule, 'Not too much', we haven't addressed yet.

At first glance, 'not too much' seems tautological — 'not too little' would be just as true. Presumably Pollan chose 'not too much' because we are in the midst of an obesity epidemic, reserving 'not too little' for a future skinniness crisis.

Now, unquestionably, *eating less energy than we expend is essential for weight loss.* But it's not sufficient to cure obesity, which is about more than merely excess fat. The strategy of eating less and moving more has been tried many times since Hippocrates recommended it in 400 B.C.[2] It often leads to hunger that requires heroic willpower to resist. Capitulation leads to weight regain. This pattern may repeat itself in yo-yo fashion.

Long experience has taught us that:

- **When the obese try to eat less on a malnourishing diet, they sooner or later become hungry and weight loss stalls or reverses.** A study in *The New England Journal of Medicine* put obese patients on a severe ten-week weight-loss diet of Optifast shakes and vegetables, followed by dietary advice. One-third of the patients dropped out during the ten weeks. The others lost an average of 13.2 kilograms. A year later, they had gained back an average of 5 kilograms and were hungrier and more preoccupied with food than before. They had hormonal changes suggestive of ongoing starvation.[3]
- **The long-term effects of eating less without improving the character of the diet are shockingly bad.** Those who experience weight fluctuations — weight loss followed by weight regain — are more likely to develop diabetes, high blood pressure, and cardiovascular disease.[4] In addition to disease and death, efforts to eat less often lead to weighing *more*. Non-obese

California teenage girls who practiced caloric restraint were three times more likely to become obese over the next four years than those who did not.[5]

In light of this experience, 'don't eat too much' is risky advice for an obese person. Advising an obese person to eat less, without explaining how this may be accomplished in a healthful way, may be no more productive of long-term health than advising a person with a cold, 'Don't cough too much.'

In both colds and obesity, the annoying outcomes (coughs and fatness) are innate responses of the body that protect against a greater harm. Attempts to frustrate these natural responses may damage health.

So: being able to consume less energy than we expend is essential if weight is to be lost. But how may this be achieved? How can we eat 'not too much' in a way that does good to our bodies rather than harm?

READER REPORTS: weight loss and health improvement

I have been on the PHD diet for over a year now. My health has improved a lot. I have lost 55 pounds [24.9 kilograms] and I now weigh about 190 pounds [86.2 kilograms] (I'm 6'1" tall). I'm probably healthier than an average person on just about any performance metric.

— Ole

I don't feel at all deprived on the *Perfect Health Diet*. Between the red meat and seafood, good fats, and safe starches, I feel so nourished and full. In two months I've lost 8 of the 11 pounds [3.6 of the 5 kilograms] I wanted to lose just by following the diet and walking.

— Abby

Nutrient Hunger and Dietary Balance

Eating less often damages health, but not because weight loss is inherently dangerous. **Hunger is the sign of danger.** Healthy weight loss occurs with minimal hunger.

We evolved appetite in order to make us well nourished. The brain's appetite system makes us hungry when it senses the body needs nourishment.

A **balanced diet** is one that gives us all the nutrients we need in the right proportions so that we reach the peak health range of every nutrient simultaneously.

An **unbalanced diet** reaches the peak health range of some nutrients while other nutrients are still deficient. Deficiency in those other nutrients will drive appetite; we'll eat more. Appetite ends when deficiencies have been relieved. But at that point, some nutrients will have been eaten in excess.

If some of the nutrients that have been eaten in excess are *macronutrients,* the diet will have an excess of energy.

So unbalanced diets lead to an excess of energy — eating 'too much' — and balanced diets lead to eating the minimum amount of energy needed to nourish the body — 'not too much'.

Carbohydrate and Protein Hunger

Let's illustrate how this works. Recall the rat study we used to illustrate how the food reward system regulates carbohydrate and protein consumption in rats. In 'The "Tastes Great!" Diet' chapter, that plot had carbs on the vertical axis, protein on the horizontal axis. Let's translate carbs into 'starch calories', assuming that starches are our carb source, and protein into 'meat calories', assuming that meat is our protein source.

Since meat typically provides about two-thirds of its calories as fat and one-third as protein, we'll translate each gram of protein into 12 calories of meat (8 calories fat, 4 calories protein) and each gram of carbs into 4 calories of starches. The result is plotted on the next page.

In these experiments, the rats could eat as much as they liked; the data points show where they voluntarily stopped eating. So at all plotted points the rats felt no hunger. We've fitted the points with two solid line segments; let's call those the 'hunger-free curve'. Any food intake below or to the left of the hunger-free curve indicates hunger, which would stimulate the rats to eat more starch and meat.

The diagonal line across the graph connects all the points at which total calorie intake (from meat plus starch) is exactly 100 calories. Let's call it a 'line of constant calories'. Any line parallel to that is also a line of constant calories, corresponding to a different number of total calories.

If we move the line of constant calories upward until it intersects the

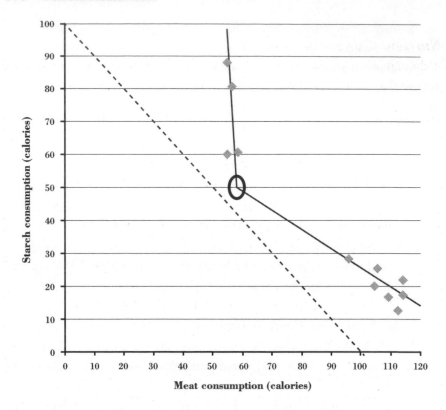

hunger-free curve, we'll find the lowest calorie intake at which hunger ceases. We've identified that point with the open circle. This lies precisely at the point we've called the 'natural carb intake' — for rats, 50 calories of starches and a meat intake of 58 calories, roughly 20 protein calories and 38 fat calories.

This is the *minimum-calorie hunger-free diet for rats*. It satisfies their need for carbohydrates and protein, eliminating their desire to eat more, at the lowest possible caloric intake — 108 total calories. It is the diet that eliminates appetite with the least amount of food.

Eating in these proportions — 50 starch calories for every 58 meat calories — is the rat recipe for eating 'not too much'. If the rats ate in a different proportion — less or more starch in proportion to meat — they would consume more calories. For instance, an 80-starch-calorie, 56-meat-calorie diet would be hunger-free, but at 136 total calories. A 20-starch-calorie, 108-meat-calorie diet would also be hunger-free, but at 128 total calories.

It's no coincidence that the diet that precisely hits the peak health range for carbs and protein is the one that makes rats hunger-free at a minimum of calories.

Nutrient Hunger in General

Although protein and carbs are important determinants of hunger, we believe that deficiency of *any* important nutrient can stimulate hunger.

SCIENCE OF THE PHD
How Does the Brain Know When Nutrients Are Deficient?

Certain nutrients are known to be closely monitored by the brain. Protein and salt are among these.

For most nutrients, however, there is no known mechanism by which the brain can monitor nutrient status.

How do we defend our belief that many distinct nutrient deficiencies can drive hunger, if the brain is only known to monitor a few? Here are two possibilities.

- The brain can directly monitor status of many nutrients, but the mechanisms are not yet known. Perhaps the sensing occurs directly within the brain — the brain senses the nutrient status of its own neurons!
- The brain cannot directly monitor nutrient status, but it can monitor whether tissues are functioning properly. When the body senses malfunctioning tissue and similar malfunctions in our evolutionary past were caused by nutrient deficiencies, the brain infers that a nutrient deficiency is present and upregulates appetite.

However sensing of nutrient status may work, we are convinced that it occurs. After all, what is the purpose of eating, but to nourish the body? What is the reason to stop eating, if not that the body is well nourished? Surely the brain would have evolved a mechanism to stimulate appetite when eating would be a beneficial act. Nourishment is too important to health and evolutionary fitness to make eating a rote act, indulged blindly without regard to the body's true nutrient needs.

There are dozens, maybe hundreds, of nutrients that the body needs for good health. If any of them may stimulate hunger, we should expect that:

1. Those who are malnourished will consume more calories.
2. Those who are malnourished will be more likely to become obese.

So we should expect that if we look at obese people, they'll typically be malnourished in multiple nutrients. The more nutrients they're deficient in, the more the brain will drive them to consume an energy excess. The greater the energy excess, the more likely that the body won't be able to burn it away and fat will be stockpiled in adipose tissue.

What do we find when we look at the nutrient status of the obese?

- Vitamin D insufficiency increases the rate of abdominal obesity by 2.57-fold in one study;[6] in another, people with low vitamin D levels were 3.2 times more likely to be obese than people with high vitamin D levels.[7]
- Intracellular magnesium levels are less than half as high in the obese than in the non-obese.[8]
- Iron deficiency is associated with obesity.[9]
- Among a set of morbidly obese patients, 73.8 per cent were zinc-deficient and 67.8 per cent were copper-deficient.[10]
- Selenium is also depleted among the morbidly obese.[11]

Yes, indeed: the obese are often malnourished.

If our theory is right, relieving malnourishment should reduce the incidence of obesity. So it does. In the Iowa Women's Health Study, use of multivitamins and other supplements was associated with lower rates of obesity.[12] In a clinical trial in China, obese women who took multivitamin and multimineral supplements lost 3.6 kilograms over six months and enjoyed reduced waist size and lower blood pressure, while those who took a placebo lost only 0.1 kilograms.[13] In a prospective study of 15,655 individuals, long-term use of supplements was associated with significantly lower levels of weight gain over a ten-year follow-up period.[14] Even when supplements don't lead to weight loss, they reduce appetite and make fasting more comfortable.[15]

If nutrient deficiencies drive appetite and consumption of excess energy drives weight gain, *the recipe for the perfect weight-loss diet is going to be the same as the recipe we've been using to construct the Perfect Health Diet:* get every nutrient into its peak health range simultaneously, so that none is deficient and none is consumed in excess. This will eliminate hunger at the lowest possible caloric intake.

READER REPORTS: easy weight loss

When you're well nourished, you're never hungry. I've been following the PHD coming up on one year next month and can honestly say, I have no cravings and am never hungry. When I see one of my former nemeses like hazelnut biscotti, while walking the aisles of the grocery store, I need only remember that I have visible ribs now and have moved down from size 16 to size 6, to smile and move on. It took a while, but the trip is well worth it . . . I'm 77 and over the years, I've tried to lose weight by going low carb. The weight losses were successful, but I didn't stop craving high carb/sugary stuff and would always gradually go back to the bad old ways and gain the weight back. One year later strictly following the PHD, I lost almost 40 lbs [18 kilograms] and not only don't I crave carbs and sugar, I am actually repelled by the smell of a bakery. Yeast and cinnamon are off-putting. When grocery shopping, just knowing that I have a visible rib cage is enough to keep me moving out of the cookie aisle. Whether it's self-hypnosis or balanced nutrition, I say thank you to Paul and Shou-Ching and all the people who comment here.

— E.R.P.

PHD is a weight-loss diet. I've lost about 15 lbs. in the past year. My primary health problem had been sleep apnea, which I've had for many years/decades. PHD got my attention because it was primarily about good health. I started following it a year ago and can say that it has significantly improved my health. In addition, I also began to lose weight, a welcome side benefit.

— Gary Wilson

Weight Loss Plateaus and Reversals

Our nutrient hunger theory of obesity can explain plateaus and reversals of weight loss. Nutrient hunger can make weight loss plateau and then reverse, even if the diet never changes.

How can the same diet produce weight loss and then weight gain? Surprisingly, it's easy. All we need is three or more nutrients that can drive hunger, one of which is stored in the body. That way, a diet lacking in the stored nutrient won't immediately produce a deficiency and won't immediately produce hunger.

Let's choose as our three nutrients carbs, protein, and fat. If we redraw our plot from the rat model, this time using pure protein in place of meat, it will look like this.

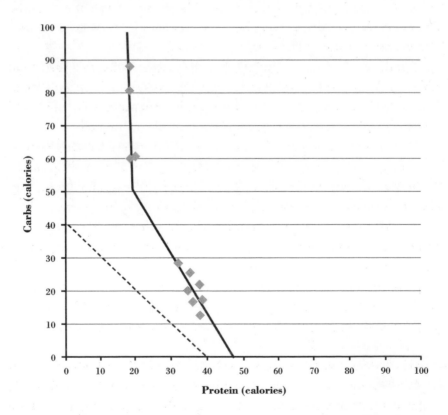

Without any fat mixed with the protein, the minimum-calorie hunger-free diet is now at zero carbs and a mere 48 protein calories. This dietary strategy — zero carbs, zero fat, and enough protein to eliminate protein-carbohydrate hunger — is called a **protein-sparing modified fast.** It is the lowest possible caloric intake that eliminates protein-carbohydrate hunger.

But, for our purposes, it doesn't really matter which point on the hunger-free curve we choose. We could equally well choose a **zero-fat high-carb diet** with 90 carbohydrate calories and 18 protein calories. All we're going to need to produce yo-yo weight loss is a low-fat diet that eventually generates a deficiency of fat or some fat-associated nutrient, such as vitamin A or choline.

Whichever diet we choose — a low-fat vegetarian diet or a low-carb protein-sparing modified fast — will still be calorie restricted and will generate weight loss at first.

But as time goes on, supplies of fat and fat-soluble nutrients are dissipated. Eventually, some fat-related nutrient becomes scarce. Maybe it's a type of fatty acid, such as omega-3 fats. Maybe it's a fat-soluble vitamin, such as vitamin A. Maybe it's a phospholipid component, such as choline. Whatever it is, it starts to drive hunger.

Hunger can start at any weight. Say the hunger is due to a scarcity of choline and omega-3 fat. There can still be any amount of saturated, mono-unsaturated, and omega-6 fats in adipose tissue. But the missing lipids will generate hunger and increase the number of calories consumed.

As long as the dietary deficiency is not remedied, hunger will keep increasing and appetite will go up. Weight loss may stop entirely; weight plateaus. Maybe at this higher calorie intake, there is enough of the missing nutrients to prevent the deficiency from getting worse. Weight may stabilise here.

But if the diet is very low in some nutrient, such as choline, simply eating more food won't solve the deficiency. Doubling food intake on a zero-choline diet still provides zero choline.

So in most cases, hunger continues despite the higher food intake. As long as the deficiency remains, the brain drives more and more food consumption and weight goes higher. Ultimately, the dieter must abandon the diet and switch to a different one.

That different diet is probably still unbalanced. But if it is deficient in a *different nutrient,* it may relieve existing deficiency conditions and enable weight loss for a time — until bodily stores of the next missing nutrient are depleted and a new deficiency condition develops.

Sometimes people alternate among extreme diets. They do a low-fat diet, and it works great until a fat-associated nutrient becomes scarce and hunger returns. Weight starts to rebound due to hunger for the fat-associated nutrient. Disturbed by weight regain, they shift to the opposite diet — low-carb, high-protein, high-fat. Now weight loss resumes until they become deficient in some plant-associated nutrient that, on their low-carb diet, they no longer obtain. Then weight loss stops, hunger increases, and weight comes back.

Jay Wright's Weight Fluctuations

One of our readers, Jay Wright, shared his dieting history with us. It looked like this.

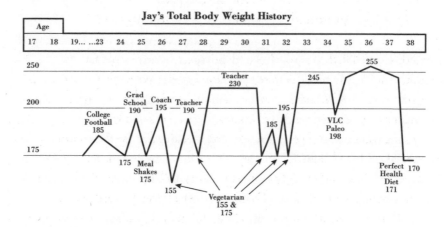

On meal shake and vegetarian diets, which have many deficiencies, he was never without hunger, though he would lose weight easily for a time. But the hunger always became unbearable after a while.

When Jay tried very-low-carb Paleo, he experienced hunger-free weight loss for a few months. But then hunger revived and he wasn't feeling well. The weight came back on — until he found the Perfect Health Diet. On PHD, he lost 36 kilograms in seven months, reached his optimal weight of 77 kilograms, and has maintained it without difficulty for a year.

Hunger-Free Weight Loss on the Perfect Health Diet

If the 'nutrient-hunger hypothesis of obesity' is correct and nutrient deficiency hunger drives calories in, and if we've properly designed the Perfect

Health Diet so that every nutrient gets into its peak health range and there are no deficiencies at all, everyone on PHD should be hunger-free, and calorie intake should be near the minimum.

This should lead to easy weight loss with minimal hunger.

We're pleased to say that nearly all of those who have reported results on our diet have experienced a reduction in hunger and cravings and relatively easy weight loss.

READER REPORTS:
eliminating food cravings and bingeing

I discovered PHD this year. I was afraid of 'safe starches' and fat, but thought I'd give it a try. At first I actually gained some weight because I was adding coconut oil snacks and the plain Greek yogurt and my favorite safe starch — sweet potatoes — all became trigger foods and I couldn't stop eating them. So I stopped the coconut oil snacking and the Greek yogurt and the sweet potatoes for a while and focused on getting enough Omega 3 and reducing my Omega 6. (My ratios were not optimal.) Now, I'm doing the Intermittent Fasting too (fast 16 hours, feed 8 hours — eating 3 times and eating coconut oil for my breakfast). It's amazing — I'm not hungry and it feels great! I've reintroduced yogurt, kefir and a daily sweet potato, but now those 3 items that had been my trigger foods are no longer and I feel satisfied very easily and don't overeat them as before. Maybe it was because my Omega 3/Omega 6 ratio was out of whack? Maybe it was because my body had to get used to safe starches after so long without them? Maybe the IF helps? Maybe after several months of PHD supplements that I'm finally not malnourished? I'm not saying that I don't ever eat sweets and don't ever eat too many. But it's a lot easier and happens only rarely.

So, my problem of overeating isn't totally gone, but my diet and weight maintenance is so much better and easier than ever before because of the PHD! And I feel better and happier and more satisfied than ever before!

— Connie

(continued on next page)

I've been adding starches to my diet for the past 6 months and find that I am more satisfied and eat far less 'treats' — just 1–2 squares of 85% dark chocolate most days. I definitely agree that food just isn't that big of a deal any more.

— Elyse

I've been doing paleo for 2 years now and this year my weight had been yo-yo-ing due to my binge eating. After my thanksgiving binge I finally decided to get serious and add in about 50–100g of carb per your recommendation and my cravings for sweets decreased a lot. Being able to eat starch got rid of the feeling of deprivation and I no longer feel the need to eat dessert after every meal. After starting the PHD, I've also been less neurotic with food.

— P.wen

Since I started PHD I no longer crave sweets. I used to eat chocolate almost every day and haven't had it for weeks now. :)

— S.E.

When doing very low carb Paleo, I was sucking down 2-3 glasses of wine a night. I've bumped up my carbs to the PHD level, and have been able to stay off alcohol entirely for the last couple of months. I've also lost about 5 more lbs since upping my carbs and quitting alcohol. Now when I get a strong craving for alcohol, I can 'satisfy' it by having a few starchy carbs. Since going off alcohol and upping carbs I've seen improvements in my mental function and sleep pattern.

— C.T.

Takeaway

Weight loss should be easy and hunger-free. It is essential to be well nourished — not just to get enough of every nutrient, but to consume nutrients in the right proportions so that there is *a deficiency of nothing and an excess of nothing.*

Achieving that — getting every nutrient into its peak health range simultaneously — is the design goal of the Perfect Health Diet. We designed it that way as a strategy for optimising health, but it turns out that the diet that optimises health is also the most effective diet for weight loss.

The fact that nearly everyone who has reported results has said that the Perfect Health Diet reduced hunger and cravings and made it easy to fast and easy to limit their food intake — that tells us we got our peak health ranges right. Their weight-loss success gives us confidence that the Perfect Health Diet is the best path to long-term, sustainable, enjoyable weight loss and good health.

Part III

....

Foods to Avoid

....

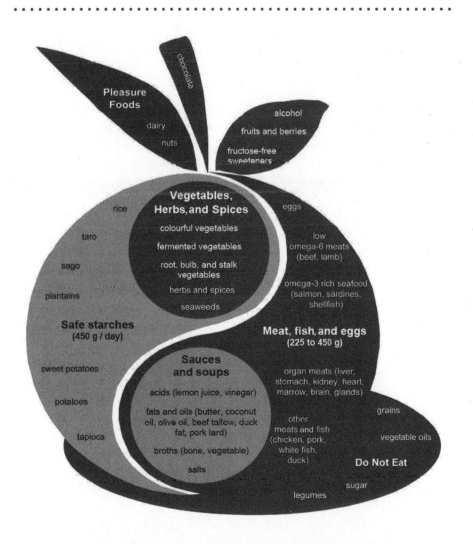

Pleasure Foods

chocolate

dairy

nuts

alcohol

fruits and berries

fructose-free sweeteners

rice

taro

sago

plantains

Vegetables, Herbs, and Spices

colourful vegetables

fermented vegetables

root, bulb, and stalk vegetables

herbs and spices

seaweeds

eggs

low omega-6 meats (beef, lamb)

omega-3 rich seafood (salmon, sardines, shellfish)

Safe starches
(450 g / day)

sweet potatoes

potatoes

tapioca

Sauces and soups

acids (lemon juice, vinegar)

fats and oils (butter, coconut oil, olive oil, beef tallow, duck fat, pork lard)

broths (bone, vegetable)

salts

Meat, fish, and eggs
(225 to 450 g)

organ meats (liver, stomach, kidney, heart, marrow, brain, glands)

other meats and fish (chicken, pork, white fish, duck)

grains

vegetable oils

Do Not Eat

sugar

legumes

18
Food Toxins

• •

Natural toxins in plant foods may have a big effect on human health.

• •

T he world is full of toxins. Almost anything is toxic in high enough doses: 6.6 litres of water, 2.3 kilograms of table sugar, or 225 grams of salt are lethal if they are ingested quickly enough.[1] Paracelsus, the medieval 'father of toxicology', wrote:

> All things are poison, and nothing is without poison; only the dose permits something not to be poisonous.

This is known today as the 'toxicologists' rule': 'The dose makes the poison.'

Toxins, we believe, have a large impact on human health. But the toxins that matter most may surprise you.

The Toxins That Matter

People worry a lot about pesticide residues on food, and rightly so: we should be confident that our food is safe. But the doses people actually receive from human-made pesticides are tiny compared to the doses of *natural* pesticides produced by plants to defend themselves against insects and mould.

Notes for this chapter may be found at www.perfecthealthdiet.com/notes/#Ch18.

Bruce Ames and Lois Gold estimate that Americans eat 5000 to 10,000 different natural plant pesticides, totaling 1.5 grams per day, but only 0.00009 gram of synthetic pesticide residues per day.[2] That works out to 99.99 per cent natural toxins, 0.01 per cent synthetic toxins.

Cooking generates another 2 grams per person per day of toxins. High-temperature cooking capable of burning food is the most likely to generate toxins.

If 'the dose makes the poison', perhaps we should worry a bit more about natural food toxins and toxins generated in cooking.

READER REPORT:
weight loss through elimination of food toxins

I continue to shed off some more fat even after I've increased my carb intake to 30% last week. I am definitely losing some body fat and no muscle loss! My trainer was very impressed when she weighed me last week. I am definitely seeing positive results since I started the PHD! The elimination of wheat, sugar, and cheese which I used to eat a lot every day has done great wonders in my body.

— S.E.

Most Toxins Are Unknown

Identifying which foods are poisonous and which compounds within them are toxic is not easy because:

- The ill effects of a toxin may not show up for many years.
- In foods, toxins are combined with beneficial nutrients. Beneficial compounds may conceal the harms of the toxins.
- Poisons may be good for us in small doses — even though large doses seriously damage our health. This pattern is known as 'hormesis'.

SCIENCE OF THE PHD
Hormesis

Hormesis is a beneficial response of the body to small doses of a toxin. Some examples: fasting may improve health, but starvation kills; exercise improves health, but running the first marathon killed Pheidippides; moderate alcohol intake may have health benefits, but alcoholism is devastating; various poisons, such as botulinum toxin,[3] are used as medicines in small doses.

Hormesis may or may not occur from any given food toxin — a review found that only 1 per cent of scientific articles showing a dose-response function reported hormesis[4] — but it is thought that low doses of some toxins stimulate the body's repair mechanisms, which then proceed to repair other defects.

The most famous experimenter with hormesis was Mithridates VI, the king of Pontus from 119 to 63 B.C. One of the most successful leaders ever to oppose the Romans (in the three Mithridatic Wars), Mithridates made himself resistant to poisons by regularly consuming small doses.

When, in his seventies, he was finally defeated by the Romans, he tried to commit suicide by poison but failed because of the immunity he had built up. He prevailed upon a friend to kill him with a sword.

If it's hard for scientists to identify toxins, how can we tell which foods to avoid?

A few principles from toxicology and evolutionary biology can help us.

Principles of Food Toxicology

Five principles are key to understanding food toxins.

First Principle: *animal foods are generally non-toxic.*
Animals receive no benefit from harbouring in their flesh compounds toxic to humans. Animal biology is very similar to human biology, so any compounds poisonous to humans would also be poisonous to their host. Even snake venom can be eaten — it is undigested venom that poisons.

When toxins are found in animal food, they usually come from bacteria. For instance, every once in a while there's a report of ground beef contamination with subtilase cytotoxin from *E. coli* bacteria. But most meats have very low toxin levels.

Second Principle: *all plants make toxins.*
Plants, on the other hand, have a very different biology. They can make compounds toxic to us but safe for them, or disable their toxins at critical times such as germination.[5] Plants make toxins because they are in danger of being eaten — and *they can't run away.* Becoming poisonous to insects, fungi, and herbivores is their best defence.

. . . .

> *The disabling of plant toxins by special enzymes during germination is why some plants that are normally quite toxic, such as beans, have edible sprouts.*

. . . .

Third Principle: *beware of plants eaten by mammals.*
Though all plants generate toxins — recall the estimate of Bruce Ames and Lois Gold that the American diet includes 5000 to 10,000 different natural plant pesticides — not all toxins are equally dangerous.

Many plant toxins are designed to poison insects. But a dose that would kill an ant weighing 3 milligrams may have hardly any effect on a human who weighs 20 million times more.

The situation is different for plants that are eaten by mammals. Plants can evolve toxins that are biologically specific to their major predators, and any toxins designed to poison herbivorous mammals will poison us too, as they are our close relatives.

Since herbivorous mammals graze in grasslands, it is among grassland plants that we should look for toxins that endanger us.

Fourth Principle: 'the dose makes the poison', so make doses low.

Because small doses of a toxin are harmless, but large doses can be lethal, the trick to healthful eating is not to eat too much of any one plant. Rather, we should eat a wide array of plant foods.

Recently, an 88-year-old Chinese woman was taken to the emergency department at New York University's Tisch Hospital by her family. She had been unable to walk or swallow for three days and soon entered a coma. Her life was saved by intravenous thyroid hormone, but she needed four weeks in the hospital before she could be moved to a nursing facility. The cause of her trouble? She had been eating 900 grams to 1.4 kilograms of raw bok choy daily for several months in the hope that it would help control her diabetes.[6]

Fifth Principle: beware of seeds.

Seeds are always the part of a plant most strongly defended by toxins. Evolutionarily, it is okay if a plant is eaten as long as its seeds are sown.

Thus, fruits are designed to be eaten, and their flesh is nourishing, but their seeds are poisonous and protected from digestion. The tasty fruit is meant to entice animals to spread their seeds.

The Four Most Dangerous Foods

Since 'the dose makes the poison', perhaps it should be no surprise that the most dangerous foods in Western diets are among the most popular:

1. cereal grains
2. legumes
3. vegetable seed oils
4. sugar

Now let's examine the evidence for the toxicity of these foods.

19
The Most Toxic Food: cereal grains

- *Because grasses were eaten by mammals throughout their evolutionary history, they evolved toxins that specifically target mammals.*
- *Cereal grains — the seeds of grasses — are rich in toxins that poison humans. They are the most dangerous foods.*

The cereal grains — wheat, corn, rice, barley, sorghum, oats, rye, and millet — are the seeds of grasses. They are the staple crops of the modern human diet. Wheat, corn, rice, and barley together account for nearly 70 per cent by weight of the world's agricultural crops — 76 per cent with sorghum, oats, rye, and millet. These eight cereal grains provide 56 per cent of the food calories and 50 per cent of the protein consumed by humanity.[1]

Grasses evolved in concert with grazing mammals: both originated at the same time and they became common together. Grasses, unlike other plants, grow their leaves from the base rather than the tip, and so are less damaged by grazing. Grasses are killed by shade, but grazers trample and eat saplings, so that land cleared by fire can remain savannah, steppe, or prairie.

To reproduce successfully despite being regularly eaten, grasses evolved two innovations. First, they generate a multitude of seeds per plant — tens of thousands annually — so that many seeds can be eaten, as long as a few scatter and take root. This fecundity is what makes the grains so attractive for

Notes for this chapter may be found at www.perfecthealthdiet.com/notes/#Ch19.

SCIENCE OF THE PHD
Grains Suppress Digestion

The ability of grains to sabotage digestion is well illustrated by this fact: for every gram of wheat bran eaten, fecal weight increases by 5.7 grams.[2]

Eating wheat causes large amounts of food to be excreted instead of digested!

---

agriculture: much of the harvest can be consumed while plentiful amounts of seed are retained for next year's crop.

The second innovation was a set of toxic compounds specifically designed to sabotage digestion in mammals. The plant's strategy is to pass its seeds intact through the digestive tract of grazing animals so that they emerge (with manure!) to take root in a new location.

Grazing mammals have evolved defences for these toxins — for instance, digestive organs such as rumens that allow the brunt of the toxins to be taken by bacteria. Humans, lacking such organs, are comparatively defence-less; our best defence is to cook and ferment grains outside our digestive tracts, as in the brewing of beer, for partial detoxification.

Grain toxins are proteins and are most abundant in the bran, but present in all parts of kernels. White wheat flour is about 10 per cent protein by weight, while crude wheat bran is about 16 per cent protein by weight.[3]

We'll focus on wheat, which seems to be the most dangerous of the grains, and on three wheat toxins in particular:

- **Gluten,** a compound protein that triggers autoimmune disease and promotes cancer, heart disease, and neuropathy
- **Opioids,** which make wheat addictive and triggers schizophrenia
- **Wheat germ agglutinin,** a protein that damages the intestine and interferes with vitamin D action, thus sabotaging the immune system and promoting chronic infections

---

SCIENCE OF THE PHD
Why Drinking Beer May Be Better than Eating Bread

We can detoxify grains the way cows do: by replacing rumens with vats and fermenting grains into alcohol. In medieval Europe, alcoholic beverages such as mead and ale often made up nearly half of calories. We would never recommend obtaining half your calories from alcoholic beverages, but it may be more healthful than eating bread!

Those are not the only toxins in cereal grains, but we hope they'll be enough to scare you!

Gluten Sensitivity and Celiac Disease

Gluten makes up 80 per cent of the protein in wheat, rye, and barley grains. Wheat gluten is compounded of two protein types: the more toxic alcohol-soluble gliadins, and the less toxic alcohol-insoluble glutenins.[4]

SCIENCE OF THE PHD
Gluten Is Toxic to Human Cells

Gluten is directly toxic to intestinal cells: it inhibits cell proliferation, increases cellular oxidation products, and changes membrane structure.[5] In the body, gluten changes the structure of the intestine: it reduces the height of villi, decreases the depth of crypts, and decreases enterocyte surface.[6]

Gluten sabotages the gut, reducing its surface area and impairing digestion.

As all toxins do, gluten inspires an immune response. This immune response helps to clear the gluten from the intestine, preventing a build-up of toxins; however, in the process it makes the intestine inflamed. This inflammation **kills intestinal cells** and **makes the gut leaky.**[7]

There appear to be four levels of immune response to wheat:

1. About 83 per cent of the population may have an inflammatory reaction to partially digested wheat gluten.[8]
2. About 30 per cent of the population develops anti-wheat-gluten antibodies locally in the intestine.[9]
3. About 11 per cent of the population develops systemic (circulating throughout the body) antibodies to wheat gluten.
4. About 0.4 per cent of the population develops systemic auto-antibodies that attack not only wheat gluten but also human cells in the intestine, thyroid, pancreas, and elsewhere.

This last group is diagnosed with celiac disease. With the immune system attacking and killing gut cells, the intestine can be damaged to the point that sufferers have difficulty absorbing needed nutrients.[10]

Here's what you really need to know: (1) Nearly everyone has an immune response to wheat. (2) The immune response to wheat can result in damage throughout the body, but usually most severely to the gut and thyroid. (3) The response to wheat varies across persons, but (4) at any time, a person may acquire antibodies against wheat, which may generate auto-

READER REPORTS: celiac disease

I have battled Celiac disease for some time and got about 80% better with a Paleo diet . . . but the Perfect Health Diet was the first book that could finally answer that last 20% with science-based logic.

— Jordan Reasoner

immune attacks and severe health effects. Finally, (5) the only way to avoid wheat-generated health problems is to remove wheat from the diet.

Consequences of Gluten Sensitivity

The immune attack against wheat not only damages the gut, but other tissues too. Wheat can trigger autoimmune disease, heart disease, neuropathy, or cancer.

Autoimmune Diseases

We mentioned that wheat consumption often triggers autoimmune attacks against the thyroid, leading to hypothyroidism.[11] Wheat can also trigger autoimmune attacks against pancreatic islet cells, inducing Type I diabetes in both rats and humans. The cause has been tracked down to a wheat protein we haven't discussed, globulin 1.[12]

Fortunately, both diabetes-related and hypothyroid-related auto-antibodies tend to disappear after wheat is removed from the diet.[13]

Wheat can even destroy the heart. Heart transplant patients usually have celiac disease, and when scientists investigated they found that antibodies against wheat gliadin also attack the heart, leading to destruction of heart tissue.[14]

Wheat can also promote autoimmune disease by other mechanisms. Wheat makes the intestine more leaky, allowing intestinal bacteria and their

. . . .

READER REPORTS:
wheat, migraines, and ulcerative colitis

I am a longtime migraine (chronic migraine 16 years) and ulcerative colitis sufferer, and also had platelet fluctuations. Six weeks ago I eliminated all packaged food, alcohol and 2 weeks ago I eliminated gluten. Since eliminating gluten I have not had a single headache. That is truly amazing!!

— Lauren

. . . .

proteins to enter the body.[15] Some bacterial proteins are 'molecular mimics' of human proteins, and production of antibodies against these bacterial proteins is thought to lead to autoimmune diseases such as lupus, rheumatoid arthritis, and type I diabetes.

Probably due to their leaky guts, celiac disease sufferers acquire auto-immune disorders — including multiple sclerosis, lupus, type I diabetes, Sjögren syndrome, and Hashimoto's thyroiditis — at a high rate. One paper says, 'The comorbidity between celiac disease and other autoimmune disorders has been clearly established . . . [T]he loss of the intestinal barrier function typical of celiac disease could be responsible for the onset of other autoimmune disease.'[16]

Cancer

There is an association between cancer and gluten sensitivity. People diagnosed with celiac disease have a higher overall risk of cancer, but mostly in the first year after diagnosis.[17] This suggests that wheat is causing or promoting the cancer, and the removal of wheat from the diet after diagnosis ends the cancer promotion.

The cancer association is most dramatic for lymphomas. People with gluten sensitivity have a 40- to 100-fold higher incidence of lymphomas.[18]

Neuropathy

Gluten can cause neuropathy even in the absence of intestinal distress, and in neuropathy patients with circulating antigliadin antibodies, a gluten-free diet continued for one year significantly improves neurophysiology.[19]

Increased Mortality Rates

People with gluten sensitivity die earlier.[20]

Epidemiological evidence suggests that *nearly everyone* who eats wheat dies earlier. The China Study was a huge undertaking: beginning in 1976, the Chinese government interviewed hundreds of millions of Chinese about their diet, gathered millions of blood and urine samples, and correlated diet with disease rates. We've blogged about how remarkably well the China Study correlations support the Perfect Health Diet.[21] Perhaps the most remarkable correlations in the China Study are those involving grains.

People in different areas of China eat different staple grains, so the China

Study correlations give a good measure of the impact of different grains on health. The correlations were:

- Wheat had a **+67 per cent** correlation with heart disease mortality rates.
- Rice had a **–58 per cent** correlation with heart disease mortality rates.
- Other grains had a **+39 per cent** correlation with heart disease mortality rates.

Wheat was by far the most toxic food found in the China Study. The relative safety of rice fits with our classification of rice among our safe starches.

Opioid Peptides, Wheat Addiction, and Schizophrenia

Many people have subclinical gluten sensitivity, characterised by acid reflux and bowel inflammation, yet continue to eat wheat.

One reason they don't quit may be that *wheat is addictive.* Wheat contains opioid peptides, and if the gut is leaky these may reach the brain with pleasure-stimulating effects like that of morphine.

Opioids and Schizophrenia

The discovery of opioid peptides in wheat was first reported by Dr Christine Zioudrou and colleagues at the National Institutes of Mental Health in 1979.[22] They looked into the matter because of the strong association between wheat and schizophrenia.[23] A brief summary of this association:

> Schizophrenics maintained on a cereal grain–free and milk-free diet and receiving optimal treatment with neuroleptics showed an interruption or reversal of their therapeutic progress during a period of 'blind' wheat gluten challenge. The exacerbation of the disease process was not due to variations in neuroleptic doses. After termination of the gluten challenge, the course of improvement was reinstated. The observed effects seemed to be due to a primary schizophrenia-promoting effect of wheat gluten.[24]

One scientist suggests that schizophrenia is rare if grain is rare: 'Epidemiologic studies demonstrated a strong, dose-dependent relationship between grain intake and the occurrence of schizophrenia.'[25] In one case, long-standing schizophrenia was cured by a low-carb diet. Wheat removal may have been key to the cure.[26]

Since these early studies, evidence has continued to finger opioid peptides as wheat toxins that promote schizophrenia.[27]

Opioids, Cancer, and Hormones

In test tubes, wheat opioids cause tumour cells to multiply. This suggests that wheat opioids may stimulate cancer growth and may be partly responsible for the association between wheat and cancer.[28]

Wheat opioids may also feminise male bodies by promoting unusual hormones. 'Man-boobs' may result from prolactin secretion stimulated by wheat opioids.[29]

Opioid peptides can be generated from other foods besides wheat. Incomplete digestion of milk proteins, rice albumin, and other food proteins can create peptides with opioid activity.[30]

Wheat Germ Agglutinin

Wheat germ agglutinin (WGA) is a lectin, a protein that bonds strongly to certain sugars. Whole wheat flour has about 30 to 50 milligrams of WGA per kilogram; many Americans, Australians, and New Zealanders consume 10 milligrams of WGA per day. WGA specifically binds to certain glycoproteins found in the human gastrointestinal tract, immune system, blood vessels, and nerves. Similar lectins are found in other grains and legumes.

WGA in the Gut

WGA is toxic to intestinal cells. It damages the integrity of the gut lining and makes it permeable, allowing gut bacteria, partially digested food fragments, and bacterial waste to enter the body. At extremely low concentrations, only a few parts in a billion, WGA stimulates immune cells in the gut to release inflammatory cytokines, further loosening the gut barrier.[31]

WGA causes shedding of the intestinal brush border and shrinkage in the surface area of the intestine.[32] In addition to promoting the shedding of mature gut cells, WGA increases the rate of cell division in the cells lining the intestine, leaving the intestinal lining in an immature state that doesn't digest food well. After ingestion of WGA, rats develop celiac disease.[33]

WGA in the Body

Some dietary WGA is transported across the gut wall into the blood, where it is deposited onto immune cells, vessel walls, and later into nerves.

In the body, WGA shrinks various organs, notably the thymus.[34]

WGA in the brain may trigger leptin resistance,[35] which could lead to **obesity.**[36] (Leptin is a hormone released by fat cells that quickens metabolism. Obese people are leptin resistant while thin people are not; mice with mutated leptin — equivalent to complete leptin resistance — become extremely obese.)

WGA binds to insulin receptors, triggering an insulin-like effect. It is as effective as insulin at pushing glucose into cells and stopping the release of fat from fat cells. This means that eating wheat may block weight loss and promote weight gain, regardless of how many calories are eaten overall.[37]

WGA helps trigger **autoimmune disease** by acting as an adjuvant to other molecules. In other words, WGA binds to proteins and causes the body to generate antibodies against them, even though the body would not form antibodies against that protein in isolation. For instance, one study found that antibodies against the egg protein ovalbumin are generated if it is accompanied by WGA.[38]

WGA is inflammatory,[39] promotes clotting, and induces the release of proteins called matrix metallopeptidases that cause clots to break free[40] — all features that increase the likelihood of a **heart attack.**

WGA promotes **kidney disease** by binding IgA, triggering IgA nephropathy.[41]

WGA, as well as other grain and legume lectins such as kidney bean phytohaemagglutinin, have been shown to denude the small intestine of mucus, stimulate stomach acid production, and promote overgrowth of bacteria, including *H. pylori.* These are conditions that lead to **acid reflux** and **stomach ulcers.**[42]

Interference with Vitamin D

Rickets is a softening of the bones in children that leads to fractures and deformity. In the early 20th century, rickets was common and was associated with mortality. Ninety per cent of children who died before the age of four had rickets, and the death rate among children was three- to tenfold higher where rickets was prevalent than in areas where it was rare.

Wheat Contributes to Vitamin D Deficiency Disease

Rickets is said to be a vitamin D deficiency disease, yet it has always been associated with grain consumption. In Edward Mellanby's pioneering experiments, he induced the disease by feeding dogs a diet of oats or wheat bread and then cured it by adding cod liver oil (which contains vitamin D). Either dietary fats or sunlight cured rickets; a cereal-based diet combined with confinement indoors caused rickets.[43]

However, it seems that rickets can be caused by cereal grains even when sun exposure and blood vitamin D levels are high.[44] Today, rickets is found mainly in sunny countries such as Nigeria, South Africa, and Bangladesh, where it is the result of 'cereal-based diets with limited variety and little access to dairy products', and is cured by the addition of dairy products, not vitamin D.[45] In Ireland in 1942, a rickets epidemic was caused by a switch from white to whole wheat flour, suggesting the presence of a rickets-inducing agent in the bran.[46]

In animals, rickets is known to occur with adequate vitamin D and calcium due to food toxins. One study of rickets in farm turkeys concluded: 'Because the feed contained adequate vitamin D, calcium, and phosphorus, the cause of this outbreak of field rickets is thought to be a toxic feed contaminant.'[47]

Another link with wheat is that rickets patients frequently have celiac disease. Possibly the immune response to gluten contributes to rickets.[48]

Feeding wheat bran to infants creates mineral deficiencies, a shift in gut flora to protein-digesting species, and early signs of rickets.[49] The likely explanation for the mineral deficiencies is phytic acid in wheat, which binds minerals such as calcium and can deplete them from the digestive tract and body.[50] The resulting calcium deficiency might contribute to rickets.

Wheat Interferes with Vitamin D

There are two known ways in which wheat consumption interferes with vitamin D production.

1. By an unknown mechanism, wheat causes people to burn through their vitamin D stores. One study found that eating just 20 grams per day of wheat bran caused vitamin D to be depleted 43 per cent faster.[51]

2. Japanese researchers found that WGA can prevent the vitamin D receptor (VDR) from entering the cell nucleus.[52] That would prevent the VDR from fulfilling its function as a transcription factor for genes involved in the innate immune response.

The Japanese result suggests that those who eat wheat may be vulnerable to infectious disease. Some bacteria and viruses (including *Mycobacterium tuberculosis*,[53] *Borrelia burgdorferi*,[54] and Epstein-Barr virus[55]) block or downregulate the VDR in order to protect themselves from the immune system. If wheat also does this, it must obstruct immune function.

Cumulatively, the evidence suggests wheat-eaters have impaired vitamin D function and higher vitamin D needs than those who don't eat wheat and may as a result be vulnerable to chronic infections and more frequently subject to premature ageing, autoimmunity, atherosclerosis, Alzheimer's disease, and multiple sclerosis.

READER REPORTS: wheat and dental plaque

Among many of the benefits of giving up gluten completely has been the disappearance of a life-long dental plaque problem (I'm currently 52); previously my problem was so bad I needed to have my teeth cleaned every four months to keep my dental hygienist happy.

— Ray M., Orange, California

Wheat's Mystery Toxins

Sometimes we can observe negative effects, but don't know which toxin to blame.

Wheat Consumption May Reduce IQ;
Rice Consumption Does Not

In Japan, most families eat rice as their staple grain, but some families eat wheat.

Japanese children who eat rice for breakfast have 'larger regional gray matter volumes of several regions' of the brain and higher IQ scores than Japanese children who eat wheat for breakfast. The IQ difference was substantial: verbal IQ was 3.4 points higher in the rice group and total IQ was 3.8 points higher.[56]

The difference between eating rice and wheat could account for most of the IQ difference between Asians and Americans!

Wheat Consumption Promotes Obesity;
Rye Consumption Does Not

In a comparison of two grains, wheat and rye, mice eating wheat ended up with a body fat percentage of 20.2 per cent, versus 13.7 per cent in mice eating rye; fasting insulin was 126 pM in the wheat-eating mice, 90 pM in the rye-eating mice; fasting cholesterol, triglyceride, and free fatty acid levels were higher in the wheat group; and the wheat-eating mice had much larger fat cells.[57]

In short: **wheat made mice fatter, more insulin resistant, and more dyslipidemic than rye did.**

Other Grains

We have focused on wheat, because that seems to be the worst of all the grains. However, all of the grasses share similar toxins. Many grains cause peculiar toxic effects.

Just to give one example, corn (maize), the domesticated form of the grass teosinte, is able to induce pellagra by mechanisms that are not understood. Pellagra was unknown until the introduction of maize into Europe from the

New World.[58] Much as vitamin D supplementation cures wheat-induced rickets, niacin supplementation cures corn-induced pellagra.[59]

Finally, some people are starch-sensitive, possibly due to toxins produced by pathogenic gut bacteria as they digest starches.[60] Grains seem to be particularly good at provoking this reaction, and association of starch sensitivity with ancestral gene alleles suggests that the provoking foods have only recently entered the human diet.[61]

Takeaway

Cereal grains damage the intestine and impair digestion. They impair immune defences and make people vulnerable to chronic infections. They can be addictive and cause or worsen schizophrenia and other mental illnesses. They trigger autoimmune disease. They promote cancer growth. They reduce IQ and brain volume. They promote obesity. They measurably increase mortality rates in gluten-sensitive and diseased populations. They are the food most strongly associated with mortality in the China Study.

We know how hard it is to give up bread. Yet there may be no single step that can do more to improve health.

20
Almost-Grains: legumes

. . . .

- *Beans and peanuts — the high-calorie seeds of legumes — are just as dangerous as grains when eaten raw and still risky after cooking.*

. . . .

Common food legumes include soybeans, the fifth largest global agricultural product and the largest nongrain crop; kidney beans; lentils; and peanuts.

Many legumes are highly toxic in their raw state: raw kidney beans at 1 per cent of diet can kill rats in two weeks. Most of those toxins can be destroyed in cooking, but not all. Let's take a look.

Grainlike Legume Toxins

Legumes are toxicologically similar to grains. Like grains, they are eaten by herbivores and have developed toxins against mammals, including humans. Important legume toxins include lectins (similar in function to grain lectins such as WGA) and alpha-amylase inhibitors (which are also found in grains).

Here is a sample of known toxicity effects from legumes.

- **Leaky gut, bad digestion, diarrhoea, bloating.** Kidney beans make rat intestines leaky, allowing bacteria and toxins to enter the body.[1] The kidney bean lectin phytohemagglutinin (PHA)

Notes for this chapter may be found at www.perfecthealthdiet.com/notes/#Ch20.

blocks production of stomach acid. This prevents proper digestion, especially of proteins.[2] PHA induces overpopulation of
the gut with immature cells that do not digest food well. Immature gut cells are easily exploited by diarrhoea-inducing bacteria such as *E. coli*. Thus, PHA ingestion 'was accompanied
by a reversible and PHA dose-dependent overgrowth with *E.
coli*'.[3] High doses of PHA disturb the mucus and shorten villi.[4]
Feeding rats the alpha-amylase inhibitor found in kidney beans
leads to extreme gut bloating:

> As starch digestion . . . was negligible . . . the cecum
> was practically blocked by solidified digesta . . . [A]s
> the distension was not always sufficient, **the [intes-
> tine] was occasionally ruptured** and the rats had to
> be killed.[5]

- **Retarded body growth and shrinkage of organs.** Rats fed
  legume alpha-amylase inhibitors show impaired digestion and
  retarded growth.[6] Feeding soybeans to rats alters organs: the
  'pancreas was significantly heavier while the liver was lighter in
  soyabean-fed rats'.[7] Kidney bean lectin (PHA) given to human
  volunteers caused their gallbladders to contract to two-thirds of
  their normal size.[8]
- **Heart disease and tendon damage.** The human body has two
  enzymes called sterolins devoted to removing plant phytosterols from the body by pumping them back into the gut. People
  with mutations in their sterolin genes that allow phytosterols
  to accumulate in the body have a disease called phytosterol-
  emia, which results in premature atherosclerosis, early death
  from heart attacks, and tendon and liver damage. Soy and other
  legumes have high levels of phytosterols.[9]

Typical legume toxicity effects include acid reflux and gut bloating, but
poorly cooked batches of legumes can trigger more severe reactions. A British hospital in 1988 offered a 'healthy eating day' in its staff cafeteria and
served a dish of red kidney beans. Within a few hours, 11 staff had suffered

profuse vomiting, some with diarrhoea. A surgical registrar vomited in the operating room. The trouble was traced to high levels of PHA.[10]

Indestructible Legume Toxins

Many legume toxins can be destroyed with overnight soaking and thorough cooking, but not all. One legume toxin that resists destruction is the amino acid canavanine, found in legumes such as alfalfa sprouts, broad beans (also known as fava beans), jack beans, and sword beans.

No human protein should contain canavanine, but canavanine resembles the human amino acid arginine and can be incorporated into proteins in arginine's place. Unfortunately, the resulting proteins don't work.

Canavanine can:[11]

- block the synthesis of nitric oxide, an important vascular, immune, and nervous system molecule
- interfere with ammonia disposal
- prevent reproduction in animals and possibly humans
- induce the autoimmune disease lupus (systemic lupus erythematosus)[12]

Legume Allergies

Peanut and soybean allergies are among the most common allergies.

Legume allergies can be quite serious. People with celiac disease who aren't healed by removal of wheat often turn out to have antibodies to soybeans or other legumes and need to remove legumes from their diet as well:

> Circulating antibodies to soya-derived protein antigens have been measured in patients with duodenitis, Crohn's disease, ulcerative colitis and coeliac disease. Significantly raised antibody titres were found frequently in the coeliac group, particularly those patients showing a suboptimal response to a gluten-free diet.[13]

Takeaway

Legumes are rich in toxins, and their dangers are not yet fully understood.

Traditional cuisines that make heavy use of legumes, such as Indian cuisine, used very long cooking times, as well as lengthy detoxification methods — overnight soaking, sprouting, and fermentation. Even with such methods, not all toxins are removed.

But with the hasty pace of modern living, few people soak their beans overnight or cook them for hours. It may be no coincidence that with India's modernisation, its rates of diabetes and obesity have soared. The country's traditional foods may be unsafe when hurriedly prepared.

Since human carbohydrate needs can easily be met with safer and more nutritious foods, we believe there is little reward and much risk to eating toxin-rich legumes such as beans and peanuts. The only legumes we eat are peas and green beans.

21
Liquid Devils: vegetable seed oils

. . . .

- *Their omega-6 fats are bad enough, but vegetable seed oils often carry other toxins too.*

. . . .

B
eginning in the 1950s, and especially after promotion of vegetable seed oil by the U.S. government in the 1970s, many scientists embraced the idea that omega-6-rich vegetable oils were healthful because of their cholesterol-lowering effect.

That turned out to be a fateful mistake. Dr William E. Lands later wrote:

We had been looking at essential . . . fatty acids as 'angels' but **in excessive amounts they turn into devils.**[1]

Vegetable oils are cheap. Unfortunately, they have two major problems:

- Vegetable oils are loaded with **omega-6 fatty acids,** which are toxic in high doses. The omega-6 content of soybean oil is 55 per cent; corn oil, 54 per cent; safflower oil, 75 per cent; canola oil, 18 per cent.[2]
- Vegetable oils, especially grain and legume oils such as soybean oil, peanut oil, corn oil, and wheat germ oil, also contain **plant toxins.**

Notes for this chapter may be found at www.perfecthealthdiet.com/notes/#Ch21.

The Problem of Excess Omega-6

We've already presented evidence that omega-6 fats become toxic above about 4 per cent of calories. We won't repeat all the evidence, just two key facts.

1. Most Americans get 9 per cent of their dietary calories from omega-6 fats, triple the safe level; Australians and New Zealanders get nearly as much. This excess is causally linked to increased mortality rates, cardiovascular disease, cancer, mental illness, and obesity.
2. The omega-6 excess is primarily caused by excessive intake of vegetable oils.

A casual look at the items on supermarket shelves will show how prevalent the use of vegetable seed oils is in industrially prepared foods. From salad dressings to cookies, soybean oil and other dangerous oils are almost always early in the list of ingredients.

READER REPORTS:
trouble from nuts (omega-6) and honey (fructose)

All four people in my family experienced a variety of new symptoms (seasonal allergies, constipation, worsening of heartburn, bladder spasms, dry eyes, increasing tiredness and low energy) when we did [a Paleo-style diet that excludes starches and recommends honey and nuts]. These problems didn't resolve until we luckily stumbled upon PHD and added back safe starches.

— Angie, Portland, Oregon

Plant Toxins in Omega-6-Rich Vegetable Oils

Nearly all plants that contain abundant omega-6 are also full of toxins. Given our earlier discussion of grain and legume toxicity, you may not be surprised to hear that grain and legume oils are some of the most dangerous to human health.

Peanut Oil and Cardiovascular Disease

Giving rhesus monkeys 40 per cent of fat calories from peanut oil induces atherosclerosis in all monkeys and heart attacks in one-third in 16 months. The culprit appears to be either the lectin peanut agglutinin (PNA) or toxic phospholipids that have a specific combination of a peanut molecule with omega-6 fats.[3]

Tree-nut oils and cocoa butter do not have this effect. Therefore, we recommend eschewing peanut butter and instead eating tree nut butters such as cashew butter, almond butter, and macadamia nut butter.

Corn Oil and Cardiovascular Disease

Corn oil, another oil that probably contains plant toxins, is about as atherogenic as peanut oil.[4] Corn oil could be the most lethal intervention ever tested on humans in a randomised trial. In the Rose Corn Oil Trial, the death rate was 364 per cent higher in the group eating corn oil than in the control group eating animal and dairy fats.[5]

Soybean Oil and Liver Damage

Some babies are born with 'short bowel syndrome' and need to be given parenteral nutrition, or nutrition delivered intravenously directly to the blood, until their digestive tracts grow and heal.

Since 1961, parenteral nutrition has used soybean oil as its source of fat.[6] And for decades, babies on parenteral nutrition have suffered devastating liver and brain damage. The death rate on soybean oil is 30 per cent by age four.

Finally, doctors at Boston's Children's Hospital investigated whether the liver and brain damage might be due to vegetable oils. After studies in mice showed that the liver damage was due to soybean oil, they tried substituting a fish oil–based formula. The results were 'freaking amazing', according to a Children's Hospital doctor; parents called it 'a miracle'.[7]

In a clinical trial, of 42 babies given fish oil, three died and one required a liver transplant; of 49 given soybean oil, 12 died and six required a liver transplant.[8] The death-or-liver-transplant rate was reduced from 37 per cent with soybean oil to 9 per cent with fish oil.

SCIENCE OF THE PHD
The Slow Pace of Medical Progress

Why did it take 43 years to figure out that soybean oil was killing these babies? An explanation was offered by Dr Mark Puder of Children's Hospital:

> In trying to figure out what was causing PN [parenteral nutrition] to damage the liver, some researchers, like Children's Judah Folkman, MD, and Robert Shamberger, MD, hypothesized that the injury was due to a missing nutrient that is present in regular food. Others thought that individual components of the solutions themselves might be to blame. Over the years, each theory was ruled out . . .
>
> Fortunately for Puder, he's not an expert on PN, or he might have ruled out the lipid as the problem from the beginning . . . 'One of the things I didn't do was read the literature to find out what everyone else was already thinking.'
>
> In fact, Puder didn't realize what everyone else was thinking until he began telling people about his observations, and they, in turn, began telling him he was wrong.
>
> 'When researchers took the lipid out of PN, and it still caused liver injury, they probably assumed that some other part of the PN preparation was the culprit,' he says. 'They never thought to question the type of lipid they were using.'[9]

Basically, supplying all calories as carbohydrates causes fatty liver disease through sugar poisoning. Replacing some of the sugar with soybean oil maintains fatty liver disease, this time due to a mix of sugar and omega-6 toxicity. The solution was to reduce sugar *and* omega-6 fats, but that was never tried.

Other studies in parenteral nutrition have noted that soybean oil kills immune cells. To reduce this destruction of lymphocytes, researchers are considering switching from a 100 per cent soybean oil formula to one with 80 per cent olive oil, 20 per cent soybean oil. The new formula still kills immune cells, but less prodigiously.[10]

Takeaway

Americans consume at least three times more omega-6 fats than is safe and have a tissue omega-6 to omega-3 ratio about nine times the optimum. Australians and New Zealanders also have excessively high tissue omega-6 to omega-3 ratios. The foods primarily responsible for excess omega-6 intake, vegetable seed oils, also contain natural plant toxins and artificial toxins introduced during industrial processing. Vegetable oil consumption is associated with higher rates of heart disease mortality, depression, violence, cancer mortality, bowel disease, and liver damage.

Vegetable oils should be replaced in the diet by healthful fats and oils: animal fats such as beef tallow, dairy fats such as butter and cream, and low-omega-6 plant oils such as coconut oil, palm oil, cocoa butter, nutmeg butter, tree nut butters, olive oil, and avocado.

22
The Sweet Toxin: fructose

· ·

- *High fructose intake is harmful. Don't eat products with added sugar.*

· ·

T able sugar and high-fructose corn syrup — the two ubiquitous modern sweeteners — are composed of two sugars, glucose and fructose. Glucose, the 'good' sugar, is healthful in moderation. Fructose is more dangerous.

Fructose in the diet comes from two main sources:

- **fruit, berries,** and **sugary vegetables,** such as carrots and beets
- **sweeteners,** such as sugar and high-fructose corn syrup, and sweetened products, such as candies and colas

In a talk the University of California posted on YouTube, where it gar-nered 2.5 million views, Dr Robert H. Lustig declared that two traits of fructose — the ability to inflict damage on the body and shunting to the liver (the body's detoxification organ) for disposal — compel a verdict: '[F] ructose is a poison. It's not about the calories, has nothing to do with the calories. It's a poison by itself.'[1]

Most scientists would not go so far. We'll meet Dr Lustig halfway: fruc-tose is a poison, but only in high doses or in combination with omega-6 polyunsaturated fats.

Notes for this chapter may be found at www.perfecthealthdiet.com/notes/#Ch22.

Agricultural Production of Sweeteners

High-fructose corn syrup is manufactured from corn, the world's second-largest crop with 21.6 per cent of agricultural production. Table sugar is obtained from the cane sugar plant, the world's sixth-largest crop with 3.3 per cent of agricultural production, and from beets, the twelfth-largest crop with 1.7 per cent of agricultural production.

But since omega-6 is so prevalent, both in human and laboratory rodent diets, it's no surprise that fructose causes much trouble.

Problems Caused by a High-Fructose Diet

In rodents, high fructose consumption leads to insulin resistance, obesity, type 2 diabetes, and high blood pressure.[2] In humans, similar syndromes develop, but less consistently than in rodents. Fructose appears most problematic when study subjects are obese or overweight and when they are eating diets high in polyunsaturated fat.

Fructose Creates a Risky Blood Lipid Profile
Fructose consumption brings about a blood lipid profile associated with high risk for cardiovascular disease and promotes visceral fat gain. For instance, in a group of overweight human subjects, shifting 25 per cent of dietary calories from glucose to fructose raised small, dense LDL levels by 45 per cent, increased postmeal triglyceride levels 100 per cent, and increased abdominal fat fourfold more.[3]

In a comparison of rats fed a diet of 60 per cent fructose with rats fed conventional chow, in only five weeks the fructose-fed rats had 15 per cent higher blood pressure, 198 per cent higher blood triglyceride levels, and 90 per cent higher blood cholesterol levels.[4]

Fructose Promotes Gout and Kidney Disease

The first step in fructose detoxification is its conversion to fructose-1-phosphate. The phosphate is drawn from the energy molecule ATP (adenosine triphosphate), creating a shortage of phosphate and excess of adenosine. The adenosine is disposed of by conversion to uric acid, which is released to the blood. High levels of fructose consumption beget high levels of uric acid.

This is problematic because humans, along with dogs and apes, are the only species lacking the enzyme uricase, which breaks down uric acid. High fructose intake therefore leads to an accumulation of uric acid crystals in the joints, causing intense pain, a condition called gout.[5] People with impaired fructose metabolism get gout at a high rate.[6]

Fructose, by way of uric acid, may be a major cause of kidney disease.[7]

Fructose Causes Metabolic Syndrome and Diabetes

Partly through its elevation of uric acid and partly through liver poisoning, fructose increases the risk of high blood pressure and metabolic syndrome.[8]

Fructose intake is proportional to diabetes rates in countries worldwide,[9] and the 8.7-fold rise in diabetes incidence since 1935 coincided with a sixfold to 20-fold rise in fructose consumption.[10]

The main mechanism by which fructose causes metabolic syndrome and diabetes appears to be through induction of *metabolic endotoxemia*. Endotoxemia is a high level of endotoxins in the body. Endotoxins are compounds found in the cell walls of gut bacteria. When gut bacteria die, their cell walls disintegrate and release endotoxins. Some of them enter the body — a lot if the gut is leaky.

Blood endotoxin levels are higher in mice consuming fructose than in mice on any other diet. The endotoxins generate fatty liver disease, and 'treatment of fructose fed mice with antibiotics . . . markedly reduced hepatic lipid accumulation'.[11]

Endotoxemia by itself causes metabolic syndrome and fatty liver disease, plus systemic inflammation, which induces adipose tissue to accumulate fat and is thought to promote a host of diseases, from cancer to Parkinson's.[12] Endotoxemia is closely associated with all the metabolic disorders; one highly cited paper states, 'metabolic endotoxemia controls the inflammatory tone, body weight gain, and diabetes'.[13] In the FinnDiane study, blood levels of endotoxins closely track the severity of all components of the metabolic syndrome, leading the authors to conclude, 'Bacterial endotoxins may thus play an important role in the development of the metabolic and vascular abnormalities commonly seen in obesity and diabetes-related diseases.'[14]

Germ-free mice — mice lacking gut bacteria — are protected from metabolic syndrome, obesity, and liver injury; antibiotic treatment reduces the endotoxemia and controls inflammation and metabolic syndrome.[15] Probiotics can help.[16] So it looks as though anything that reduces endotoxin flux into the body is protective against metabolic syndrome.

Both high-fructose and high-omega-6 diets can induce endotoxemia.[17] In the literature, it is usually stated that high-fat diets induce endotoxemia, but nearly all of the high-fat diets used in scientific research are high-omega-6 diets.[18] For instance, a paper we mentioned earlier used corn oil (57 per cent omega-6) and industrial lard (33 per cent omega-6) to cause metabolic endotoxemia.[19] Most of these endotoxemia-inducing diets are high in sucrose, which is half fructose.

Endotoxemia, in turn, induces fructose malabsorption. When LPS is injected into animals, their digestive tracts reduce absorption of fructose, making it more available to gut bacteria.[20] The extra fructose causes the bacteria to multiply and more endotoxins are released.

So a diet high in fructose and omega-6 fats creates a vicious circle. It causes endotoxemia, which causes fructose malabsorption, which multiplies endotoxin production in the gut, which worsens endotoxemia. The endotoxemia causes metabolic syndrome, diabetes, liver disease, and other ailments.

- -

READER REPORTS:
improved health with fructose elimination

My gut feels better, I have better digestion with less bloating from fruit/sugar. If I eat some organic dairy I don't get as many pimples as I used to, and if I do they are noticeably smaller, they barely become inflamed and they heal more quickly.

— Wyatt

- -

Heart disease is probably another result of this vicious circle. Cardiovascular disease rates are highest in those who follow low-fibre, low-saturated-fat (and thus high-sugar, high-polyunsaturated-fat) diets, lowest in those whose diets have a high saturated fat and high fibre content together.[21]

Fructose and Obesity

Fructose consumption is associated with obesity. Each additional daily fructose-sweetened soft drink increases the rate of obesity by 60 per cent,[22] and reduction of soft drink consumption in British schoolchildren by only one-fifth of a glass (50 millilitres) per day reduced the number of overweight and obese children by 7.5 per cent.[23] A review of 88 studies found that higher intake of soft drinks was associated with greater caloric consumption, higher body weight, lower intake of other nutrients, and worse indicators of health.[24]

A possible mechanism was discovered when it was shown that eating fructose causes leptin resistance. Leptin is a hormone that normally causes fat reduction, quickened metabolism, and weight loss; leptin-resistant people tend to become obese.[25]

Fructose Can Damage Both Brain and Body

Very large intakes of fructose can spill past the liver and poison the body, a problem that is especially severe in diabetics. This is bad: fructose is far more likely to glycate proteins and oxidise fats than glucose.[26] The brain is impacted upon: a high-fructose diet impairs memory in rats.[27] Fructose also increases the blood pressure and shortens the life span of rats.[28] Fructose consumption by diabetics is strongly associated with retinopathy — a major cause of blindness.[29]

Takeaway

Fructose from normal quantities of low-calorie plant foods such as fruits, berries, beets, and carrots is healthful, even for diabetics. The PHD prescription is to consume at most 25 grams of fructose per day, at most 10 grams per meal.

Higher doses of fructose can be dangerous. The large quantities of sugar and high-fructose corn syrup that most Americans consume are probably quite dangerous, especially in combination with omega-6 vegetable oils. Fructose-induced liver damage and endotoxemia, aggravated by excess omega-6 vegetable oils, may be at the root of the current epidemic of metabolic syndrome, obesity, and diabetes.

23

Toxins Introduced by the Industrial Food System

· ·

- *Industrial producers have made food cheap but unhealthy.*

· ·

Many consumers pay little heed to the quality of their food but a great deal of attention to its price. So food companies have worked to give them what they want: the cheapest possible food. Unfortunately, *cheap* is often at odds with *healthful*.

Toxic Ingredients

One of the easiest ways to make food cheap is to start with freely available waste products.

In 1793, Eli Whitney invented the cotton gin for separating cotton fibres from their seeds. That enabled the cotton textile industry to grow tremendously, but led to huge waste piles of seeds. Natural cottonseeds could not be eaten due to their high toxin content; for instance, gossypol, a cotton phenol, induces potassium deficiency, paralysis, and infertility.[1]

Chemists began studying how to make something useful from these seeds. By the 1870s, they were used as fertiliser; by the 1880s, as cattle feed.[2] In 1899, David Wesson of the Southern Oil Company developed a method for

Notes for this chapter may be found at www.perfecthealthdiet.com/notes/#Ch23.

removing toxins and unpleasant odours from cottonseed oils. All those waste cottonseeds began to be used to make high-omega-6 (52 per cent) liquid cooking oils such as Wesson Oil and hydrogenated shortenings such as Crisco.

Today, cotton grown for seed oil extraction is one of the 'big four' genetically modified food crops, after soy, corn, and rapeseed (for canola oil). Cottonseed oil appears in a wide array of industrial foods, including cereals, breads, and snack foods.[3]

Toxins Introduced During Detoxification

The methods for removing toxins from naturally poisonous plants can themselves introduce new toxins.

Canola oil (an oil developed in the 1970s and named for 'Canadian oilseed, low-acid') is rapeseed oil bred and processed to remove erucic acid and glucosinolates. During processing, the oil is treated with the solvent hexane and very high temperatures; it may also be subject to caustic refinement, bleaching, and degumming.[4] Soybean oil, corn oil, peanut oil, safflower oil, and other vegetable oils undergo similar processing to remove toxins and odours and improve taste.

Unfortunately, such processing can introduce toxins.

Formation of Trans Fats
Industrial food processing can lead to hydrogenation of polyunsaturated fats, generating highly toxic trans fats.

Until recently, it was common for supermarket breads, cakes, cookies, crackers, potato or corn chips, French fries, and pizza crusts to contain 10 to 40 per cent of fat calories as trans fats.[5] Commercial liquid canola oil had trans-fat levels as high as 4.6 per cent.[6]

With growing awareness of the dangers of trans fats and the requirement that trans-fat content be labelled, most industrial foods now contain less than 0.5 gram of trans fat per serving, which permits them to be labelled as having zero trans fat.

However, serving sizes are sometimes quite small; the serving size for a well-known brand of crackers is one cracker.[7] If a processed food has an unusually small serving size, it may be because it has a lot of trans fat!

Transformation of Nutrients into Toxins

All that processing can convert beneficial plant compounds into toxins.

In many prepared foods, oils are intentionally hydrogenated to extend the shelf life. During hydrogenation of soybean and canola oils, the plant form of vitamin K is hydrogenated into dihydrophylloquinone. Dihydrophylloquinone is a sort of antivitamin: it competes with vitamin K in the body but is incapable of activating vitamin K–dependent proteins. Dihydrophylloquinone intake was associated in the Framingham Offspring Study with lower bone mineral density.[8]

High-Temperature Processing

Even if chemical treatments are not required, high-temperature processing of commercial foods may introduce toxins.

A clever way to test for the presence of food toxins is to feed lab animals a protein-free diet (or as protein-free as possible if the toxins are proteins) and see how soon they die. On protein-deficient diets, the liver loses half of its proteins and most of its ability to detoxify. Toxic foods given without protein, then, may actually shorten life span compared to a total fast.

Sally Fallon of the Weston A. Price Foundation recounts two remarkable stories:[9]

- One, originally reported in the biochemist Paul Stitt's book *Fighting the Food Giants,* was conducted in 1942 by a cereal company. The study compared rats consuming extruded puffed wheat, water, and vitamins and minerals with rats consuming whole wheat grains, water, and vitamins and minerals. The rats receiving whole wheat grains lived more than a year, but the rats receiving extruded puffed wheat died in two weeks — less than rats that received only water and vitamins and minerals.
- The second, reported to her by Loren Zanier and conducted at the University of Michigan in 1960, gave a control group chow and water, another group cornflakes and water, and a third group the cardboard box the cornflakes came in plus water. The control group did normally, the rats eating the card-

board boxes died of malnutrition, but the rats eating the cornflakes died the quickest — the last cornflake-fed rat was dead
before the first box-fed rat.

Fallon's interpretation is that the extrusion process, which treats grains
with heat and pressure, denatures proteins and other biological compounds
to create toxins.

Apart from their potential to create new toxins, industrial processing
methods have another defect: they fail to destroy natural food toxins. Some
of the most dangerous natural toxins in cereal grains, such as wheat germ
agglutinin, can be destroyed by boiling in water, but are unaffected by dry
heat. As a result, industrially prepared grain-based foods have much higher
levels of natural food toxins than would home-cooked meals prepared from
the same foods.[10]

Reconstituted and Chemically Processed Food

Often, industrial food processing separates foods into isolated ingredients
and then recombines them. For instance, factory milk is separated in centri-
fuges into fats, protein, and miscellaneous solids and liquids; the ingredients
are then recombined in new proportions to make skim, 1 per cent, 2 per
cent, and 'whole' milk; leftovers are used to make butter, cream, cheese, and
other milk products.[11]

Chemical and heat treatments during these steps hold the potential to
alter natural food compounds and create toxins. Dr John Briffa describes
how soy foods are created:

[A] slurry of soy beans is treated with acid and alkali solutions to
get the protein to precipitate out. In this process the product can
be tainted with the metal aluminum (aluminum exposure has been
linked with an increased risk of degeneration of the nervous system
and Alzheimer's disease). The resultant protein-rich 'curd' is spray
dried at high temperature to produce a powder . . . [and] heated
and extruded under pressure to make a foodstuff known as textured
vegetable protein (TVP) . . . TVP will often have monosodium
glutamate (MSG) added to it to impart a 'meaty' flavour before it

is fashioned into products such as vegetarian burgers, sausages and mince.[12]

Toxins Introduced at the Farm

Toxin introduction is not limited to factory settings.

Nicholas Kristof of *The New York Times* recently reported on two papers that assessed commercially produced chickens for toxins and found arsenic, caffeine, Benadryl, Tylenol, and antibiotics.[13]

Apparently 90 per cent of commercially produced chickens are fed low doses of arsenic because it reduces infections and makes their meat look more attractively pink.[14] One-third of feather meal samples — probably a smaller fraction of chickens, since the samples draw feathers from many birds — contained the antihistamine in Benadryl, given to reduce anxiety in chickens; a majority of feather meal samples contained acetaminophen; and feather meal samples from China contained the antidepressant in Prozac.[15]

Processed Meats

All (uninfected) meats are safe to eat in their natural state, fresh from the animal. However, processed meats may have some risk.

An epidemiological study reports that although beef, pork, and lamb do not increase disease rates, the consumption of a daily hot dog or equivalent weight of processed deli meat raises the risk of heart disease by 42 per cent and of diabetes by 19 per cent. The lead author noted that 'processed meats contained, on average, 4 times more sodium and 50% more nitrate preservatives . . . [D]ifferences in salt and preservatives . . . might explain the higher risk of heart disease and diabetes seen with processed meats, but not with unprocessed red meats.'[16] If nitrates are responsible, supplemental vitamin C would help prevent toxicity, since vitamin C inhibits nitrosation.[17]

Other authorities argue that nitrates, which are abundant in leafy green vegetables, are beneficial, and that a more likely culprit is the sugar used in curing to impart flavour and colour. Toxic advanced-glycation end products (AGEs) are abundant in sugar-cured processed meats.[18]

Fresh meats are preferable to processed meats. Eat uncured bacon and smoked salmon, and steer clear of meats cured with sugar.

Genetically Modified Foods

Breeding has made some plants less toxic. Wild almonds contain amygdalin, a chemical that turns into cyanide in the body. Eating only a few wild almonds may be lethal. However, breeding has eliminated amygdalin from domesticated almonds, making them relatively safe.[19]

Genetic engineering holds the promise to improve upon breeding as a means for removing plant toxins. Removal of lectins, alpha-amylase inhibitors, and opioids and modification of gliadin to reduce its immunogenicity might eventually turn wheat into a safe starch.

Unfortunately, to date genetic modifications of agricultural crops have not been made to increase their safety to humans but rather to *increase their toxicity to pests* and thus increase crop yields. Such modifications may reduce the price of food but are unlikely to improve human health.

There are valid concerns that genetically modified cereal grains may be more toxic to humans than their (already toxic) wild ancestors.

SCIENCE OF THE PHD
The Uncertain Safety of Genetically Modified Foods

One strategy in genetic modification efforts has been to protect crop plants from insects by incorporating pesticides from other plant species into crop plant genomes.

Most genetically modified crops have been tested in animals for only 90 days, which may be too little time to detect negative health effects.

Such is the complexity of biology that seemingly innocuous genetic alterations can have far-reaching effects. A good example of this is provided by the 'Pusztai affair'.[20]

In the 1990s, an English biotechnology company developed a genetically modified potato by adding the gene for a lectin from the

(continued on next page)

snowdrop plant. Snowdrop lectin is highly toxic to insects but, by itself, safe for mammals.

Árpád Pusztai, a leading expert on plant lectins, tested the new genetically modified potatoes. Rats fed ordinary potatoes mixed with snowdrop lectin remained healthy, but rats fed the genetically modified potatoes developed damage to their intestines and immune systems. The damage was not due to snowdrop lectin, but to derangement of potato biology from alterations to gene expression. The modification had triggered much higher expression of native potato toxins.

No biologist would be shocked at this result: gene networks are intricately connected, and seemingly minor changes to regulatory sequences can have far-reaching effects.

What was shocking, however, was the response to Pusztai's findings. Pusztai and his research team lost their jobs at a British government research institute. A House of Commons committee attacked Pusztai. He was blocked from publishing his work, though after new data were collected the results appeared in *The Lancet* after an extraordinary review process. He found employment in the United States, his collaborator Stanley Ewen was pushed to retirement, and the editor of *The Lancet* was threatened. Allegedly, pressure had been applied by Prime Minister Tony Blair and U.S. President Bill Clinton to suppress the findings on behalf of the genetically modified food industry. The biotech company went out of business.

What's the best way to detoxify genetically modified grains? Let animals eat them first. In Ohio before the steamboat, when it was prohibitively expensive to carry corn to market, pigs were called 'walking corn' since they could profitably be driven to market. We could with equal justice say that pork is 'healthful corn'.

Takeaway

The 20th century brought a great deal of ingenuity to food production. Food became cheaper, but its character changed.

Food scientists resemble the sorcerer's apprentice: meddling with things they do not fully understand, with consequences we cannot confidently predict.

Industrial food production introduces toxins into food. Each of these toxins individually is not known to be dangerous at the doses in which they are present. However, that shouldn't comfort us, because it is difficult to prove that toxins impair health and a great many toxins are being introduced. Some are bound to do harm.

If our food is to be reliably healthful, consumers must, first, be willing to cook at home and, second, be willing to spend time and money to obtain low-toxicity foods. Food producers will respond to a demand for healthful foods. For this reason, we ourselves try to purchase from local organic farmers.

This needn't be expensive. We found that switching from restaurant and prepared food to home cooking dramatically reduced our food budget, even though we began buying more expensive ingredients.

There are also creative ways to trim a food budget while increasing the healthfulness of food. Our local grassfed-beef farmers sell steaks for $25 per pound [450 grams] but organ meats such as liver, kidney, heart, tongue, and tripe for $3 or $4 per pound. It's possible to save money by buying more nourishing cuts of meat!

24
Four Steps to a Low-Toxicity Diet

. . . .

To achieve a low-toxicity diet:

1. *Eliminate grains, legumes, added sugars, and vegetable seed oils.*
2. *Maintain the safety of safe starches with proper storage and cooking.*
3. *Cook foods gently but thoroughly.*
4. *Eat Paleo, not toxic, by consuming a diversity of vegetables.*

. . . .

Removing the four major toxic foods — grains, legumes, sugars, and vegetable oils — is the first step to a low-toxicity diet. Three further steps will make your diet very low in toxins.

Let Your Starches Be Safe

Starchy foods, attractive to insects and herbivores due to their calorie content, often generate toxins. However, some — the ones we call 'safe starches' — become nearly toxin-free with proper preparation.

Our safe starches include taro, white rice, sweet potatoes, yams, well-handled potatoes, sago, and tapioca. Safe starches are a nutritious and important part of the Perfect Health Diet. They provide glucose without

Notes for this chapter may be found at www.perfecthealthdiet.com/notes/#Ch24.

fructose; resistant starch, which improves gut health; and useful minerals such as potassium.

Cooking can eliminate toxins by rendering proteins digestible. Starchy plants that are rendered safe by cooking include:

- **Taro.**[1]
- **Cassava.** Cassava contains toxic cyanogenic glucosides, and improper preparation causes a disease called *konzo*. Cooking destroys most cassava toxins. **Tapioca** is made from cassava.
- **White rice.** 'Antinutrition factors in the rice grain . . . include phytin (phytate), trypsin inhibitor, oryzacystatin and haemag-glutinin-lectin . . . All the antinutrition factors are proteins and all except phytin (phytate) are subject to heat denaturation. Phytin . . . is responsible for the observed poorer mineral balance of subjects fed brown rice diets in comparison to that of subjects fed milled rice diets.'[2]

We recommend avoiding brown rice because of the phytin, mentioned above, and because rice protein — found primarily in the bran — has been found to provoke an immune response, implying toxicity. No antibodies to rice proteins have ever been identified, however, so it appears that rice toxicity cannot progress to severe disease in the way wheat toxicity can.[3]

Other plants can be kept safe with proper handling. **Potato** toxins solanine and chaconine are generated under exposure to heat and light. At low doses, these toxins are efficiently cleared from the body. Thus, potatoes kept continuously in cool, dark conditions are safe. Discoloured potatoes should be discarded.

Some alternative starch sources, such as quinoa, buckwheat, and amaranth, have been little studied, so it is difficult to judge their toxicity. Of the three, **buckwheat** is probably the safest.

Thanks to the 'gluten-free' movement, it's easy to find familiar products such as noodles and crackers made from safe starches. Look for:

- gluten-free bread and baked goods made from rice flour, potato starch, and tapioca starch
- rice noodles for pasta dishes
- rice crackers rather than wheat crackers

- -

READER REPORTS:
diabetes recovery with non-toxic Paleo foods

My stepdad was diagnosed with type 2 diabetes and had to take high doses of Metformin. I convinced him that Metformin was just a Band-Aid. I managed to get him to read Sisson's articles at Mark's Daily Apple and follow the Primal Blueprint. This was NOT easy — he is very stubborn. But Mark does have a way with words and now my step dad — in 8 months — has great blood sugar readings and does not take any medication. His best friend is also T2D and used to take 6 'mega shots' (his words) of insulin every day and now, after about 6 months, he is down to one shot per day. They both have lost weight and both are in their late 50's. Don't give up! The PHD or Primal Blueprint are actually perfect to handle diabetes.

— Daniel

- -

Cook Food Gently but Thoroughly

Gentle but thorough cooking creates the healthiest food.

Cook Gently to Avoid Toxin Formation

A variety of toxins can form when foods reach high temperature. In meats that are grilled, barbecued, or pan-fried, heterocyclic amines (HCAs) form from amino acids, sugars, and creatine. Formation of HCAs is substantial at temperatures around 200°C.[4] HCAs can cause cancer.[5]

No, this doesn't mean you should give up barbecuing meat. But cook it longer at lower heat; don't char your meat or let it get coated with smoke particles (another toxin).

In plant foods cooked at high heat, a common group of toxins is the Maillard reaction products produced by reactions between sugars and proteins and derivative compounds such as acrylamide. Acrylamide is formed when starches are cooked above 120°C — which happens with roasting, grilling, or frying but not boiling. Interestingly, potato fibre protects the intestine from acrylamide damage.[6]

The health effects of eating food cooked at high temperatures are measurable. A 53 per cent carbohydrate diet of grilled, fried, and roasted foods was compared to a similar diet of steamed foods. After one month, the high-heat diet reduced insulin sensitivity, increased triglyceride levels, and lowered serum levels of omega-3 fatty acids and vitamins C and E.[7]

Plant foods become vulnerable to toxin production when they are dry. For instance, acrolein, which binds to guanine in DNA, promoting mutations, is formed from the dehydration of glycerol or cleavage of dehydrated carbohydrates.[8] This may be another reason why water-rich starches such as white rice and potatoes are more healthful than dry starches such as wheat; and why industrial wheat products, which are subject to high-heat extrusion, are toxic. It may also be a reason to favour cooking starches in water or steam rather than dry heat.

Cook Food Thoroughly to Destroy Pathogens

Internationally, pork consumption is more highly correlated with liver cirrhosis than is alcohol consumption.[9] It's also correlated with liver cancer and multiple sclerosis.[10]

The likely reason: most farm-raised pigs in Asia and Europe, and many in the United States, are infected with hepatitis E virus. Hepatitis E virus can be destroyed in cooking, but it takes an hour at a meat temperature of 70°C. Medium-cooked pork may reach a temperature of only 60°C.[11]

Hepatitis E viral titers are highest in pork liver, intestine, and blood, and highest in raw meat. In Europe, a majority of people who eat raw figatellu, a sausage made from pig liver, have hepatitis E infections.[12]

Because of the risk of infectious disease, not to mention pork's higher

· ·

READER REPORTS: better body temperature regulation

I have noticed my temperature has increased since starting PHD. I used to be always cold and being warmer feels much, much better — being constantly cold is a miserable way to live.

— H. Riley, Brighton, England

· ·

omega-6 content, we grade pork as less healthful than other red meats such as beef, lamb, and goat. For safe pork consumption, we would recommend avoiding liver, intestine, or gut products; washing pork carefully to rid it of blood; and cooking it thoroughly to a temperature of 70°C.

Eat Paleo, Not Toxic: get a diversity of plant foods

Our Paleolithic ancestors ate a low-toxicity diet in general — though they did eat some toxic foods. Clear evidence for the grinding of cereal grains has been found at a site in Israel dating to 21,500 B.C.,[13] and sorghum grain residues have also been found on stone tools at a site in Mozambique, Africa, dating to 103,000 B.C.[14] Middle Stone Age Africans used sorghum grasses for bedding, kindling, and (possibly) baskets and may have prepared and cooked sorghum grains, though there is no direct evidence of this.

However, Paleolithic diets were much less toxic than modern diets for several reasons.

1. Paleolithic hunter-gatherers ate a much wider variety of plant foods — hundreds of species[15] rather than a handful as in Western diets — so the quantity of any one toxin was far lower. Since 'the dose makes the poison', this reduces the toxicity of the diet.
2. The most toxic foods in the modern diet were not available.

   • Grains and legumes were eaten seasonally, not stored for year-round consumption. Nor were they eaten in quantity even when in season: since grains require laborious processing and cooking, they may have been backup or 'starvation' foods.
   • Aside from honey and fruits, there were no available sources of fructose. The discovery of how to crystallise sugar cane was not made until A.D. 350, and as late as 1500 imports of sugar into Europe were only a few tonnes.[16]
   • High-omega-6 vegetable oils did not enter the human diet until industrial processing methods were available to remove toxins and concentrate the oils. Paleolithic fats were overwhelmingly from animals, though some plant oils — palm

oil, coconut oil, tree nut oils, olive oil — were probably extracted. Mesolithic American Indians extracted hickory nut oil.[17]

3. Paleolithic hunter-gatherers, like modern hunter-gatherers, probably prepared plant foods in ways that reduced the toxin load. For instance, seeds may have been soaked in water overnight to start the germination process, or fermented. Modern industrial food processing, on the other hand, tends to be optimised for speed rather than health.

Eating Paleo-style — excluding grains, legumes, vegetable oils, and sugars and including a diverse array of plant foods — generates a diet very low in food toxins.

25

A Traditional Pacific Islander Diet

· ·

*The Perfect Health Diet closely resembles traditional diets of
the Pacific Islands, whose inhabitants were noted for their
exceptional health and beauty.*

· ·

Now that we have designed the diet, it may be helpful to summarise
the differences between the Perfect Health Diet and Western diets.

Americans in 2005 obtained 23 per cent of calories from cereal
grains, 3 per cent from legumes, 23 per cent from vegetable oils, and 17 per
cent from sugar and high-fructose corn syrup.[1] Americans get two-thirds of
their calories from foods the Perfect Health Diet eliminates!

To adopt the Perfect Health Diet, Americans will have to find healthful
foods to replace the two-thirds of calories from grains, legumes, vegetable
oils, and sugars. Specific foods the Perfect Health Diet recommends eating
more of include:

- **Safe starches such as sweet potatoes, taro, and white rice.**
  These should increase from about 3 per cent of calories in the
  American diet to about 20 to 30 per cent of calories.
- **Fruits and berries.** These should increase from 2.9 per cent of
  calories to 5 to 10 per cent of calories.
- **Sea vegetables.** Negligible in the American, Australian, and
  New Zealand diets; should be common.

Notes for this chapter may be found at www.perfecthealthdiet.com/notes/#Ch25.

- **Ocean fish and shellfish,** which provide omega-3 fats. Less than 0.6 per cent of calories in the American diet; should provide about 7 per cent of calories.
- **Coconut oil and coconut milk,** which provide short-chain fats. Negligible in the American diet; should provide up to 6 per cent of calories.
- **Meat, eggs, and healthful fats and oils.** These should rise from 23.6 per cent of calories in the American diet to about 55 per cent of calories.

Looking over the foods that should be increased in the diet, we noticed something interesting: these are precisely the staple foods of traditional East Asian and Pacific Islander diets. The Perfect Health Diet is a Pacific Islander diet!

Let's look at traditional Pacific Islander diets and what they did for the islanders' health.

The Okinawan Diet

The traditional diet of Okinawa consists of white rice, sweet potatoes, fish, pork, eggs, and vegetables, including seaweed. All parts of pigs were eaten ('tails to nails'), and lard was used for cooking. The gerontologist Kazuhiko Taira described traditional Okinawan food as 'very, very greasy'.[2]

On these foods Okinawans had the longest life expectancy in the world, with numerous centenarians. The age-adjusted death rate from heart disease was 82 per cent lower than in the United States, from cancer 27 per cent lower, and from all causes 36 per cent lower. Hormone-dependent cancers, such as breast, ovarian, and colon cancer, were 50 to 80 per cent less frequent in Okinawa than in the United States.[3]

Centenarians had the highest intake of milk, meat, fish, eggs, fat, and oils.[4]

Unfortunately, Okinawans recently began to eat vegetable oils, grains, and industrially prepared foods. Okinawans now have widespread obesity, rising rates of heart disease, cancer, and diabetes, and shortening life span.[5]

The Kitavan Diet

In 1989, a global search for aboriginal peoples eating in their traditional manner discovered the islanders of Kitava, off the coast of New Guinea. The residents of Kitava lived on safe starches (yam, sweet potato, taro, tapioca, cassava), fruit (banana, papaya, pineapple, mango, guava, watermelon, pumpkin), fish, coconuts, and vegetables. Lauric acid, the 12-carbon SaFA found in coconut oil, was the dominant dietary fatty acid.[6]

Despite the presence of a fair number of elderly, with ages up to 95, a research team led by Staffan Lindeberg was unable to find a single person who had ever had a heart attack, based on EKG examinations and community interviews. The Kitavans were entirely free of heart disease. They were also free of stroke, diabetes, and dementia. No one was overweight, no one had acne, and no one had high blood pressure. Infections — primarily malaria — and accidents — drowning and falling from coconut trees — were the leading causes of death.[7]

The Hawaiian Diet

The traditional diet of the native Hawaiian consisted of taro (often prepared as poi), sweet potatoes, breadfruit, coconut, fish, squid, shellfish, pork, fowl including chicken, taro leaves, seaweed and *limu* (algae), and a few sweet fruits.

A famous festival hosted by King Kamehameha III in 1847 served '271 hogs, 482 large calabashes of poi, 602 chickens, 3 whole oxen, 2 barrels salt pork, 2 barrels biscuit, 3125 salt fish, 1820 fresh fish, 12 barrels *lu'au* and cabbages, 4 barrels onions, 80 bunches bananas, 55 pineapples, 10 barrels potatoes, 55 ducks, 82 turkeys, 2245 coconuts, 4000 heads of taro, 180 squid, oranges, limes, grapes and various fruits'.[8] Except for the biscuits — hardly a food that would have been available 70 years earlier — these are all foods we can highly recommend. As this menu suggests, most calories came from meat, fish, taro, and coconut.

Early European explorers remarked on the beauty, strength, good nature, and excellent physical development of the native Hawaiians and other Pacific Islanders. The chronicles of Magellan (1521) and Quiros (1606) refer to

Pacific Islanders as 'singularly tall, muscular and well-proportioned people'. Of the Tahitians the French explorer Louis de Bougainville said, 'I never saw men better made,' and in the 1770s Captain James Cook noted the good diets and health of Pacific Islanders.[9]

Takeaway

We did not know when we began writing that we would be recommending the foods traditionally eaten by Pacific Islanders. We are reassured that the Perfect Health Diet, which we arrived at from our study of the scientific literature, is very similar to traditional diets known to produce superb health.

26
Food Toxins Matter

· ·

Reducing the number of food toxins in your diet may do more
for your health than any other single step.

· ·

Food toxins may do a lot more damage to health than most people realise. The good news: removing food toxins may bring dramatic health improvements.

Clinical Trials

Most dietary trials examine alternative macronutrient ratios (low-fat or low-carb diets) or food types (plant-based or animal-based diets). But Paleo diet pioneer and Swedish doctor Staffan Lindeberg has conducted trials of Paleo-style diets that remove most toxins.

The results are remarkable: dramatic improvements in health.

One of Lindeberg's trials found that 'a Paleolithic diet improved glycemic control and several cardiovascular risk factors compared to a diabetes diet in patients with type 2 diabetes'.[1] A Paleo diet outperformed the standard diet recommended to diabetics.

Paleo-style eating seems to rapidly cure metabolic syndrome, induce weight loss in the obese, and improve biomarkers in diabetics. One paper concludes:

Notes for this chapter may be found at www.perfecthealthdiet.com/notes/#Ch26.

It is difficult to refute the assertion that if modern populations returned to a hunter-gatherer state then obesity and diabetes would not be the major public health threats they now are.[2]

These early trials suggest the importance of eliminating food toxins for good health.

One study, which included lots of carbs (1000 carb calories per day) and high levels of fructose from honey and carrot juice, is helpful because both the Paleo arm and the control arm consumed the same macronutrient ratios. So the improved lipid profiles, glucose tolerance, and blood pressure seen in the Paleo arm were likely due to the elimination of food toxins from grains and legumes. The improvements came quickly — in days:

> Even short-term consumption of a paleolithic type diet improves BP and glucose tolerance, decreases insulin secretion, increases insulin sensitivity and improves lipid profiles . . . in healthy sedentary humans.[3]

Another trial, comparing a Paleolithic diet with a Mediterranean diet among type II diabetes patients, similarly found that elimination of toxic foods benefits health even if macronutrient ratios are unchanged. The authors concluded:

> The larger improvement of glucose tolerance in the Paleolithic group was independent of energy intake and macronutrient composition, which suggests that *avoiding Western foods is more important than counting calories, fat, carbohydrate or protein.* The study adds to the notion that healthy diets based on whole-grain cereals and low-fat dairy products are only the second best choice in the prevention and treatment of type 2 diabetes [emphasis added].[4]

Note that the diet containing whole-grain cereals, though described as 'healthy', was inferior to the diet that had no grains at all.

Toxin elimination works in pigs too: pigs on a grain-free Paleo-type diet weighed 22 per cent less and had 43 per cent less subcutaneous fat around their middles than pigs on conventional cereal-based swine feeds. Their insulin sensitivity was much better, their blood pressure was 13 per cent lower, and their levels of C-reactive protein (a marker of inflammation) were 82 per cent lower.[5]

READER REPORTS: improved sleep and skin

One of the things I immediately noticed after doing PHD is that it improved the quality of my sleep (used to keep waking up several times at night and that is now a thing of the past because I now sleep uninterrupted for 7–8 hours); and no more cramps in my calves (that used to happen occasionally after a heavy work out); no more menstrual cramps either. Also, today is the first time I had my monthly period that I didn't get a pimple in my face. I usually get a big, really deep and hard to get rid of pimple just before or during my monthly period and my husband or a dermatologist would actually help me get it out especially if I had an important function to attend to . . . So yes at least in my experience, a great improvement in my overall health since I incorporated the principles that I learned from the PHD. And btw, I have a very sensitive skin and I usually get itchy and/or red spots in my skin all the time but in the last 4 weeks the anti-itching cream which I carry everywhere has never been used even once. And to top it all off, I lost 3 lbs [1.4 kilograms] in the last 4 weeks (losing the 15 lb [6.8 kilograms] excess weight is not even on top of my list because I am trying to get pregnant). I don't have any health problems and hardly get sick. I simply want to eat healthy and trying to figure out what diet works best for me. And I found it! Thanks to PHD. Thanks to the Jaminets! At 42, 5'6" height, 125 lbs [11.3 kilograms] weight, and doing PHD on 20% carbs, I feel great! And yes, I am sticking with PHD for the rest of my life.

— S.E.

Dietary Transitions

If adopting a low-toxicity Paleo-style diet improves health, we should see that going the other way, from a low-toxicity Paleo-style diet to a Western diet, should damage health.

Pacific Islanders

A good test case is provided by Pacific Islanders, who were so healthy on their traditional diets. The traditional Pacific Islander diet was:

- low in polyunsaturated fat (less than 2 per cent of energy on Kitava)[6]
- low in sugar, high in starch
- entirely composed of safe starches (taro, cassava, yams) and devoid of wheat or beans

Pacific Islanders have mostly abandoned their native diets and adopted Western diets high in vegetable oil, sugar, and wheat. The result has been a huge increase in obesity rates.

In Kosrae, a district of the Federated States of Micronesia, 88 per cent of adults are overweight, 59 per cent obese, and 24 per cent extremely obese.[7] Yet half a century ago, obesity was nonexistent. The U.S. Navy's survey of health in Micronesia after World War II noted almost a complete absence of obesity, hypertension, or diabetes. Obesity first appeared with the introduction of the U.S. Department of Agriculture supplementary feeding program in the 1960s and 1970s.[8]

Today, the more Western the diet, the more obesity. A comparison of American and Western Samoans found that the American Samoans, who ate a more modern diet, had an average BMI of 35.2 compared to 30.2 for Western Samoans.[9] In Papua New Guinea also, the more modern the diet, the higher the BMI.[10] The body weights of Cook Islanders increased by 21.8 kilograms between 1966 and 1996.[11]

Other Peoples

In other parts of the world, too, shifts from traditional diets to modern Western diets brought about declines in health and increases in obesity.

Pima Indians living a modern lifestyle near Phoenix, Arizona, have an average BMI ten points higher, and higher rates of diabetes, than Pima Indians living a traditional lifestyle in rural Mexico.[12] In *Western Diseases: their emergence and prevention,* Hubert C. Trowell and Denis Burkitt gathered a number of accounts of transitions from healthful traditional diets to unhealthy Western diets.[13] Based on a survey of doctors at 200 hospitals in developing countries, Burkitt deduced that a host of diseases — diverticular disease, appendicitis, bowel cancer, ulcerative colitis, varicose veins, deep vein thrombosis, pulmonary embolism, and hemorrhoids — were 'rare or unknown in communities who still adhere to their traditional way of life'.[14]

READER REPORTS: hypothyroidism, joint inflammation

I had soft tissue recovery issues, joint inflammation, skin issues etc. After endless doctor visits, a smart dermatologist suggested I had a leaky gut and gluten sensitivity. At one point Hashimoto was also thrown into the mix. Paleo and GAPS took care of most of the joint inflammation and skin problems, but my T3 and some of my thyroid symptoms got worse while I was on the (unintentional) ketogenic healing diet. Your posts on this issue have been helpful, and I am now upping my carb intake. I have bought the book for a few people in my family and my best friend.

— Edle Tenden

Takeaway

Scientists are only beginning to study the effects of natural food toxins on human health. However, it is clear that Paleolithic and traditional diets are more healthful than modern diets, and lower levels of food toxins are probably the reason.

Reducing the toxicity of your diet is an effective way to bring about rapid health improvements. Start by excluding the four major toxic food groups: grains, legumes, sugars, and vegetable seed oils. Avoid industrially processed foods, cook using gentle moist cooking methods such as boiling and steaming, and eat a variety of healthful foods with a focus on safe starches and low-omega-6 meats and oils.

Part IV

How to Be Well Nourished

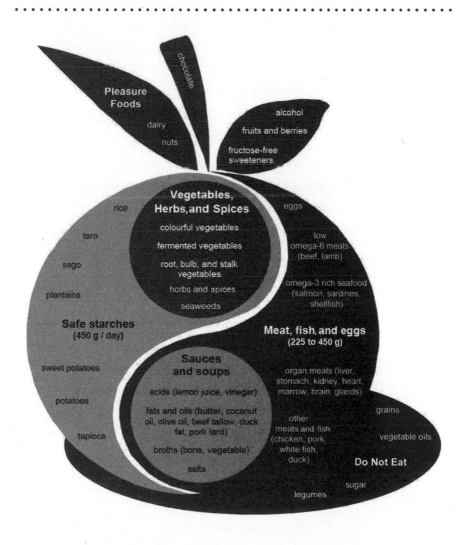

27

Why Most People Are Malnourished

· ·

- *In the modern world, nearly everyone is malnourished.*
- *Malnourishment has dangerous, long-lasting — even transgenerational — effects.*

· ·

Good health doesn't only depend on removing toxins and getting the right macronutrients. The human body also needs micronutrients such as vitamins and minerals. This raises several questions. Are people on modern diets malnourished? What is the peak health range of each nutrient? Which ones are we deficient in? Which ones are we getting in excess? Should we repair deficiencies with food or supplements?

Six Reasons Most People Are Malnourished

Modern people are malnourished compared to our Paleolithic ancestors — and Paleolithic people were not always well nourished. Here are six reasons we should expect that most moderns are malnourished.

First: modern life is sedentary. Inactivity may reduce appetite and therefore reduce nutrient intake.

Our Paleolithic ancestors were hunter-gatherers, and hunter-gatherers are much more active than modern Australians and New Zealanders. Hunter-gatherers also eat more food per kilogram of body mass: a study found that !Kung and Ache hunter-gatherers eat 50 per cent more calories per 450 grams of body weight than modern office workers, and a recent high-quality study of the Hadza found that they eat about 15 per cent more calories per 450 grams of body weight than Westerners.[1] Consuming more calories per kilogram of body weight, other things being equal, implies consuming more nutrients per kilogram of body weight.

Second: modern foods are nutrient-poor compared to Paleolithic foods.

Modern plant foods such as wheat, rice, corn, and sugar have around 1300 to 1500 calories per 450 grams and relatively few nutrients per calorie. Paleolithic plant foods such as starchy tubers, fruits, and vegetables average around 200 calories per 450 grams and are nutrient-rich.

Paleolithic humans ate the whole carcass of animals, including nutrient-rich tissues such as liver and bone marrow. Modern Australians and New Zealanders eat only skeletal muscle.

If, in addition to consuming more calories, Paleolithic people were getting several times more nutrients per calorie than modern Australians and New Zealanders, they must have been obtaining vastly more nutrients.

Third: water treatment and agricultural food production diminish the mineral content reaching consumers.

Minerals are lost in the treatment of drinking water. Water was the largest source of calcium and magnesium in Paleolithic diets, but modern water treatment removes most dissolved minerals.

Repeated plantings of a single crop on the same plot of land diminish the mineral content of the soil and ultimately the mineral content of the plants, unless fertiliser adequately replaces the minerals.

Mineral deprivation in pastureland leads to deficiencies in animal meats, eggs, and dairy products. A study found that copper levels in U.K. foods have declined by 90 per cent in dairy products, 55 per cent in meat, and 76 per cent in vegetables.[2]

The biggest factor in reduced mineral content in agricultural foods was the 'Green Revolution'. Norman Borlaug won the Nobel Peace Prize for inventing fast-growing dwarf cultivars that doubled wheat yields. However, the fast-growing varieties deplete soil of minerals. A study of the mineral content of archived soil and grain samples dating back to 1845 found that a dramatic fall in mineral content coincided with the adoption of dwarf varieties in the 1960s.[3]

Fourth: modern cooking methods often leave nutrients behind.

Traditional cuisines made soups or broths when cooking in water and sauces or dressings from cooking oils and drippings, thus retaining water-soluble and fat-soluble nutrients. Traditional diets also added inedible organic matter, such as bones, to soups, allowing minerals and other nutrients to leach into the broth. But modern cooks don't use bones and discard cooking water, oils, and drippings.

Fifth: modern foods contain antinutrients that lock up nutrients as well as toxins that impair intestinal absorption of micronutrients.

Antinutrients such as phytic acid lock up minerals and prevent their absorption, and toxins in grains and legumes impair digestion. Many of these toxins specifically target protein digestion; for instance, trypsin inhibitors prevent the breakdown of proteins into amino acids. This impairs micronutrient status, because many minerals are chelated to proteins or bound in enzymes.

Sixth: even on their low-toxin, high-nutrient diets, Paleolithic humans may have been malnourished.

Anthropologists have detected occasional signs of malnourishment, such as tooth hypoplasia, in Paleolithic skeletons.

Moreover, on theoretical grounds we should not expect Paleolithic nutrition to have been optimal for individual health. Though Paleolithic diets were undoubtedly largely non-toxic, Malthusian population growth would have increased the population above the level optimal for individual human health. Widespread slight malnourishment was probably the norm, especially after the Last Glacial Maximum.

Cumulatively, these factors suggest that micronutrient deficiencies are widespread today. But how harmful are they?

The Perils of Malnourishment

Although we have a good understanding of acute diseases arising from severe nutrient deficiencies, such as scurvy, rickets, beriberi, and pellagra, little is known about the long-term effects of chronic deficiencies. Long-term effects may be insidious and hard to trace.

Chronic Disease

A plausible theory, proposed by Bruce Ames of the University of California at Berkeley and called 'triage theory', holds that when nutrients are scarce, the body prioritises functions needed for reproduction and short-term survival — such as the ability to hunt — while short-changing maintenance functions that sustain a long, healthy life.[4] Triage theory predicts that the chronically malnourished will die younger and be less healthy in their older years.

Support for this idea comes from studies of the effects of famines, such as the Dutch famine during World War II and the famine during the Chinese Great Leap Forward, on children born before, during, and after the famine. Those studies show that malnourishment in the womb is associated with high rates of chronic diseases such as obesity and diabetes. The same effects occur in animals.[5] What's surprising is that the worst health — especially, the worst mental health — belonged to children conceived *after the famines had ended*:

- Pregnant women's exposure to the Dutch famine *prior to conception* doubled the risk of adult depression in the offspring, but exposure to the famine *during pregnancy* had no effect.[6]
- In rural China, as a result of the famine during the Great Leap Forward, 'the post-famine cohort had the highest risk of developing schizophrenia, and there was virtually no difference in schizophrenia risk between the pre-famine and the famine cohort'.[7]

Apparently it is crucial for women to be well nourished *before conception* if their babies are to be entirely healthy.

Because pregnant women donate nutrients to their developing babies, mothers may become malnourished during pregnancy. Postpartum depression, for instance, is linked to iron deficiency.[8]

Facial Structure and Tooth Quality

Weston A. Price was a Cleveland dentist who travelled the world to find dietary causes of tooth decay. He found that in premodern cultures eating traditional diets, cavities were rare: fewer than 5 per cent of teeth had decay,

READER REPORTS: fibromyalgia

I started feeling terrible in the winter of 2007. I went to five doctors, none of them knew what was wrong with me. I had blood drawn about 15 times for various lab tests. I was afraid I would be bedridden one day because of the pain.

The first doctor who helped me diagnosed me with fibromyalgia. He started me on Savella 50 mg/day. I improved on Savella, and was told to do a cleanse diet to detect food sensitivities. Many people with fibromyalgia have food sensitivities as well. I did not have the will power to execute this plan properly. However, I was not going to rely on doctors anymore, so I began my search for healing on my own.

I tried a few different things, natural supplements, and diets. Some gave no help, some gave a bit of help, then I plateaued. Most importantly, with regard to the food restrictions I tried, I had such cravings that I did not care about my fibromyalgia pain and just indulged. Then, when I was full, I cared about my fibromyalgia pain again.

I learned of the *Perfect Health Diet* from a friend in the summer of 2011. I did not think I would be able to do it all, knowing my failures in the past. So, I started small. I had a friend with celiac and was most convinced by the section on the toxicity of wheat and other cereal grains. Thus, I began by eliminating these. I noticed an improvement within a few weeks: I could type! No more Dragon NaturallySpeaking for me!

In light of my previous failures, the key that made the avoidance of wheat and company successful was that I could eat a lot of fat. After a few weeks, I had some cravings for bread, but nothing as strong as my cravings for things excluded in other trial diets. Now I have no cravings for bread.

I decided I would put more effort into the other parts of the PHD. Next in line was vegetable oil. I had been eating a lot of salads, and I loved ranch dressing. With a few false starts, I finally broke the habit of vegetable oils, and was encouraged by some weight loss.

Next, I went half in on the supplements. I noticed the magnesium had significant effects on my muscle soreness and neck stiffness. I read

(*continued on next page*)

the post on constipation and decided to add selenium, vitamin C, NAC, copper, etc. Finally, I got started on working up to high dose iodine, with the recommendation of starting low and doubling every month. In the last two weeks I have been at 12 mg/day iodoral, and I have recently noticed a great uptick in my mood and lowered occurrence of stiffness in my neck. I have been getting much more done at work, and have not had as much 'brain fog'.

In fact, it took some forced thinking to recall how far I've come. I used to stand up very slowly, and limp for a bit afterward because of pain in my hips. I used to try to play volleyball, but could not move suddenly or land the wrong way lest I feel great pain. I used to accept that I would always be stiff and have difficulty moving in the morning. I used to get random pains in the bottom of my foot which made me limp. I used to take a lot of fiber and was still not regular. I used to be 25 pounds [11.3 kilograms] heavier. I used to have strong cravings for sugar, bread, chicken strips, and chips, just to name a few. I used to have acne flare ups all the time. In the past I had to stop typing every five minutes and massage my elbows for ten minutes; it usually hurt to turn my neck; my shoulders were frequently sore; I could not throw a baseball, a football, or a frisbee. Frequently, I could not remember details of things I knew a lot about. I would get confused and get tired easily.

Now, I do still have elbow pain and some psoriasis/rash, so all is not perfect. I am beginning to think these are unrelated to the fibromyalgia and that the fibromyalgia is gone. I am at 1/32nd of the original Savella dose, feeling fine, but will report back if I regress when taking the dose down to zero.

THREE AND A HALF MONTHS LATER:

I delayed reporting because I wanted to be sure symptoms would not flare up again. I got completely off the Savella 3 months ago. Today I ran my fastest 2 mile [3.2 kilometre] time, then played ultimate frisbee for a few hours later in the day. I feel great. I used to get extremely sore from just trying to run half a mile [0.8 kilometre], which was also pretty depressing. I am feeling strong and limber with no trace of soreness. I am almost back to where I was in my early 20's.

— Justin, South Bend, IN

whereas people in modern cultures typically had cavities in 20 to 40 per cent of teeth. Some cultures — the Eskimos and Inuit, Melanesians and Polynesians — had cavities in less than 0.4 per cent of teeth.

He also noticed differences in facial architecture. Premodern peoples eating traditional diets had broad faces with wide dental arches with straight teeth. Members of those groups who had adopted modern diets, and modern peoples all over the world, frequently had narrow faces and compressed dental arches with crooked teeth. Price estimated that 25 to 75 per cent of Americans had that facial pattern and believed that a fraction of people with it had accompanying defects in the development of the brain that manifested as reduced intelligence and alterations in character.[9]

Price found that the critical nutrients accounting for the difference in facial structure and dental health were fat-soluble vitamins contained in animal fats such as butter and cod liver oil and minerals such as magnesium, calcium, and phosphorus. Price reported that the fat-soluble vitamins A, D, and K2 (Price's 'activator X') were tenfold more abundant in primitive diets than in modern diets, magnesium was as much as 25-fold more abundant, and calcium and phosphorus were typically fivefold more abundant.[10]

Transgenerational Effects of Malnutrition

Two remarkable sets of data imply that malnutrition not only damages one's own health but is also, to borrow a biblical phrase, visited upon the sons to the third and fourth generations.

Pottenger's Cats

Dr Francis Marion Pottenger, Jr, was a veterinarian who worked in a lab producing adrenal hormones for medical use. At the time there was no good way to evaluate the strength of manufactured hormone, so the evaluation was done in cats with surgically removed adrenal glands.

Pottenger's cats had a high death rate, but he noticed that when the offal portion of the diet — liver, tripe, sweetbreads, brains, and heart — was fed to them raw rather than cooked, their health improved tremendously.

That observation led him to conduct a remarkable experiment from 1932 to 1942. The experiment evaluated five diets over four generations and included 900 cats. The work was described in his book *Pottenger's Cats*.

Cats fed raw milk and raw meat and offal maintained remarkable health through four generations. However, cats fed cooked meat and pasteurised, evaporated, or condensed milk experienced steadily deteriorating health:

- First-generation cats developed degenerative diseases late in life.
- Second-generation cats developed degenerative diseases in midlife.
- Third-generation cats developed diseases, allergies, and soft bones and succumbed to parasitic infections early in life. Most of the cats could not produce offspring.
- Not a single fourth-generation cat could reproduce. Fourth-generation cats 'suffered from most of the degenerative diseases encountered in human medicine'.[11]

It's now generally accepted that the decline of Pottenger's cats was due to nutritional deficiencies induced by cooking. Cooking destroys some nutrients, such as vitamin C. More significantly for cats, the taurine in cooked meat but not raw meat is degraded in the intestinal tract.[12] Taurine is an essential dietary nutrient for cats, and taurine deficiency in cats causes many of the symptoms seen in Pottenger's cats.[13]

We find two aspects of Pottenger's experiments especially fascinating.

- The effects of a malnourishing diet were passed down through generations, such that health deteriorated in every generation. *This reproduces the effects seen in famine studies, where malnourished mothers produced children prone to obesity and disease.*
- On the malnourishing diets, most human degenerative diseases were recapitulated. *This suggests that much human disease may be due to malnourishment.*

It's been shown that obesity advances through the generations much like chronic diseases in Pottenger's cats. In mice on an obesogenic diet, obesity becomes progressively more severe over four generations,[14] and in humans a tendency toward obesity is passed to children of obese or overweight parents.[15] Perhaps this is evidence that obesity is caused by malnutrition.

The Flynn Effect

When immigrants from poor countries came to the United States in the late 19th and early 20th centuries, their descendants' IQ increased by about 10 points per generation for three to four generations, a phenomenon known as the 'Flynn effect'. There has been a similar, but smaller, effect in Americans. The Flynn effect operates only in people with low IQs; people with high IQs have negligible IQ increases over generations. The Flynn effect seems to have ceased operating in the late 20th century.[16]

The Flynn effect has been linked to improved nutrition.[17] This is no surprise: we know from other studies that breast-fed babies have IQs six to eight points higher than formula-fed babies,[18] so there's every reason to believe that nutritional status affects IQ.

Immigrants' heights increased in parallel with their IQ,[19] supporting the nutritional explanation.

Iodine intake could be a major factor. Iodine deficiency is the leading global cause of mental retardation, and even a moderate iodine deficiency lowers IQ by ten to 15 points.[20]

Another possibility is relief of omega-3 fat deficiencies. Omega-3 deficiencies are known to build up over multiple generations. In rats fed an

READER REPORTS: a new approach to nutrition

Your book and writings have totally changed the way I think about my diet, nutrition and health. So in the past year, I have minimized grains, cut out processed food, do not eat sweets and avoid omega-6 rich cooking oils like the plague. I have increased my intake of saturated fat by several fold and use butter and coconut oil as my cooking oils. I eat eggs for breakfast and add cream/coconut milk to my coffee. I eat sardines and salmon weekly. I get plenty of sunshine and exercise several times a week. I eat just as much fruits and vegetables as I did in the past. I do however consume more sweet potatoes and potatoes. I use to avoid the "evil" potato as well! . . . I do not calorie count and eat to what I feel. I have actually lost weight and my skin has become healthier as well.

— Erik

omega-3-deficient diet, DHA levels in the brain decrease to as little as 20 per cent of normal by the fourth generation.[21] Perhaps brain DHA levels may be restored equally slowly.

Takeaway

Famine studies, Weston A. Price's observations of dental health, Pottenger's cats, and Flynn's humans all point to one conclusion: malnourishment has long-lasting, even transgenerational, effects on health and may be a primary factor in human disease.

To be well nourished, it is not enough to relieve only *macronutrient* deficiencies. It is common for children of obese mothers to experience stunted growth.[22] The children are malnourished, but not for lack of calories. They lack micronutrients: vitamins, minerals, and other biological compounds.

So let's learn how to optimise micronutrients: how to eat and supplement so as to bring all micronutrients into their peak health ranges.

28
Multivitamins: good or bad?

· ·

- *Multivitamins may do as much harm as good.*

· ·

Multivitamins are extremely convenient — just one pill per day. Almost 20 per cent of Australians routinely supplement with a multivitamin.

It seems logical that if most people are malnourished, as we believe they are, multivitamins should deliver health benefits. Some deficiency diseases — rickets (vitamin D), scurvy (vitamin C), beriberi (vitamin B1), and pellagra (vitamin B3) — plus many mineral deficiencies can be *fatal*. Even subclinical deficiencies can have large but insidious effects on health. The health improvement from repairing deficiencies should be substantial.

Yet studies have generally been unable to detect any benefits from taking multivitamins:

- A study of 161,808 women followed over eight years as part of the Women's Health Initiative found that the 42 per cent of women who regularly used multivitamins had no difference in rates of cancer, heart attack, stroke, or mortality from those who did not take multivitamins. The multivitamin users were 2 per cent more likely to die, a result that was considered insignificant.[1]
- A meta-analysis of eight clinical trials conducted in the elderly found 'weak and conflicting' evidence for benefits from multi-

vitamins. Multivitamin users had the same number of infections as nonusers, but got over them in about half the time, experiencing 17.5 fewer days per year with infections. The study was unable to analyse death rates, which had not been adequately reported.[2]

It's a puzzle: if most Americans are malnourished and malnourishment injures health, why don't multivitamins improve health?

Adding to the puzzle: while multivitamins have little effect, individual supplements generally improve health. Here are hazard ratios — the relative probability of dying if you take the supplement — for supplements in at least 500 users from the Iowa Women's Health Study:[3]

Supplement	Hazard Ratio (Adjusted for Age and Energy)
Multivitamin	1.02
Vitamin A	0.99
Vitamin B6	1.04
Folic acid	1.09
Vitamin B complex	0.93*
Vitamin C	0.96*
Vitamin D	0.92*
Vitamin E	0.92*
Calcium	0.83*
Iron	1.03
Magnesium	0.97
Selenium	0.97
Zinc	0.97

*Statistically significant.

The results are adjusted for energy intake, which is unfortunate because it makes supplements look worse than they are. Supplements suppress appetite, and lower energy intake reduces mortality rates; adjusting for energy intake takes credit for this away from the supplement. However, even so, individual supplements look beneficial: nine of the 12 decreased mortality rates; **every one of the five that reached statistical significance reduced mortality rates.** But multivitamins increased mortality rates by a statistically insignificant 2 per cent.

How big might the benefits of supplementing properly be? If the benefits of the various micronutrients are independent of one another, we can just multiply their hazard ratios to see their combined effect. Supplementing vitamin B complex, vitamins C, D, and E, calcium, magnesium, selenium, and zinc would reduce the mortality rate by 43 per cent. Pretty good!

Why do multivitamins do so much worse than individual supplements? We believe that multivitamins:

- Provide too little of bulky nutrients such as magnesium and vitamin C and of fat-soluble nutrients such as vitamin D and vitamin K2
- Provide large amounts of some potentially risky nutrients, including vitamin A, manganese, and folic acid, and in some cases iron and selenium, thus potentially contributing to toxicity

Even if the levels provided by multivitamins, when combined with levels in food, are not intrinsically toxic, multivitamins may exacerbate an *imbalance of nutrients.*

Just like omega-6 and omega-3 fats, some micronutrients need to be in proportion to one another. Vitamins A and D are an example. Many Australians get a sufficiency of vitamin A from food but are low in vitamin D because they don't expose their skin to the sun. Until recently multivitamins provided about 4000 IU of vitamin A and little vitamin D — increasing an already high vitamin A to vitamin D ratio.

Because of their flawed formulas, multivitamins are not the best way to relieve nutritional deficiencies. A strategy of eating more nourishing foods and supplementing individual nutrients has a better chance to achieve optimal nourishment.

We'll therefore discuss micronutrients individually — actually, in groups of micronutrients that collaborate and need to be taken in proportion with one another — to find their peak health ranges. We'll provide detailed discussions of 14 nutrients that are crucial for health and easy to get wrong:

1. Fat-soluble vitamins: **vitamins A, D,** and **K2**
2. Thyroid minerals: **selenium** and **iodine**
3. Electrolytes: **potassium** and **sodium**
4. Water-soluble minerals: **calcium** and **magnesium**
5. Vascular antioxidants: **zinc** and **copper**
6. Collagen repair: **vitamin C**
7. Methylators: **choline** and **folate**

We'll add very brief assessments for others — the B vitamins, vitamin E, and trace minerals.

Finally, we'll conclude Part IV with a recommended set of supplements and supplemental foods to be eaten in designated amounts weekly or daily.

29
Vitamins A, D, and K2

· ·

- *Eat egg yolks, liver, and organic butter for these fat-soluble vitamins.*
- *Get sunshine for vitamin D, and supplement if necessary to reach 40 nanograms per millilitre of 25OHD.*
- *Supplement vitamin K2.*
- *Vitamin D optimisation cuts mortality rates in half; vitamin K2 optimisation cuts mortality rates by 26 per cent.*

· ·

Vitamins A, D, and K2 are fat-soluble vitamins that collaborate in many functions: immunity and bone health, to name two. It was vitamins A, D, and K2 that Weston A. Price identified as the key nutrients for skeletal and dental health.

Vitamin A has various forms:

- In animal foods, vitamin A is present as **retinol,** a yellow fat-soluble antioxidant.
- In plants, vitamin A precursors are present as **carotenoids,** which give colour to many vegetables.

Vitamin D is mainly manufactured in the skin under exposure to sunlight; it is present in some animal foods such as cod liver oil.

Vitamin K comes in a plant form, K1, which is common in green leafy vegetables and in animal and bacterial forms, collectively called K2. The main forms of K2 are MK-4, which the liver manufactures from dietary K1, and MK-7, which bacteria manufacture. Both MK-4 and MK-7 are functional and nourishing in the human body. Most people get MK-7 from gut bacterial fermentation of fibre and from fermented foods such as aged cheese, kimchi, and natto, and MK-4 from animal foods such as liver, butter, cream, and eggs.

All three vitamins are extremely important to health:

- Vitamin A is needed for vision, immune function, bone remodelling, skin health, creation of new blood cells, protection of fats from oxidation, and other functions.
- Vitamin D is needed for bone mineralisation, immune function, and other functions.
- Vitamin K2 is needed for activation of certain proteins, including proteins controlling mineralisation of bone and preventing calcification of arteries.

Vitamin A deficiency leads to blindness and impaired immunity, often resulting in death from infectious disease. Vitamin D deficiency leads to rickets, a potentially fatal bone-softening disease, and immune impairment.

Because these three nutrients interact, it's somewhat tricky to find their peak health ranges. Let's start by looking at evidence from human population studies and intervention trials.

At First Glance: too much vitamin A, not enough vitamins D and K2

Many studies have found negative effects from high intakes of vitamin A and its precursor, β-carotene. A review and meta-analysis of seven high-quality clinical trials covering 131,727 persons found that supplementation with β-carotene and vitamin A together increased mortality rates by 29 per cent; β-carotene alone increased mortality rates by 5 per cent.[1]

A prospective observational study of 72,000 nurses found that those ingesting more than 10,000 IU per day of vitamin A from food and supplements had a 48 per cent higher risk of hip fractures than those ingesting about 3000 IU per day.[2] Unfortunately, the study did not report death rates.

The high-fracture group obtained about half their vitamin A from multi-vitamins. The low-fracture group took neither multivitamins nor beta-carotene supplements, obtaining almost all their vitamin A from food. Carrots supplied about two-thirds of the food-sourced vitamin A in the study, with liver and milk the next most abundant food sources.

Yet it seems clear that many Australians are deficient in vitamins D and K2. Let's find the optimal levels of those two, then revisit the situation with vitamin A.

Optimal Vitamin D Levels

Three forms of vitamin D are important:

- Cholecalciferol, or **vitamin D3,** is produced by sunlight acting on cholesterol in the skin. It is biologically inactive — a storage form of the vitamin.
- The liver converts cholecalciferol into 25-hydroxyvitamin D. This is an active form of vitamin D that circulates throughout the body and crosses cell membranes. We'll call this form **25OHD** for short.
- All human cells can convert 25OHD into a still more active form, 1α,25-dihydroxyvitamin D. We'll call this **1,25D** for short. This form does not cross cell membranes, so every cell has its own level.

25OHD has the same level throughout the body and provides a universal baseline level of vitamin D activity in every cell. Cells finetune their level of vitamin D activity by converting more or less 25OHD into 1,25D, which is about 500 times more potent than 25OHD at activating the **vitamin D receptor (VDR).**[3]

Dr Robert Heaney has found that healthy men need about 3000 to 5000 IU of vitamin D3 a day from all sources to maintain a 25OHD level of 30 nanograms per millilitre through a Nebraska winter.[4] Women may need a little less. More may be needed if illness or food toxicity depletes vitamin D.

It is likely that under regular sun exposure, the body limits average daily vitamin D production to about these levels. Although up to 20,000 IU can be made in a single day,[5] with regular sun exposure daily vitamin D production is reduced.

Another way of estimating an optimum is by circulating 25OHD level. It seems fairly clear that a 25OHD level below 32 to 35 nanograms per millilitre indicates a deficiency, at least in people of European descent. A number of diseases become more prevalent when 25OHD levels fall below 32 nanograms per millilitre.[6] For instance, bone density is highest and fracture rates lowest with 25OHD levels over 32 nanograms per millilitre. Cancer rates are reduced above this level, as are rates of many other diseases.

Biokinematic studies also support establishing the lower boundary of the plateau range at about 35 nanograms per millilitre. One study reported:

> One could plausibly postulate that the point at which [the liver's] 25(OH)D production becomes [saturated] constitutes the definition of the low end of normal status. This value . . . is at a serum 25(OH)D concentration of 88 nmol/L (35.2 ng/mL) . . . It is interesting that this estimate is very close to that produced by previous attempts to define the lower end of the normal range from the relations of serum 25(OH)D to calcium absorption and to serum parathyroid hormone concentration (ie, 75–85 nmol/L, or 30–34 ng/mL).[7]

So four independent methods agree: 25OHD levels below 35 nanograms per millilitre are inadequate; levels above 35 nanograms per millilitre are within the optimal range.

It is more difficult to assess the 25OHD level at which vitamin D toxicity begins, because few people attain high vitamin D levels. A recent review of the literature found few contraindications for vitamin D supplementation below 10,000 IU per day and a paucity of reports of toxicity for serum 25OHD levels below 200 nanograms per millilitre.[8] However, there are reasons to think the maximum safe level of serum 25OHD is 50 nanograms per millilitre:

- Once adequate vitamin D is provided, most people seem to reach a stable equilibrium 25OHD level around 40 to 45 nanograms per millilitre. At this level, nearly all additional vitamin

D3 is placed into storage.[9] African hunter-gatherers are around this level: the Hadza of Tanzania average 43.6 nanograms per millilitre.[10]

- 25OHD levels after abundant summer sun exposure, as in lifeguards, peak between 45 and 80 nanograms per millilitre. Outdoor workers in the tropics typically have 25OHD levels between 48 and 80 nanograms per millilitre.[11] These tropical outdoor workers get too much vitamin D.

  - People in South India with 25OHD levels of 89 nanograms per millilitre have a threefold higher rate of heart attack.[12]

  - Lifeguards in Israel develop kidney stones 20 times more often than the general population.[13]

- Human cells destroy vitamin D by turning on the vitamin D–degrading gene CYP24A1 at 25OHD levels below 100 nanograms per millilitre.[14] This indicates that optimal 25OHD levels are well below 100 nanograms per millilitre.

Another sign that the optimal 25OHD level is below 50 nanograms per millilitre: bone mineral density peaks in the range 32 to 45 nanograms per millilitre and then falls as 25OHD rises above 45 nanograms per millilitre. For blacks, the fall in bone mineral density begins at 40 nanograms per millilitre.[15]

Because the body tries to defend a 25OHD level around 40 nanograms per millilitre by placing extra vitamin D3 in storage, there is a risk that persistent supplementation may build up a reservoir of stored vitamin D3. Then, if storage room runs out or stored vitamin D is released due to weight loss, 25OHD levels could spike to toxic levels. One study notes the risk:

> Deposition in body fat almost certainly occurs in cases of vitamin D intoxication, and persistence of hypercalcemia for months has been attributed to sustained release of vitamin D from such body stores.[16]

For optimal health, then, the 25OHD level should be 40 nanograms per millilitre — a level that is normally achieved with vitamin D3 intake from sun and supplements of about 4000 IU per day.

Most Americans Suffer from Vitamin D Deficiency

In modern life, with indoor work, most people rarely expose their skin to the sun.

No wonder, then, that many Americans are deficient in vitamin D, especially at northern latitudes during the winter. If 25OHD below 35 nanograms per millilitre is the measure of deficiency, about 80 per cent of Americans are deficient:

- 69 per cent of U.S. children have 25OHD levels below 30 nanograms per millilitre.[17]
- 77 per cent of U.S. adults have 25OHD levels below 30 nanograms per millilitre.[18]

Most American adults would have to supplement with at least 2000 IU per day and most children with 1000 IU per 22.7 kilograms of body weight to bring 25OHD readings into the optimal range.

Vitamin D deficiency is extremely damaging to Americans' health. Among other things, it contributes to the following diseases:

- **Cancer.** The farther north one lives, the more likely one is to die of cancer. This is true of a host of cancers, including breast, colon, and ovarian cancers. The National Cancer Institute offers online maps illustrating the pattern, which we recommend perusing.[19] Increasing 25OHD levels by 20 nanograms per millilitre can be expected to decrease breast cancer rates by 41 per cent[20] and other cancers by similar amounts. The simple step of optimising vitamin D levels could cut U.S. cancer rates in half.
- **Cardiovascular disease.** Levels of vitamin D predict who will die of stroke: the lower the vitamin D level, the more likely a fatal stroke will occur.[21] Heart disease deaths in Europe are correlated with the level of solar radiation: the more sun, the fewer deaths.[22]
- **Mortality rates.** People with higher vitamin D levels are less likely to die of any cause.
  - In a study of 3258 persons followed for 7.7 years, those in the third quartile (median 25OHD level 13.3

nanograms per millilitre) had a 53 per cent higher chance of dying than patients in the highest quartile (median 25OHD level of 28.4 nanograms per millilitre), and those in the lowest quartile (median 25OHD level 7.6 nanograms per millilitre) had a **108 per cent higher chance of dying.**[23]

- Elderly in the lowest 25OHD quartile were **124 per cent more likely to die** over a 6.2-year follow-up period.[24]
- In the LURIC study, only 8 per cent of subjects had 25OHD level above 30 nanograms per millilitre. Those lucky ones had only one-quarter the risk of dying of those who were severely deficient.[25]

- **Diabetes.** Higher vitamin D status is associated with lower rates of diabetes.[26]
- **Infectious diseases.** When rickets was rampant, victims frequently died of respiratory infections, such as pneumonia, tuberculosis, and the flu. The flu and other respiratory infections strike primarily in the winter, when people's vitamin D levels are low.

   These associations are not coincidental. Low vitamin D levels increase the risk of tuberculosis fivefold.[27] In a randomised trial of Japanese schoolchildren, supplementation with 1200 IU per day of vitamin D reduced the risk of influenza A by 42 per cent.[28]

   Cellular studies have shown that vitamin D is essential to the innate immune response to intracellular pathogens — viruses and cell-wall-deficient bacteria. Vitamin D is essential for transcription of antimicrobial peptides such as cathelicidin. Such peptides are important killers of intracellular, gut, and skin pathogens.[29]

- **Dementia.** Vitamin D is highly effective in improving cognition in Alzheimer's patients.[30] In one case, a Georgia doctor reported that an Alzheimer's patient who had not spoken in a year regained her ability to converse a few months after starting vitamin D at 5000 IU per day.[31]

   A possible reason: Alzheimer's may be caused by a chronic

bacterial infection of the brain, perhaps by *Chlamydophila pneumoniae*.[32] The bacteria steal glucose and pyruvate from neurons, starving them. The amyloid plaques that litter the brain of Alzheimer's patients may have an antibacterial function.[33] A strong immune response, activated by vitamin D, may kill the bacteria or drive them into a dormant state that allows neurons to regain function.

- **Multiple sclerosis.** It has long been known that multiple sclerosis (MS) has a strong latitude dependence — disease rates are much higher at northern latitudes. MS is strongly associated with low vitamin D levels.[34]

  Recently, evidence has begun to accumulate that vitamin D improves the course of MS. For instance, in a clinical trial giving MS patients 10,000 IU per day, 'treatment group patients appeared to have fewer relapse events and a persistent reduction in T-cell proliferation compared to controls'.[35]

  MS is associated with simultaneous infection by the parasitic bacteria *Chlamydophila pneumoniae* and the Epstein-Barr

READER REPORTS:
mood, cognitive function, joint noises, and aches

A couple of months after starting PHD there was an obvious improvement in mood and cognitive function. Now 12 months later the mental improvements persist.

I've had joint 'noises' for about 20 years (I'm 72yo) but have ignored this 'crepitude' as being an unavoidable aging effect until recently, when my manageable back/neck aches spontaneously improved and that happened about 3 months after adopting the PHD diet . . . I can sleep on my back for the first time in 8 years and turn my neck 90 deg without any discomfort . . . Pre-PHD, with the same exercise effort, if I increased calories my fat would easily but slowly increase, but not now. I feel great.

— Morris Goruk

virus (sometimes the *Varicella zoster* virus). Vitamin D's effectiveness against Epstein-Barr infections may explain the latitude dependence of MS.[36]

Sun or Supplements?

Most Americans could improve their health and cut mortality risk by up to half simply by optimising their vitamin D levels. The best way to optimise vitamin D levels is to get a half hour of sun exposure on bare skin daily, preferably in the morning or at midday. Anyone who gets limited sun exposure should have his or her serum 25OHD level tested and supplement to reach a serum level of around 40 nanograms per millilitre. Supplemental D3 doses that may be appropriate with infrequent sun exposure are in the table below.

Location	Winter Dose	Summer Dose
Alaska	4000 IU	2500 IU
Northern continental United States	2500 IU	1000 IU
Southern United States	1000 IU	—

However, serum 25OHD levels should be monitored and the supplemental dosage adjusted to produce optimal serum levels year-round.

Optimal Vitamin K Levels

Vitamin K2 is an extremely important fat-soluble nutrient that is needed to activate various proteins through a process called *carboxylation*. Without vitamin K, blood doesn't clot, leading to **hemorrhage;** bones don't calcify properly, leading to **fractures;** soft tissues do calcify, leading to **atherosclerosis** and **joint disease;** and **cancer** runs rampant.

Most Americans Suffer from Vitamin K2 Deficiency

One measure of vitamin K2 deficiency is the percentage of circulating osteocalcin that has not been activated. The EPIC-Heidelberg study found that for every 10 per cent of osteocalcin that is undercarboxylated, advanced-stage prostate cancer cases increase by 38 per cent.[37]

If 10 per cent osteocalcin undercarboxylation is proof of K2 deficiency, most Americans are deficient. The Framingham Offspring Study found that American men average 17 per cent undercarboxylated osteocalcin and American women 19 per cent. The rate of undercarboxylation was highest in postmenopausal women, and estrogen replacement improved vitamin K2 status.[38] A majority of 11- and 12-year-old Dutch girls have over 20 per cent of their serum osteocalcin undercarboxylated.[39] In children ages eight to 14, the range of osteocalcin undercarboxylation was 11 to 83 per cent.[40] Another study in the Netherlands found 43 per cent undercarboxylation in Dutch adults and 67 per cent in Dutch children.[41] Vitamin K2 deficiency is severe in children because growing bones consume more vitamin K2.

Vitamin K has no significant storage pool in the body, so deficiencies develop quickly. Infants on vitamin K–free formula develop vitamin K2 deficiency in seven to ten days.[42]

The consequences of vitamin K2 deficiency are quite serious.

- **Loss of bone strength.** Vitamin K2 is required for bone mineralisation. Seven clinical trials studying vitamin K2 supplementation at 45 milligrams per day consistently observed reduced fracture rates. On average, vitamin K2 supplementation reduced the risk of vertebral fractures by 60 per cent, hip fractures by 77 per cent, and nonvertebral fractures by a remarkable 81 per cent.[43]

- **Atherosclerosis and heart disease.** Vitamin K2 prevents calcification of soft tissues, which causes a host of problems (kidney stones, arthritis, cataracts, heart valve insufficiency, wrinkled skin, bone spurs, senility) but, above all, coronary atherosclerosis. Calcification of coronary arteries — in which the arterial walls are turned bony and stiff — is a direct measure of atherosclerosis and a highly accurate predictor of heart attacks and mortality.[44]

  The Dutch Prospect arm of the EPIC study found that vitamin K2, but not vitamin K1, reduces the risk of coronary calcification[45] and heart disease.[46] Every additional 10 micrograms per day of vitamin K2 reduced the rate of heart disease by 9 per cent.

- **Mortality rates.** In the Rotterdam Study, vitamin K2 intake, but not vitamin K1 intake, was inversely proportional to the mortality rate.[47] Over a period of seven to ten years, people in the upper third of vitamin K2 intake, consuming just 41 micrograms per day of vitamin K2, were:

- 26 per cent less likely to die of any cause
- 57 per cent less likely to die of heart disease
- 52 per cent less likely to suffer aortic calcification

Périgord, France, is the world capital of foie gras, or fatty goose liver, which is rich in vitamin K2. Périgord has the lowest rate of cardiovascular mortality in France.[48]

- **Cancer.** It has been known for 30 years that vitamin K2 kills cancer cells, including liver, colon, lung, stomach, breast, and mouth cancers as well as leukemia and lymphoma cells. Vitamin K2 also induces leukemia cells to differentiate into more normal blood cells and prevents cancer cells from multiplying.[49]

In the EPIC-Heidelberg study, being in the top quartile of dietary vitamin K consumption produced a 24 per cent reduction in the risk of prostate cancer and a 75 per cent reduction in the risk of advanced-stage prostate cancer.[50]

The ECKO trial supplemented elderly women with 5 milligrams per day of vitamin K1 for up to four years to see if it reduced bone loss and fractures. **It did reduce fractures** — there were nine fractures among the vitamin K group and 20 among the controls — but **it reduced cancers even more:** there were three cancers in the vitamin K group compared to 12 in the control group, a **75 per cent reduction in cancer incidence.**[51]

Perhaps significantly, all the cancers in the vitamin K group appeared early in the trial; not a single new case of cancer appeared in the vitamin K group in the final two years of the study.

Clinical trials also indicate that vitamin K can help heal cancer. In a trial of acute myeloid leukemia patients, an MK-4 dose of 45 milligrams per day led to regression of the cancer in 71 per cent of patients.[52] Several clinical trials have found that vitamin K2 reduces the occurrence and recurrence of hepatocellular cancer (HCC, a form of liver cancer).[53] This disease normally results in death within three to six months.[54]

A Japanese trial found that 45 milligrams per day of vitamin K2 with a blood pressure drug 'markedly inhibited the cumulative recurrence of HCC'.[55] Vitamin K2 inhibits metastasis and invasion.[56] The best predictor of survival is a measure of vitamin K status.[57]

Based on this evidence, we would advise anyone with cancer to take high doses of vitamin K2 as well as enough vitamin D to optimise serum 25OHD.

SCIENCE OF THE PHD
Vitamin K2 for Patients on Coumarin

In rats, blocking vitamin K2 with warfarin produces calcified arteries in only three weeks. However, supplemental vitamin K2 then reverses arterial calcification.[58]

As with rats, so with humans: patients who take coumarin experience arterial calcification.[59] Such patients should supplement with vitamin K2. This will improve bone and vascular health and, with adjustment of coumarin dose, stabilise INR levels.

- **Reduced neurological and cognitive function.** Vitamin K2 is required for embryos to develop a healthy brain and nerves. Use of the vitamin K antagonist warfarin during the first six weeks of pregnancy causes severe birth defects and, during the second and third trimesters, causes neurologic abnormalities, spasticity, and seizures.[60]

  Vitamin K2 activates enzymes that produce constituents of the brain and nerves.[61] Higher serum vitamin K2 levels lead directly to higher brain levels of *myelin sulfatides,* which protect against cognitive decline with age.[62] Vitamin K2 also protects cells that manufacture myelin, which sheaths nerves and is essential for their proper function.[63]

- **Vitamin D toxicity.** Large doses of supplemental vitamin D can cause improper tissue calcification and an array of symptoms including anorexia, lethargy, growth retardation, bone loss, and death.

  Vitamin K2 protects against all of these effects, suggesting that vitamin K2 prevents vitamin D toxicity. Indeed, it has been argued that vitamin D is toxic *only if it induces a vitamin K2 deficiency.*[64]

  It is known that vitamin D depletes vitamin K2.[65] Therefore, to avoid vitamin D toxicity and vitamin K2 deficiency, vitamin D should be cosupplemented with vitamin K2.

Our Take: a case for supplementation

There is no known toxicity from supplementation of either vitamin K1 or vitamin K2. Japanese trials lasting three years and testing large supplemental doses of vitamin K2 — 45 milligrams per day, 1000 times the common intake — have not detected toxicity.

Although vitamin K2 deficiency leads to hemorrhaging,[66] high doses do not lead to excess clotting as long as the dose is adjusted gradually. Because vitamin K2 activates procoagulation and anticoagulation factors in parallel, high serum levels of vitamin K2 are generally consistent with normal blood clotting.[67]

Vitamin K2 supplementation appears to have substantial benefits — reducing mortality rates by 26 per cent in one ten-year study. It has no reported negative effects, even at doses a thousand times greater than most Australians obtain. Vitamin K2 is a necessary companion to vitamin D; the two are especially effective against cancer.

We therefore recommend *both* eating vitamin K–rich foods such as green leafy vegetables, organic butter and cream, fermented vegetables, aged cheese, liver, and egg yolks, *and* supplementing. Available supplements are bacterial-produced MK-7, available in 100-microgram doses, and synthetic MK-4, available in high doses. We would suggest supplementing either 100 micrograms of MK-7 daily or mixed formulations of several milligrams of vitamin K2 at least weekly.

Optimal Vitamin A Levels

Now we can revisit the question of optimal vitamin A levels.

The results of high vitamin A intake — bone fractures and cancer — are precisely the same as the results of vitamin D and vitamin K2 deficiency.

This is not a coincidence. Vitamins A and D need to be in balance with one another, because they act in concert to control gene expression in the nucleus of human cells. An improper ratio of vitamin A to vitamin D in the body distorts gene expression.

If *balance* between vitamins A and D is what matters for health, the ratio of vitamin A to vitamin D matters more than the amounts, and an excess of vitamin A will look the same as a deficiency of vitamin D. Optimal intake of vitamin A may look excessive if vitamin D is deficient.

The vitamin A toxicity that the clinical trials and prospective cohort studies observed in Americans with high vitamin A intake may be due to vitamin D deficiency.

The primacy of vitamin A and vitamin D balance is suggested by several studies. Irwin Spiesman in 1941 published a study of vitamins A and D as treatments for the common cold. He found, first, that vitamins A and D together were effective at preventing colds, but either individually was useless. Only a combination worked. Second, he found that toxicity was common when either was given individually: four of seven vitamin A–only recipients experienced toxicity, and two of seven vitamin D–only recipients did so, but none of 40 persons receiving both together experienced toxicity.[68]

Support for the balance view is provided by Tufts University researchers. They followed up on a suggestion by Chris Masterjohn[69] and assessed the relation between vitamin A and vitamin D status and the activation state of the vitamin K–dependent protein MGP. Their findings:[70]

- Vitamin A alone did nothing to improve the status of MGP.
- Vitamin D alone increased the amount of activated MGP but increased the amount of uncarboxylated MGP — a probable toxin — even more.
- Vitamin A and D together increased the amount of activated MGP even more than vitamin D alone, but completely eliminated the increase in toxic uncarboxylated MGP.

Thus a balanced intake of vitamins A and D amplifies the benefits of vitamin D while eliminating its side effects.

The Optimal Amount of Vitamin A

If it's the ratio of vitamin A to vitamin D that matters most, what's the optimal ratio?

Earlier we saw that Americans who are deficient in vitamins D and K2 experience toxicity from vitamin A at an intake of 10,000 IU per day, which people taking multivitamins commonly reach. The typical American (and some Australians in southern states) probably gets about half the optimal amount of vitamin D3, or 2000 IU of vitamin D. We infer that the optimal vitamin A–to–vitamin D ratio in IU should be less than five to one. Let's estimate it at two and a half to one.

Since the optimal vitamin D intake is 4000 IU, this suggests that the optimal vitamin A intake is about 10,000 IU, if vitamin D has been optimised.

Although this amount of vitamin A is dangerous in a state of vitamin D and K2 deficiency, both vitamin D and vitamin K2 protect against vitamin A toxicity, and quite large doses of vitamin A (as in Dr Spiesman's experiments) have been given safely with beneficial effects when vitamin D and vitamin K2 were at high enough levels.

Our Take: get vitamin A from foods only, but eat vitamin A–rich foods

Given the potential danger of vitamin A toxicity, we recommend avoiding supplemental vitamin A. This is another reason to avoid multivitamins; it was those who took multivitamins who developed vitamin A toxicity in the Nurses' Health Study.

However, we believe that a high intake of vitamin A–rich foods is probably beneficial in the context of optimal levels of vitamins D and K2. Therefore, we recommend eating vitamin A–rich foods, especially **egg yolks** and **liver** (and giblets) among animal sources, and colourful vegetables such as carrots, pumpkin and squash, peppers, sweet potatoes, and green leafy vegetables for carotenoids that are vitamin A precursors.

Takeaway

Our prescription for vitamins A, D, and K2 is as follows.

Nutrient	Primary Source	Supplements
Vitamin A	Three egg yolks per day, 115 grams of liver per week, organic butter, colourful vegetables	None
Vitamin D	30 minutes of sunshine on bare skin per day	Vitamin D3 as necessary to bring serum 25OHD to 40 ng/dl
Vitamin K2	Three egg yolks per day, 115 grams of liver per week, organic butter, fermented vegetables, aged cheese	100 mcg MK-7 per day *or* 1 mg MK-4 and MK-7 per week

30
Selenium and Iodine

· ·

- *Eat kidneys, beef, eggs, fish, and shellfish for selenium.*
- *Supplement iodine starting at 225 micrograms per day, working up to 1 milligram per day.*
- *Benefits: optimising selenium may reduce cancer rates by 30 to 50 per cent; optimising iodine may reduce cancer rates by 20 to 30 per cent and infectious disease rates substantially.*

· ·

S elenium and iodine are two more nutrients that must be kept in balance, since they collaborate for thyroid and immune functions.

Functions of Selenium and Iodine

Among the most important hormones for human health is the thyroid hormone triiodothyronine (T_3). With its partner the thyroid receptor, T_3 activates transcription of many genes. Its primary effect is to fire up the metabolism: T_3 increases oxygen and energy consumption, increases the rate at which glucose is produced and released into the blood, increases the rate at which fats are taken up into cells for energy, and increases the heart rate and the force of heartbeats. T_3 also stimulates production of myelin, neurotransmitters, and axon growth, and is essential for development of the nervous system in embryos and infants.

Notes for this chapter may be found at www.perfecthealthdiet.com/notes/#Ch30.

A deficiency of T_3 is called *hypothyroidism.* Hypothyroidism makes its sufferers weak and puffy and exacerbates nearly all human diseases, including obesity.

In order to make T_3, the body needs two minerals: selenium and iodine. Thyroid hormones are composed of iodine: the precursor to T_3, thyroxine or T_4, has four iodines attached to a peptide, and T_3 is created by the action of the selenium-containing deiodinase enzyme, which removes an iodine atom.

Selenium is also needed by a few dozen other enzymes. Two are *glutathione peroxidase* and *thioredoxin reductase,* which are important for maintaining the key cellular antioxidants glutathione and thioredoxin.

A deficiency in selenium strongly impacts three organs that use antioxidants heavily — the thyroid, the gut, and immune cells.

- Glutathione and thioredoxin protect the thyroid against damage from hydrogen peroxide and ROS produced during the creation of thyroid hormone. If goitrogens from toxic foods such as soy are eaten, ROS production is particularly high; if poor antioxidant function is also present, there will be thyroid damage. Thus, selenium has a double effect on thyroid function — it enables the creation of active T_3, and it protects the thyroid from harm.
- Glutathione is especially important for the gut, where most of the immune cells in the body are located and where ROS produced to control gut bacteria are common. Repairing a selenium deficiency can be extremely helpful for gut health.
- White blood cells kill pathogens by releasing reactive oxygen species (ROS); their supply of protective antioxidants, especially glutathione, determines how much ROS they can safely manufacture and release. Low selenium levels imply poor white cell function.

Iodine is also important for immune function. Neutrophils, a type of white blood cell, kill bacteria and fungi with a 'respiratory burst' of enzymes, ROS, and acid. To make this burst, the myeloperoxidase enzyme needs a halide partner.[1] Iodide is the most effective partner.

Neutrophils draw their iodine from thyroid hormones.[2] To support neutrophil function, thyroid hormones concentrate in diseased tissue, where thyroid hormone is consumed at a rapid pace.[3] So a deficiency in thyroid hormone impairs immune defences by depriving neutrophils of iodide. An ordinarily adequate intake of iodine can lead to hypothyroidism during chronic infections, if thyroid hormone is consumed by immune cells faster than it can be replenished from a limited iodine pool.

Iodine was widely prescribed for infectious diseases in the 19th century. The Nobel laureate Dr Albert Szent-Györgyi, the discoverer of vitamin C, recounted this anecdote:

> When I was a medical student, iodine in the form of KI was the universal medicine. Nobody knew what it did, but it did something and did something good. We students used to sum up the situation in this little rhyme:
>
> > If ye don't know where, what, and why
> > Prescribe ye then K and I.[4]

A standard dose of potassium iodide was 1 gram, containing 770 milligrams of iodine.

Since immune cells obtain iodine by stripping it from thyroid hormone using selenium-containing deiodinase enzymes, a deficiency of *either* selenium *or* iodine will impair immune function.

Selenium

Selenium inadequacy is associated with a number of human diseases: Keshan disease, Kashin-Beck disease, cancer, impaired immune function, neurodegenerative and age-related disorders, and thyroid disorders. Selenium deficiency also exacerbates conditions caused by inadequate iodine, such as cretinism.[5]

Higher Selenium Intake Is Often Beneficial
Many people experience improved thyroid function upon supplementation of selenium. In French women, the size of the thyroid is inversely proportional to selenium intake.[6]

Selenium supplementation often improves immune function. Both healthy and immunosuppressed individuals supplemented with 200 micrograms per day of selenium for eight weeks showed an enhanced immune response to foreign antigens.[7]

Supplementation of selenium with CoQ10 reduced all-cause mortality by 24 per cent and cardiovascular mortality by 53 per cent in elderly Swedes.[8]

Selenium supplementation may help prevent cancer.

- Four supplementation trials showed that 'selenium showed significant beneficial effect on the incidence of gastrointestinal cancer'.[9]
- More than two-thirds of over 100 published studies in 20 different animal cancers found that selenium supplementation significantly reduces tumour incidence.[10]
- An intervention trial of selenium supplementation in China in areas with high rates of liver cancer found that selenium supplementation reduced the rate of liver cancer by 35 per cent. In a smaller subgroup of chronic hepatitis B–infected patients, none of 113 selenium-supplemented patients developed liver cancer, while seven of 113 placebo-supplemented patients did.[11]
- In American men with a history of skin cancer, supplementation with 200 micrograms per day of selenium decreased prostate cancer incidence over the following 7.4 years by 49 per cent.[12]

Selenium Toxicity

Selenium is dangerous in high doses. Fatal toxicities have occurred with accidental or suicidal ingestion of gram quantities of selenium. Clinically significant selenium toxicity was reported in 13 individuals after they took supplements that contained 27.3 milligrams per tablet due to a manufacturing error.

Chronic selenium toxicity may occur with smaller doses of selenium over long periods of time; the symptoms are hair and nail brittleness and loss, gastrointestinal disturbances, skin rashes and acne or rosacea, fungal infections, a garlic breath or body odour, fatigue, irritability, hypothyroidism, and nervous system abnormalities. The Food and Nutrition Board has set the tolerable upper intake level (UL) for selenium at 400 micrograms per day in adults based on the prevention of hair and nail brittleness.[13]

However, there are subtleties to selenium toxicity:

- Animal foods, such as kidney and shellfish, which deliver selenium primarily as selenocysteine, are probably the safest sources of selenium. Very high intakes of selenocysteine by Greenland Inuit were not found to be toxic.[14]
- Plant foods, which deliver selenium primarily as selenomethionine, are probably less safe; selenomethionine is less useful to humans and may be toxic in ways selenocysteine is not. For instance, selenomethionine suppresses DNA repair[15] and distorts DNA methylation;[16] it also replaces methionine in proteins such as albumin with unclear effects. High levels of selenomethionine intake in people on the Lower Tapajós River of the Amazon Basin in Brazil cause 42 per cent of the population to display fingernail damage and 24 per cent to have general irritation or fungal infections on the skin — both symptoms of selenosis.[17]
- Inorganic forms such as sodium selenite or selenate, which are commonly found in supplements, are the most dangerous. Developing embryos are sensitive to selenite poisoning: in zebrafish, excess selenite induces loss of neurons from brain, trunk and tail, defects in heart function, and embryonic death, but supplementation with folic acid can relieve the cardiac and neuronal defects.[18]

Based on these considerations, we favour obtaining selenium mainly from animal sources, secondarily from plant sources, and not at all from inorganic supplements.

Another factor contributing to a risk of inadvertent selenium toxicity is that selenium content of foods can vary dramatically depending on the selenium content of local soils.

Livestock raised in western Canada have four times more selenium than livestock raised in eastern Canada.[19] In the U.S. upper Midwest, due to very high selenium levels in the high plains of Nebraska and the Dakotas, the selenium content of wheat varies from 14 to 803 micrograms per 100 grams, a 57-fold range, and the selenium content of beef varies by 11-fold, from 19 to 217 micrograms per 100 grams.[20] Four hundred and fifty grams of beef might provide anywhere from 86 to 985 micrograms of selenium!

Variability means that stated values of selenium in nutritional databases are not reliable. In the USDA nutritional database, Brazil nuts are listed as having 1917 micrograms of selenium per 100 grams due to their provenance from high-selenium Brazilian soils. Brazil nuts from other locations may have much less selenium.

Optimal Selenium Levels

Given uncertainty regarding the amount of selenium any person is actually obtaining from food, the importance of maintaining adequate selenium for health, and the dangers from selenium toxicity, we need to attend both to the risk of deficiency and the danger of toxicity.

In general, selenium is low in plants except in grains, nuts, and seeds, which are not major parts of the Perfect Health Diet. Meat commonly has about 180 micrograms per 450 grams, but kidneys, the organ richest in selenium, have about 750 micrograms per 450 grams. Eggs may have 150 micrograms per 450 grams. Fish and shellfish typically range from 360 to 720 micrograms per 450 grams.

Our peak health range for selenium is 200 to 400 micrograms per day. Since most selenium on the Perfect Health Diet comes from meat, fish, and eggs, your intake will depend on how much of these you eat.

- If you are at the high end of our protein range, 450 grams of meat, fish, and eggs per day mostly from ruminants and seafood, you are probably getting over 200 micrograms per day from food. Do not supplement selenium.
- If you are at the low end of our protein range, 225 grams of meat per day, your dietary selenium intake will be around 100 micrograms per day when you eat low-selenium muscle meats — a bit low, in other words — but in the peak health range when you eat kidneys, fish, or shellfish. There are many ways to ensure that you average over 200 micrograms per day: (a) eat eggs regularly, (b) eat fish and shellfish regularly, (c) add some Brazil nuts to your diet — two or three per day, *or* (d) supplement occasionally — perhaps once or twice a week. Be sure to supplement with organic forms of selenium, not selenite.

How can we deal with the risk of selenium toxicity?

Excess selenium, along with other minerals, is excreted in urine and in sweat. Sweat excretion is why a selenium overdose can generate a garlicky body odour.

A way to avoid toxicity from selenium and many metals[21] is to **make yourself sweat.** Drink lots of water, and every day do something — strenuous exercise or a visit to the sauna — that makes you sweat.

There are other reasons to drink water and exercise, but toxin elimination is a good one. We think that obtaining selenium predominantly from animal foods, drinking copious water, and frequently generating sweat will largely eliminate selenium toxicity risk.

READER REPORTS: nutrition for hypothyroidism

I am doing quite well on PHD. I have Hashimoto's and have found there is DEFINITELY a thyroid improvement (energy levels, reduced neck swelling) when some carbs are in my diet. On PHD my thyroid medication was reduced, to one-third the previous dose. This is all thrilling. Thank you so much for all your work.

— Becky

I treat thyroid problems in my practice and have Hashimoto's . . . The longer I am on the PHD and appropriate supplements, the less desiccated thyroid I require. It used to take 2½ tabs daily and now I use ½ tab daily. I have increased my safe carb intake and feel great! Thanks Paul.

— William D. Trumbower, MD, Columbia, Missouri

Iodine

Iodine is probably one of the most widely deficient micronutrients, and yet it is one of the most important for health.

Benefits from Increased Consumption of Iodine

Iodine deficiency is the most common cause of preventable brain damage in the world. About 800 million people suffer from iodine deficiency disorders including hypothyroidism and mental retardation.[22]

Iodine deficiency impairs immune response and is associated with high rates of stomach cancer.[23] A mandatory program of iodine prophylaxis in Poland reduced rates of stomach cancer by 18 per cent in men and 29 per cent in women.[24]

Clinical trials of iodine supplementation for chronic disease are lacking, which is odd in light of the positive experiences of physicians from the 19th and early 20th centuries, as well as anecdotal accounts from many modern people who have tried high-dose iodine supplementation and seen regression of chronic diseases.

These experiences are also supported by epidemiological evidence. In general, seaweed-consuming cultures are long-lived and healthy.

The Japanese are notably long-lived, and they eat a lot of iodine-containing seaweed. Average daily iodine consumption in Japan is 1.2 milligrams per day.[25] People in the northern coastal region eat 50 to 80 milligrams per day.[26]

By contrast, the U.S. RDA is only 150 micrograms per day, one-eighth the consumption of a typical Japanese. The mean consumption of iodine in the United States is about 240 micrograms per day.[27]

Iodinisation of salt has had remarkable effects not only for prevention of mental retardation, but for prevention of cancer. Poland had the lowest iodine intake and highest stomach cancer death rates in Europe before it began a program of iodine prophylaxis in 1996. Since that date, stomach cancer rates have fallen steadily, declining 2.3 per cent per year in men and 4.0 per cent per year in women.[28]

Iodine Is Generally Non-toxic

Iodine, in its inorganic form, can be among the safest of trace minerals. In humans, doses of up to 6 grams per day of potassium iodide, containing 4.6 grams of iodine — about 40,000 times the recommended intake for Australians and New Zealanders, which is 150 micrograms per day — have been given safely for several years.[29] The Asthma Clinic of the

Free University of West Berlin treated thousands of patients with doses of 36 grams per day four days per week and found that 'the unwanted effects of potassium iodide are no more important than those of many other remedies'.[30]

The most common (apparently) negative effect from iodine supplementation is bromine toxicity, which often produces acne. Iodine displaces other halides such as bromine from chemical compounds, releasing them into the circulation. This is good; bromine is undesirable, and once bromine is circulating, the kidneys can remove and excrete it. However, eliminating bromine from the body may take months. To hasten its elimination, drink extra water, eat extra salt, and supplement extra vitamin C.

There is conflicting evidence for the value of iodine in thyroid conditions. In a Chinese study, there was a higher incidence of autoimmune thyroiditis and subclinical hypothyroidism with high iodine intake.[31] In rats, high iodine intake damages the thyroid only if selenium is deficient or in excess. In Hashimoto's patients, higher iodine intake is associated with lower antibody titers, lower TSH, and reduced goiter size.[32]

High doses of iodine are not guaranteed to be benign:

- If selenium status is sub- or abnormal, high or low iodine intake may injure the thyroid. In selenium-deficient rats, high iodine intake injures the thyroid and causes hypothyroidism; but in rats given the equivalent of 200 to 400 micrograms selenium per day, the thyroid remains healthy on a wide range of iodine intakes, including the human equivalent of 12 milligrams per day.[33]
- Iodine intake should be increased gradually to allow the thyroid time to adapt. A too-rapid increase in iodine may lead to a transient hyperthyroidism often followed by a reactive hypothyroidism. However, if doses are altered gradually, 'Normal human thyroids can adapt to excess intake of iodine by autoregulation'.[34]
- In cases of preexisting thyroid damage from thyroiditis or treatment with recombinant interferon-alpha, the thyroid may be unable to adapt to high iodine doses. In these conditions, high doses of iodine can induce hypothyroidism, which fades in two to three weeks after iodine is stopped.[35]

- Some organic compounds containing iodine, such as the drug amiodarone, have been known to poison the thyroid and induce either hypothyroidism or hyperthyroidism.[36] This danger is generally absent from natural food sources of iodine, such as seaweed, and from inorganic iodine supplements.
- Finally, because iodine strengthens the killing ability of white blood cells, people with autoimmune disease may worsen their condition by supplementing with high doses of iodine. Ironically, the organ that is most frequently the subject of autoimmune attack is the thyroid. High doses of iodine should be avoided until several months after wheat has been eliminated from the diet, to reduce the risk from autoimmunity.

However, we agree with the assessment in *The New England Journal of Medicine* by Dr Robert Utiger — 'the small risks of chronic iodine excess are outweighed by the substantial hazards of iodine deficiency'.[37]

Optimal Iodine Levels

As iodine is non-toxic and iodine insufficiency is extremely dangerous — birth defects, cretinism, cancer, hyperthyroidism, hypothyroidism, infectious disease, and bromine poisoning are some of the risks — we strongly recommend consumption of iodine.

A reasonable dose for most people is 1 milligram of iodine per day via potassium iodide tablets. Seaweed is an alternative source, but seaweeds which concentrate iodine also concentrate many toxins: naturally produced bromine compounds,[38] arsenic and mercury,[39] and even radioactive iodine.[40] Iodine is one nutrient in which inorganic supplements are best.

In some health conditions, including cancer and infectious diseases, high doses of iodine — up to 50 milligrams per day — may be therapeutic. To reduce the risk of negative effects, high iodine intake should be accompanied by (a) selenium intake comfortably above 200 micrograms per day, preferably through consumption of kidneys, shellfish, fish, and eggs; (b) high intake of water and salt, to promote excretion of bromine and excess selenium; (c) vitamin C and magnesium supplementation.

High-dose iodine supplementation should not begin until wheat has been eliminated from the diet and should be initiated gradually. A good strategy is to start at 225 micrograms per day or less and double the dose once per month: to 450 micrograms after one month, 900 micrograms after two months, 1.5 milligrams after three months, 3 milligrams after four months, and so on until the desired intake is reached.

SCIENCE OF THE PHD
Hypothyroidism

Hypothyroidism is a widespread and underdiagnosed problem.

Most doctors diagnose hypothyroidism by measuring levels of thyroid stimulating hormone, or TSH. If the body has too little thyroid hormone, the pituitary gland releases TSH in order to stimulate the thyroid to make more hormone.

However, the 'normal' levels reported on lab tests are far too wide. Most labs place the upper end of the normal TSH range around 4 mIU per litre, but health worsens dramatically as TSH increases within the 'normal' range:

- The HUNT study enrolled more than 25,000 healthy Norwegians with normal TSH levels for 8.3 years. People with a TSH level in the range 1.5–2.4 mIU per litre were 41 per cent more likely to die than people in the range 0.5 to 1.4 mIU per litre, and people in the range 2.5 to 3.4 mIU per litre were 69 per cent more likely to die.[41]
- An Italian study of 4123 pregnant women found that those who had a TSH level between 2.5 and 5.0 mIU per litre had a miscarriage rate of 6.1 per cent, while those with a TSH level below 2.5 mIU per litre had a miscarriage rate of only 3.6 per cent.[42]
- A Dutch study found that the likelihood of breech birth requiring a cesarean section was lowest with a TSH level below 0.7 mIU per litre, five times higher with a TSH level between 0.71 and 2.49 mIU per litre, 11 times higher with a TSH level between 2.5 and 2.89 mIU per litre, and 14 times higher with a TSH level above 2.9 mIU per litre.[43]

(continued on next page)

So halving the TSH level from 2.0 to 1.0 mIU per litre may reduce the risk of death by a third, and a TSH of 1.0 mIU per litre may still indicate inadequate thyroid function!

Now consider that one-fifth of Americans have a TSH level above 3.0 mIU per litre.

If you have clinical symptoms of hypothyroidism, such as lethargy or fatigue, low body temperature, cold intolerance, weight gain, coarse dry hair or hair loss, muscle cramps and aches, constipation, depression, irritability, memory loss, or abnormal menstrual cycles, it's essential to address your thyroid status. Don't let a 'normal' TSH level deter you.

And even if you lack hypothyroid symptoms, try to get your TSH level around 1.0 mIU per litre.

To fix hypothyroidism, we believe it's best to begin with a natural approach. First, eliminate grains, legumes, and vegetable oils. Then optimise intake of selenium, iodine, copper, iron, vitamin D, vitamin C, and magnesium. Vitamin A deficiency, if it exists, should also be corrected.

Iodine supplementation should start at 225 micrograms per day or less and then increase gradually, following a cycle of waiting a month or until side effects subside and then doubling the dose. It's desirable to bring the TSH level close to one.

If these steps are insufficient, your doctor can prescribe thyroid hormones. Options are levothyroxine, a synthetic T4 hormone; liothyronine, a synthetic T3 hormone; and natural thyroid extracts containing a mix of T3 and T4. Most doctors prefer to start with the synthetic T4 only, but most hypothyroid patients obtain better results from a mix of T4 and T3 than from T4 alone.[44]

Takeaway

Our prescription for selenium and iodine is:

* **Selenium** is best obtained from foods only, primarily animal foods. All meats have selenium, but the best sources are fish,

shellfish, eggs, and kidneys. Those who eat little of these foods may benefit from occasional, but not daily, supplementation. To avert any risk of selenium toxicity, drink plenty of water and exercise to produce sweat.

- **Iodine** should be supplemented via potassium iodide tablets or liquid iodine solutions. Start low at 225 micrograms per day; work up to 1 milligram per day. In disease conditions, it may be beneficial to increase iodine even further. To avoid potential negative effects, accompany high-dose iodine with extra intake of salt, water, vitamin C, magnesium, and selenium.

31
Potassium and Sodium

. . . .

- *Eat natural plant foods for potassium: potatoes and other tubers, tomatoes, green leafy vegetables, chocolate, avocado, beets, carrots, and bananas.*
- *Eat salt to taste.*
- *Optimising potassium and sodium intake reduces mortality rates by one-third.*

. . . .

These minerals are the primary electrolytes of the human body — meaning they dissolve in water and can carry an electrical charge.

Potassium is the intracellular, sodium the extracellular electrolyte. Cells constantly pump sodium outside the cell and potassium inside. So important is cellular potassium-sodium balance that fully 40 per cent of the energy usage in the brain is devoted to sodium-potassium pumping![1]

Good health depends upon a proper dietary balance between potassium and sodium.

Benefits of a High Potassium-to-Sodium Ratio

Paleolithic diets were high in potassium, low in sodium; salt was rare and highly valued. So we evolved mechanisms for protecting against the threat of low sodium levels: a food reward system that powerfully rewards salt con-

Notes for this chapter may be found at www.perfecthealthdiet.com/notes/#Ch31.

sumption and a hormonal network, the renin-angiotensin system, that shuts down urination and sweating whenever sodium is scarce. There are no similar mechanisms to protect us against low potassium levels, even though they are every bit as devastating to our health.

Much like the carbohydrate reward system that evolved to promote foraging for carbs in the Paleolithic but now overrewards consumption of sugar, it seems that in the modern world we are now overrewarded for salt consumption and underrewarded for potassium consumption. (Perhaps, since potassium is found in plant foods, reward for carbs was in the Paleolithic also a reward for potassium; but today we can easily obtain potassium-free sugar, so evolution's strategy no longer works.)

Whatever the reason, it's clear that Americans, Australians, and New Zealanders get too little potassium and too much sodium:

- The National Health and Nutrition Examination Survey found that Americans with high dietary sodium-to-potassium ratios have 50 per cent higher death rates; mortality rates decrease as potassium intake increases.[2]
- The higher the sodium-to-potassium ratio in urine, the more cardiovascular disease.[3]

It's more important to increase potassium than to decrease sodium. Increasing potassium is the key to control of blood pressure, kidney stones, and osteoporosis.[4] Higher potassium intake improves bone health[5] and reduces blood pressure.[6] Tomatoes are rich in potassium; that may be why eating 225 grams of tomatoes a day can significantly reduce blood pressure.[7]

Potassium is also important for athletes, as it protects lean muscle mass. In order to gain muscle mass, it is necessary to supply the body with adequate potassium; if potassium becomes deficient, muscle mass will be sacrificed to release potassium to other cells. For example, in a metabolic ward study, a diet of turkey only was compared to a diet of turkey plus grape juice; the turkey-only subjects lost lean tissue, but the subjects allowed grape juice maintained lean tissue.[8] The explanation turned out to be that the turkey-only subjects were potassium deprived, while the subjects allowed grape juice had adequate potassium.[9]

Optimal Potassium and Sodium Intake

The U.S. Food and Nutrition Board estimated in 2004 that 4.7 grams per day of potassium is sufficient to achieve all known benefits.[10] This still seems the best available estimate.

In addition to tomato, potassium-rich foods include avocado, potato, sweet potato, banana, green leafy vegetables, and seaweeds such as dulse. Here are the amounts of potassium (milligrams per 450 grams) in some of the foods in four plant food categories — safe starches, healthful sugary plants, fatty plants, and low-calorie vegetables.

Safe Starches		Healthful Sugary Plants	
Potato	2429	Beets	1385
Sweet potato	2156	Carrots	1453
Taro	2197	Bananas	1625
White rice	132	Blueberries	350
Fatty Plants		Vegetables	
Avocado	2202	Spinach	2533
Macadamia nuts	1671	Sun-dried tomatoes	15,558
Coconut milk	1194	Seaweed, laver	1616
Chocolate (70–85% cocoa)	3246	Asparagus	1017

Since our diet calls for eating 450 grams of safe starches, 450 grams of sugary plants, and 450 grams of other plant foods per day, meeting the potassium target of 4700 milligrams per day requires averaging 1600 milligrams potassium per 450 grams of plant foods.

The target is easily achieved as long as high-potassium plant foods are favoured. Most of the time, eat **potato, sweet potato,** and **taro** rather than white rice as safe starches; **beets, carrots,** and **bananas** as sugary plants; **chocolate, avocado,** and **nuts** for snack foods; **coconut milk** as a cooking oil; and **sun-dried tomatoes, green leafy vegetables,** and **seaweed** as vegetables.

While optimising potassium requires some conscious effort, optimising sodium does not. Our evolved food reward system, and its attention to salt, comes to our aid here: we can let it guide us to our proper salt intake.

All foods contain some sodium; and a bit of salt will supply the rest of our needs. A half teaspoon to 1 teaspoon of salt a day is usually sufficient. But rather than eat a prescribed amount, simply eat salt to taste. Try a bit of salt on your tongue: if it tastes good, eat more. If it doesn't, you don't need it.

32
Calcium, Collagen, and Magnesium

· ·

- *Don't supplement calcium — rather, make bone broths and have up to a bowl per day.*
- *Do supplement magnesium — 200 milligrams per day.*
- *Magnesium supplementation may reduce mortality rates by 24 per cent.*

· ·

Calcium and magnesium are two more electrolytes that, because they dissolve in water, are at risk for deficiency in modern diets. Water treatment has removed them from drinking water, and calcium and magnesium in food may easily be lost if cooking liquids are discarded.

Calcium

Calcium has become an extremely popular dietary supplement, especially among older women, in the hope that it might prevent osteoporosis. Huge doses, sometimes as high as 1200 milligrams per day, have been recommended.

Unfortunately, it looks as though high-dose calcium supplementation was a mistake.

Notes for this chapter may be found at www.perfecthealthdiet.com/notes/#Ch32.

Supplementation Is Dangerous

Calcium supplements don't do much to improve bone health. They don't clearly reduce fracture rates in older women and might actually increase the rate of hip fractures.[1] In people with normal vitamin D levels (25OHD above 30 nanograms per millilitre), there is no benefit to calcium supplementation. A normal dietary intake of calcium, around 600 milligrams per day, maximises bone health.[2]

SCIENCE OF THE PHD
The Right Way to Improve Bone Health

Calcium supplementation was a mistake. The true culprits in osteoporosis are deficiencies of vitamin D, vitamin K2, and magnesium.

- Bone mineral density is maximised with serum 25OHD around 40 nanograms per millilitre.[3] Most Americans are around 20 nanograms per millilitre.
- Vitamin K2 supplementation brings about a fourfold decrease in hip fractures and a fivefold decrease in vertebral fractures.[4]
- Magnesium supplementation does much more to improve bone mineral density than calcium.[5]

It gets worse.

Studies have consistently found that supplemental calcium increases the incidence of strokes and heart attacks by over 30 per cent[6] and increases the overall risk of death by 9 per cent.[7] One analysis concluded, 'Treating 1000 people with calcium or calcium and vitamin D for five years would cause an additional six myocardial infarctions or strokes and prevent three fractures.'[8]

Heart attacks and premature death aren't the only risks from calcium supplementation.

- Calcium intake is associated with brain lesions in the elderly.[9]
- In the Nurses' Health Study, supplementation of calcium increased the risk of calcium oxalate kidney stones by 20 per cent.[10]
- Calcium promotes the formation of biofilms and can aggravate infections.[11]
- Those who supplement with vitamin D may develop dangerous hypercalcemia when supplementing calcium at 1200 milligrams per day.[12]

Optimal Calcium Levels

It's fairly clear now what the optimum calcium intake is:

- Calcium balance occurs at an intake of 741 milligrams per day.[13] Above this intake, the body has an excess and tries to excrete more calcium than is consumed.
- This intake also happens to be the one that minimises bone fractures. The lowest fracture rates occur with calcium intakes between 700 and 900 milligrams per day.[14]

This amount can readily be obtained from food. Green leafy vegetables and dairy products are good sources of calcium, but the best way to obtain calcium, we believe, is from bone broth soups.

Simply buy some bones from grass-fed cattle. Simmer them for three hours to create a first soup, which will include fat, marrow, and meat — don't overcook it. Then make a second soup, simmered three to eight hours and including some vinegar in the water, to help leach minerals from the bone. This second soup will have high levels of calcium and phosphorus, the primary minerals in bone. Both soups are highly nutritious and rich in nutrients missing from other foods.

Bone broth soups also taste great. From the broth, make a different soup every night by adding vegetables.

People who don't eat bone broth soups, dairy products, or green leafy vegetables may benefit from drinking mineral water or supplementing calcium. If supplementing, the dose should be low: at most 300 milligrams per day.

SCIENCE OF THE PHD
The Right Amount of Bone Broth

There are known cases of calcium overdose from consuming too much bone broth. A young cricket player in India drank 1 to 2 litres of bone broth most days of the week and after six months developed hypercalcemia.[15]

Bone broth may contain about 1,500 milligrams of calcium per litre. A typical soup bowl holds 0.3 litre. So one bowl of bone broth soup per day will provide about 450 milligrams of calcium.

An implementation of the Perfect Health Diet that doesn't have a lot of green leafy vegetables and dairy products may contain about 300 milligrams of calcium from food. So one bowl of bone broth soup per day will generally bring calcium intake close to perfection. But one bowl is sufficient.

As always, let taste be your guide. If bone broth is tasty, you will probably benefit from the calcium. But if you feel that you've had enough of it, stop eating it for a while.

Collagen and Other Matrix Materials

More than 30 per cent of all protein in the body is in the extracellular matrix: a scaffold of proteins bonded with sugars that forms a frame upon which cells attach to form organic structures.

Some of the compounds of the extracellular matrix are well known. Collagen is the most abundant protein in the body, comprising 30 per cent of all protein in the body. Glucosamine and chondroitin sulfate have become popular as supplements. Hyaluronic acid is the most abundant polysaccharide (sugar chain) in the extracellular matrix.

Matrix is crucial to health, yet most Australians and New Zealanders rarely eat it. We eat muscle meats, which don't contain a lot of matrix material.

Yet there is evidence that eating extracellular matrix components improves the body's ability to keep its matrix in good health.

Here are a few studies in which collagen supplementation improved health:

- **Bone mineral density.** Adding gelatin (cooked collagen) to the diet of lab rats increases their bone mineral density.[16]
- **Osteoarthritis.** Supplementation of collagen improved joint function scores of osteoarthritis patients by 33 per cent, compared to a 14 per cent improvement with glucosamine and chondroitin supplements.[17]
- **Rheumatoid arthritis.** In a clinical trial of chicken collagen in rheumatoid arthritis patients, 69 per cent of those taking chicken collagen had at least a 20 per cent improvement in swollen joint counts, pain, and function, while 41 per cent had a 50 per cent improvement.[18]
- **Back pain.** Supplementation with 1.2 grams per day of collagen reduced lumbar spine pain compared to a control group.[19]
- **Skin damage.** Collagen supplements reduced skin damage from summer sun exposure.[20]

So should we supplement collagen? No!

First, we could have compiled a similar list of studies for other extracellular matrix components, such as glucosamine and chondroitin, or hyaluron. It would be better to get a complete set of matrix compounds, not only collagen.

Second, supplements are extremely expensive. But you can get large quantities almost for free from your local supermarket! Butchers are constantly discarding fresh collagen and matrix matter, in the form of bones and joints.

Buying bones and joints and cooking them yourself will give the complete range of organic matrix compounds, at very low cost. The only catch is that you have to cook them yourself.

This is easily done: we want you to make bone broth for calcium and phosphorus. Just buy bones with some joint material attached, and you'll get matrix material for free.

Ox hooves, oxtails, and chicken feet are especially rich in collagen and other matrix materials. Don't be shy about mixing them in with your bones when making broth.

Magnesium

Magnesium is a mineral essential for good health. More than 300 enzymes need it, including those needed to make the energy molecule ATP and to synthesise DNA, RNA, and proteins. Magnesium also plays a structural role in bone and in cell membranes, where it helps transport ions across the membrane.

Deficiency Is Widespread and Dangerous

NHANES surveys have shown that most Americans are deficient in magnesium. Median magnesium intake is 326 milligrams per day in white men, 237 milligrams per day in black men, 237 milligrams per day in white women, and 173 milligrams per day in black women — in all cases far below the RDA, which is 420 milligrams per day for men and 320 to 400 milligrams per day for women.[21] Paleolithic intake, by contrast, has been estimated at 700 milligrams daily.[22]

The RDA is based in part on balance studies. Under controlled dietary conditions in healthy men, intestinal absorption of magnesium begins to decrease at an intake of about 380 milligrams and is reduced by about 60 per cent at twice that intake.[23]

Magnesium deficiency can be fatal. Symptoms of acute magnesium deficiency include muscle cramps, heart arrhythmias, tremor, headaches, and acid reflux.

Chronic magnesium deficiency causes or is associated with a host of diseases: cardiovascular disease, high blood pressure, metabolic syndrome and diabetes, migraines, osteoporosis, hypothyroidism, dysmenorrhea and PMS, and asthma.[24] Actual heart attacks have been observed during magnesium-deprivation experiments.[25]

Magnesium deficiency causes mitochondrial decay and accelerated ageing.[26] Magnesium is needed for proper immune function, since it is necessary to synthesise glutathione.[27]

Vitamin D function also depends on magnesium,[28] to such an extent that magnesium deficiency can induce rickets in people replete with vitamin D.[29]

Magnesium deficiency is damaging to developing babies. In one clinical trial, magnesium supplementation by pregnant mothers reduced the risk of cerebral palsy by 30 per cent.[30]

Magnesium reduces mortality rates.

- Areas with higher water hardness (and thus higher magnesium content) have lower cardiovascular death rates.[31]
- Clinical trials have shown significant mortality reduction from giving magnesium to cardiac patients. In a study of heart attack patients, magnesium therapy given before thrombolytic therapy decreased mortality rates by 24 per cent.[32] In a Russian trial, the group given magnesium supplements was only half as likely to die during the period of the trial.[33]

READER REPORTS: magnesium for constipation

You helped my mom who has suffered with chronic constipation for 60 plus years. She had taken Senna for decades. I read your post about using Magnesium Citrate instead. It works like a charm and she is no longer taking toxic Senna. Thank you!

— Helena

Little Risk of Toxicity

Magnesium has a broad peak health range. There is no evidence that anyone has ever reached toxic levels of magnesium from food consumption.

The initial symptom of magnesium toxicity from high-dose supplementation is diarrhoea. In people with healthy kidneys, this is likely to be the only effect, which is why magnesium is generally safe as a laxative. An adult laxative dose of 2 grams of magnesium (the amount in 17 grams of magnesium citrate) typically produces loose stools.

Very high doses of magnesium — well above 2 grams — may lead to a fall in blood pressure, which in turn induces lethargy, confusion, disturbed heart rhythm, and poor kidney function. Extremely high doses can lead to cardiac arrest.

Optimal Magnesium Levels

There are tremendous health benefits from eliminating magnesium deficiency. Magnesium intake of 400 milligrams per day or more is needed to achieve this. Total (dietary plus supplemental) intake of 800 milligrams per day is unlikely to produce any toxicity if kidney function is normal. We consider 400 to 800 milligrams per day the peak health range for magnesium.

About half of Americans obtain less than 250 milligrams per day of magnesium from food, and few obtain as much as 500 milligrams per day. Magnesium deficiency is also common in Australia. This suggests that many Americans and Australians should increase their magnesium intake by about 200 milligrams per day to reach the peak health range.

Seaweed, nuts and nut butters, coffee, tea, and chocolate are good sources of magnesium. Perhaps that accounts for their health benefits; for instance, eating lots of chocolate reduces rates of cardiovascular disease by 37 per cent and stroke by 29 per cent.[34]

However, the easiest way to ensure good magnesium status is to supplement. We recommend routine supplementation of 200 milligrams per day.

33
Zinc and Copper

- *Get more copper by eating 115 grams of beef or lamb liver per week. If you don't eat liver, supplement with 2 milligrams of copper per day.*
- *Supplement zinc, but lightly: 50 milligrams per week, not per day, is optimal.*
- *Benefits: copper and zinc optimisation may significantly reduce deaths from cardiovascular disease.*

Zinc and copper are two more nutrients that need to be in balance. One reason is that an extremely important antioxidant — zinc-copper superoxide dismutase — contains both.

The importance of balance between zinc and copper was demonstrated by the Italian ilSIRENTE study, which found that the ratio of copper to zinc in the blood was a better predictor of mortality than the levels of either zinc or copper individually.[1]

Copper

Copper deficiency was first observed in animals. The effects are severe:

- Copper-deficient cattle died suddenly due to heart atrophy and scarring.[2]

Notes for this chapter may be found at www.perfecthealthdiet.com/notes/#Ch33.

- Pigs deprived of copper died of weakened and ruptured arteries and heart attacks.[3]
- Mice deprived of copper similarly died of blood clots, heart muscle degeneration, and coronary calcification.[4]
- In rats, copper deficiency shortens life span and can lead to sudden death by rupture of the heart. Disturbingly in light of the American, Australian, and New Zealand diets, fructose increases their need for copper. Rats eating sugar experienced far more sudden death in response to copper restriction than rats eating starch.[5]

In humans, a variety of negative effects from copper deficiency have been observed, including anemia,[6] hypothyroidism,[7] and greying of hair,[8] but the big concern is heart disease.

In a human copper restriction trial, a modest reduction of copper intake from 1.38 milligrams per day to 1 milligram per day produced heart trouble in four of 23 subjects, including one heart attack. The authors commented:

> In the history of conducting numerous human studies at the Beltsville Human Nutrition Research Center involving participation by 337 subjects, there had previously been no instances of any health problem related to heart function. During the 11 weeks of the present study in which the copper density of the diets fed the subjects was reduced . . . 4 out of 23 subjects were diagnosed as having heart-related abnormalities.[9]

This is a disturbing result, since the U.S. recommended daily allowance is only 0.9 milligram per day. The U.S. RDA is much too low. Fortunately, in Australia and New Zealand the recommended daily intake is higher (1.7 milligram for men and 1.2 milligram for women), but this may still be less than optimal.

It may be improper to speak of a fixed RDA for copper without reference to zinc intake. Balance studies have shown that copper needs to increase as zinc intake increases. At 10 milligrams per day of zinc, 1.1 milligrams per day of copper are sufficient to achieve balance, but at 15 milligrams of zinc,

1.35 milligrams of copper are needed, and at 20 milligrams of zinc, 1.6 milligrams of copper are required.[10]

Plausibly the reason Americans avoid heart attacks on their low copper intake is because they simultaneously maintain a low intake of zinc. The Beltsville trial that was so deadly provided 21.5 milligrams per day of zinc, almost double the zinc intake of most Americans and Australians.

Deficiency Is Widespread

According to a 2001 study, the median American copper intake is only 0.759 milligram per day, well below the RDA. A quarter of Americans get less than 0.57 milligram per day, and only a quarter get 1 milligram per day.[11] Considering that copper intake of 1 milligram per day in the Beltsville study led to heart attacks, this is an alarming deficiency rate! Deficiency has also been identified in Australian populations.

Widespread deficiency is no great surprise, since Americans rarely eat copper-rich foods such as liver, shellfish, and nuts, and lack of copper in most fertilisers has led to soil exhaustion. A British study estimated that since 1940 the copper content of dairy products has declined by 90 per cent, vegetables by 76 per cent, and meats by 55 per cent.[12]

Toxicity

Copper poisoning sometimes occurs, especially after consumption of beverages stored in copper containers. Symptoms are belly pain, nausea, vomiting, and diarrhoea, all part of the body's efforts to eliminate the excess copper. Once in the body, excess copper damages the liver and kidneys.

The U.S. Food and Nutrition Board set the tolerable upper limit for copper consumption at 10 milligrams per day.[13] Although many studies have reported no negative effects from copper in the range 6 to 10 milligrams per day, one study did observe mild negative effects from five months of copper at 7.8 milligrams per day.[14]

Although organic copper from foods is safe, inorganic copper from supplements or copper pipes, plumbing fixtures, and cookware may be much more toxic. These sources of copper are associated with cognitive impairment and neurodegenerative disorders in the elderly.[15]

Optimal Copper Intake

We estimate the plateau range of copper at 2 to 4 milligrams per day. The U.S. RDA of 0.9 milligram per day, and the Australian RDI of 1.7 milligrams for men and 1.2 milligrams for women, are both too low, as significant improvements in health have been observed with an increase in copper from 1 to 1.4 milligrams per day. Unfortunately, only about 5 per cent of Americans obtain 2 milligrams per day of copper.

The most abundant dietary sources of copper are beef and lamb liver, oysters, shiitake mushrooms, cocoa or dark chocolate, cashew nuts, squid, and lobster.

Due to evidence for toxicity from inorganic copper in supplements and the large number of beneficial nutrients (such as choline and trace minerals) in liver, we recommend obtaining copper by eating **115 grams of beef liver or lamb liver per week** as a supplemental food.

One hundred and fifteen grams of beef or lamb liver provides 12 to 16 milligrams of copper, or 2 milligrams per day — sufficient by itself to get copper into the peak health range. (Other animal livers are not nearly as copper-rich. One hundred and fifteen grams of pork liver provides only 0.8 milligram of copper and 115 grams of chicken liver only 0.4 milligram of copper.) Be careful to eat no more than about 115 grams; if you want more liver, switch to chicken liver to avert any risk of consuming excess copper.

Zinc

Zinc is an essential mineral whose deficiency can be fatal. Before zinc supplements were available, babies with acrodermatitis enteropathica, a genetic disorder that impairs zinc absorption, died in infancy.

Symptoms of severe zinc deficiency include dwarfism, delayed sexual maturation, skin rashes, hair loss, diarrhoea, immune impairment, impaired wound healing, night blindness, depression, cognitive decline, and behavioural disturbances. Mild zinc deficiencies impair immune function.[16]

Zinc shares a critical function with copper: forming the essential antioxidant, superoxide dismutase. Copper and zinc supplementation prevent atherosclerosis in one of the classic animal models of atherosclerosis, the cholesterol-poisoned rabbit.[17]

Deficiency Is Common

The U.S. RDA is 8 milligrams of zinc per day for women and 11 milligrams per day for men; median intake is about 9 milligrams per day for women, 14 milligrams per day for men. The recommended daily intake in Australia and New Zealand is similar: 8 milligrams for women and 14 milligrams for men.

Deficiency is common, even based on the RDA. About one-third of Americans get less than the RDA. In the elderly, who tend to eat less meat, zinc status is far worse. Elderly Italians get less than half the RDA.[18] About 20 per cent of pregnant mothers are thought to be zinc-deficient, and this may have long-lasting effects upon their babies.[19]

However, we believe the RDA is too low and intake should be equal to or greater than 15 milligrams per day. By that standard, most Americans, Australians, and New Zealanders are mildly zinc-deficient.

Support for the idea that the peak health range for zinc begins around 15 milligrams per day comes from clinical trials showing benefits from zinc supplementation. Benefits include improved immune function and improved physical and neuropsychological development of children.[20] Observational studies support a similar conclusion. Zinc intake below 14 milligrams per day is associated with increased mortality from prostate cancer.[21]

READER REPORTS: antioxidants for constipation

I've been following the PHD and taking the recommended supplements and many of the therapeutic supplements for several months. Last week, I just started supplementing with Zinc and NAC. This week — no more constipation for the first time in many, many years — amazing!

— Anonymous

Toxicity

The tolerable upper intake level (UL) for zinc is 40 milligrams per day. The reason is that high levels of zinc can induce copper deficiency by impairing copper absorption in the intestine. High intake of zinc therefore *reduces* levels of zinc-copper superoxide dismutase.[22]

Intakes of zinc high enough to create a copper deficiency more than double prostate cancer risk.[23]

Zinc is neurotoxic in high doses, and neurodegenerative disorders may be the most likely ill effect of chronic high zinc intake. It's been suggested that Alzheimer's may result from zinc excess and copper deficiency,[24] while high intake of zinc and copper together may promote ALS (Lou Gehrig's disease), a disease involving aggregations of zinc-copper SOD.[25]

Excessive intake of zinc might also benefit pathogens. Zinc is a key nutrient for pathogens, and during infection our immune cells attempt to deprive pathogens of zinc by releasing calprotectin, a zinc chelator. Zinc seems to be the most potent of all minerals in promoting fungal growth.[26]

Optimal Zinc Intake

It appears that it's beneficial to consume more than 15 milligrams per day of zinc as long as copper intake is sufficient to maintain the zinc-copper balance. But high doses of zinc, such as 40 milligrams per day, are positively dangerous.

Based on the copper-balance studies,[27] our recommended copper intake — around 2 to 4 milligrams per day — is optimally accompanied by a zinc intake of 15 to 30 milligrams per day.

Zinc intake from food on the Perfect Health Diet will typically be around 10 to 15 milligrams per day. Therefore, except for athletes eating larger quantities of food or those making a specific effort to eat zinc-rich foods such as oysters, we suggest supplementation of zinc, but not in large amounts — at most 10 milligrams per day.

A simple way to achieve this is to supplement with 50 milligrams of zinc once per week.

34
Vitamin C

- -

- *Supplement about 1 gram of vitamin C per day.*
- *It has many benefits and few or no risks.*

- -

Vitamin C is needed for the manufacture of body components.

- **Collagen,** the scaffolding on which all organs, bones, and tissues are built.
- **Carnitine,** which transports fats into mitochondria for energy production.
- **Norepinephrine** and **epinephrine** (adrenaline), hormones and neurotransmitters that control alertness, arousal, and motivation.
- **Enzymes** involved in the creation of peptide hormones, tyrosine metabolism, and bile acid.

Vitamin C is also needed to maintain levels of glutathione, the immune system's primary antioxidant.

Symptoms of vitamin C deficiency may include a tendency toward cavities or fractures, hair or tooth loss, bruising, bleeding gums, muscle loss or difficulty gaining muscle, slow wound healing, and joint pain and swelling. Severe vitamin C deficiency results in death unless remedied.

Notes for this chapter may be found at www.perfecthealthdiet.com/notes/#Ch34.
Notes specific to this Australian edition are indicated with †

Deficiency Is Widespread and Can Be Devastating

Analysis of the National Health and Nutrition Examination Survey (NHANES) found that 18 per cent of U.S. adults, 14 per cent of teenage males, and 20 per cent of teenage females get **less than 30 milligrams per day** of vitamin C — far below the RDA of 90 milligrams for adult males, 75 milligrams for adult females and teenage males, and 65 milligrams for teenage females.

Blood tests found that 34 per cent of men and 27 per cent of women were deficient in or depleted of vitamin C, as indicated by blood levels below 28 micromoles per litre. Australian sources note that plasma vitamin C concentrations are reduced by 40 per cent in male smokers.[†] The elderly, the sick, alcoholics, smokers, the obese, and other persons under stress are most depleted of vitamin C and probably have an increased need for it.[1]

Vitamin C deficiency is devastating — and potentially fatal.

- Without carnitine, the body becomes fatigued and weak, and mitochondrial impairment accelerates ageing.
- Without collagen, all tissues waste away — including the heart, blood vessels, muscle, gut, and bone — and wounds cannot be repaired.
- Without glutathione recycling, oxidative stress increases and immune defences are weakened, leading to infections and inflammation.

If vitamin C deficiency is combined with other nutrient deficiencies, effects are even more severe. For instance, combined selenium and vitamin C deficiency results in severe muscle cell death.[2]

Optimal vitamin C intake is probably far above the RDA. Healthy young people need to supplement with at least 400 milligrams per day before blood cells — and presumably other cells — cease to take up vitamin C.[3]

In sickness, much higher doses of vitamin C may be beneficial. Vitamin C is helpful against many viral infections. We have blogged about the New Zealand man whose doctors considered his case hopeless and wanted to terminate life support; he was cured by 100 grams per day of vitamin C.[4] Dr Robert Cathcart treated more than 12,000 patients with high-dose vitamin C and found it was effective against many infections.[5]

Clinical trials, too, have found benefits from extra vitamin C. High-dose vitamin C supplementation can significantly reduce mortality, especially cardiovascular mortality:

- The First National Health and Nutrition Examination Survey (NHANES I) Epidemiologic Follow-up Study in the U.S. found that among those supplementing with vitamin C to achieve a total intake of 300 milligrams per day or more, the risk of death from all causes was decreased 35 per cent in men and 10 per cent in women. The cardiovascular disease mortality rate was 42 per cent lower in men and 25 per cent lower in women and the cancer mortality rate 22 per cent lower in men and 14 per cent lower in women. Men who took 800 milligrams per day of vitamin C lived six years longer than those consuming only the recommended daily allowance.[6]
- The Nurses' Health Study (NHS) in the U.S., which followed the health of 85,000 women over 16 years, found that vitamin C supplementation was associated with a 28 per cent lower risk of heart disease.[7]
- A pooled analysis of nine prospective cohort studies, which followed 290,000 adults for an average of ten years, found that those who took more than 700 milligrams per day of supplemental vitamin C had a 25 per cent lower risk of coronary heart disease than those who did not take vitamin C supplements.[8]

No Toxicity

It has been remarkably difficult to find negative effects from high doses of vitamin C. Intravenous doses of 120 grams per day are well tolerated and safe.[9]

Oral doses in excess of 4 grams per day may produce bowel queasiness and, ultimately, diarrhoea. This is the basis for the Upper Limit (UL) of 2 grams per day.[10] However, the limit of bowel tolerance is quite variable; sick people may not reach bowel tolerance until oral doses of 100 grams per day. It is likely that bowel intolerance begins when the body ceases to take up and utilise vitamin C. Thus, the point of bowel tolerance may indicate the dose at which vitamin C ceases to have benefits, rather than a toxicity level.

A Caution for Cancer Patients

Vitamin C protects all human cells against injury — including cancer cells.[11] As vitamin C reduces the effectiveness of chemotherapy, cancer patients should obtain vitamin C intermittently, avoiding it while on chemotherapy.

Takeaway

It is perilously easy to become vitamin C–deficient on modern, hurried diets. The consequences of chronic vitamin C deficiency are devastating but insidious, since the negative effects accumulate gradually and a deficiency may persist for years before it is diagnosed.

Vitamin C supplementation in the range of 500 milligrams to 1 gram per day does no harm and appears to offer substantial benefits, including a significant reduction of mortality rates. Therefore, we recommend that healthy people supplement vitamin C in this range.

Those who are sick or under stress should supplement with higher doses, possibly — as Dr Robert Cathcart recommended — to the limit of bowel tolerance, indicated by a sensation of queasiness.

35
Choline and Folic Acid

- *Choline optimisation prevents birth defects, liver disease, obesity, cardiovascular disease, and cancer; yet nearly everyone is deficient.*
- *Folic acid supplementation, though possibly beneficial for women seeking to conceive, is a poor way to relieve a choline deficiency. Most people should obtain folate from food only.*
- *Get choline by eating three egg yolks a day and liver once a week; get folate from liver, giblets, egg yolks, seaweed, green leafy vegetables, and mushrooms.*

Choline is an extremely important nutrient that is needed to make the neurotransmitter acetylcholine and to make phospholipids (cell membrane fats) such as phosphatidylcholine. It is also a methyl donor, able to contribute methyl groups for methylation reactions such as the methylation of DNA for gene regulation.

Folic acid is a synthetic vitamin that in the body becomes various forms of 'folate', including tetrahydrofolate, which is able to take on a methyl group to become methyltetrahydrofolate. Methyltetrahydrofolate is extremely important: it can donate its methyl group to support many biological processes, including recycling of homocysteine along a path that leads to choline synthesis; it also supports synthesis of the neurotransmitters dopamine, serotonin, and norepinephrine.

These two nutrients, then, are important for brain and neurological function, lipid metabolism, DNA health, and many other aspects of health.

Notes for this chapter may be found at www.perfecthealthdiet.com/notes/#Ch35.

Choline is abundant in liver and egg yolks — foods that Australians eat less than ever before, thanks in part to the demonisation of cholesterol. Meanwhile, folic acid, which doesn't occur in nature, has reached extremely high dosages in the Australian diet:

- Multivitamins typically contain 400 micrograms, prenatal multis 800 micrograms.
- In the United States, flour and cereals have been enriched with folic acid since 1973; the level of enrichment was increased in 1998, and every pound of enriched flour is now required to contain 700 micrograms of folic acid. Australia introduced mandatory fortification of folic acid in wheat flour for bread-making in 2009.

Natural levels of food folate provide about 300 micrograms per day. In Americans taking a multivitamin, synthetic folic acid now accounts for 65 per cent of all dietary folate; in American women taking a prenatal multivitamin, 75 per cent. Women who eat a lot of commercial baked goods and cereals along with their prenatal multivitamin can easily obtain 1500 micrograms or more of synthetic folic acid per day — yet the tolerable upper limit of folic acid intake is 1000 micrograms per day.[1]

Folic acid provisioning is an extraordinary public health experiment. The experiment is not going well.

Folic Acid

In adults, folic acid supplements have been linked to increased risk of cancer and cardiovascular disease. For instance:

- **Cancer.** Natural folate from food seems to be protective against cancer, but 1 milligram per day of supplemental folic acid doubles the risk of prostate cancer.[2] Colon cancer rates doubled in Chile after wheat flour was fortified with folic acid.[3] In the Prostate, Lung, Colorectal, and Ovarian (PLCO) Cancer Screening Trial, taking 400 micrograms per day of folic acid raised breast cancer risk by 20 per cent.[4] When female rats are given folic acid, their pups are twice as likely to develop breast cancer and the tumours are faster growing.[5]

- **Cancer, mortality rate.** In a Norwegian trial, persons receiving 0.8 milligram per day of folic acid and a small amount of vitamin B12 were 21 per cent more likely to develop cancer and 38 per cent more likely to die.[6]
- **Heart attack, stroke, mortality rate.** A Canadian trial supplied diabetics with 2.5 milligrams per day of folic acid and small amounts of vitamins B6 and B12. The folic acid group experienced a 20 per cent higher death rate, a doubled risk of heart attack or amputation, and a sixfold higher rate of stroke, as well as greater kidney damage.[7]

Folic acid taken prenatally reduces the rate of neural tube defects, which can produce diseases such as spina bifida. However, there are hints that children of mothers who take prenatal vitamins are more likely to have **asthma** and **autism:**

- Supplementation with folic acid during pregnancy leads to higher rates of **wheezing** and **asthma** in children.[8] In mice, folic acid during pregnancy gives the pups asthma.[9]
- The correlation between use of prescription prenatal vitamins containing 1 milligram folic acid and **autism** is 87 per cent — very high.[10] (Against that, a recent study found that mothers of children with autism took slightly less folic acid than mothers of normal children.[11])

Mechanisms of toxicity from folic acid are not known. The body doesn't completely convert synthetic folic acid to natural folate, and one idea is that toxicity from low levels of circulating folic acid may be responsible for the ill effects.[12] However, the more likely explanation is that too much folate, period, is responsible for the ill effects. A likely avenue is through increased levels of gene silencing.

It seems likely that evolution optimised our biology for the levels of folate found naturally in foods — around 300 to 400 micrograms per day. Quite possibly, our genes do not cope well with the high levels of folate entering our bodies today through multivitamins and fortified foods.

SCIENCE OF THE PHD
Folic Acid and Gene Dysregulation

One of folate's most important functions is to support the 'silencing' of genes through methylation of DNA. More folate means, as a rule, greater silencing of genes.

Our genes appear to function best with the specific amount of folate contained in our evolutionary diets. Supplementing the diet with folic acid causes aberrant gene methylation, dysregulating over a thousand genes:

> We found significant dysregulation in gene expression at [folate] concentrations . . . lower than what has been achieved in the blood through folic acid fortification guidelines.[13]

> Early results from the Newborn Epigenetics Study (NEST) confirm that aberrant methylation does occur in babies of mothers who supplement folic acid.[14] Such dysregulation isn't likely to be good for us.

> Folic acid during pregnancy also produces epigenetic changes in mouse pups. For instance: folic acid given to the mum can change the pups' coat colour from yellow to black.[15]

If supplemental folic acid is bad, what about the neural tube defects that all this folic acid was meant to prevent? There's a better way than folic acid to prevent neural tube defects.

Choline

Choline was not officially recognised as an essential nutrient until 1998, 25 years after folic acid fortification began. Based on levels needed to prevent liver damage, the Food and Nutrition Board set the Adequate Intake level for choline at 425 milligrams per day for women and 550 milligrams per day for men.[16]

By these standards, nearly all Americans, and probably Australians and New Zealanders too, are choline-deficient. In the Nurses' Health Study, **less than 5 per cent** of nurses had an adequate intake of choline.[17] In the National Health and Nutrition Examination Survey, only 10 per cent of Americans had adequate intake.[18]

Yet the official adequate intake levels may be too low. High intakes of choline have tremendous health benefits:

- **Choline prevents metabolic syndrome, fatty liver, and obesity.** Choline deficiency by itself causes metabolic syndrome (insulin resistance, elevated serum triglyceride levels, and high serum cholesterol levels) and obesity. Add in a low-protein diet, and it causes fatty liver disease.[19] Choline supplementation rapidly cures fatty liver disease. In a mere 12 days, supplemental choline can reduce liver fat from 15 per cent to 4 per cent.[20]
- **Choline is anti-inflammatory.**[21] In the ATTICA study, people whose diets were rich in choline had the lowest levels of the inflammatory markers IL-6, TNF-alpha, and C-reactive protein.[22] In the Nurses' Health Study, those with the highest dietary choline intake had improved biomarkers for inflammation, including higher adiponectin levels and lower resistin and CRP levels.[23]
- **Choline prevents cancer.** Eating a choline-deficient diet for as little as a month leads to increased DNA damage.[24] Women with high choline intakes have a 24 per cent lower risk of breast cancer.[25]
- **Choline makes babies smarter.** Pregnant mothers need to take special care to get adequate choline. Maternal choline deficiency leads to lifelong memory and learning deficits in the child.[26]
- **Choline prevents folate deficiency.** Choline can perform many of the functions of folate, and relieves folate deficiency.[27]
- **Choline is better than folic acid for preventing neural tube defects.** Taking a multivitamin with folic acid cuts the risk of neural tube defects in half.[28] But in California mothers, the

incidence of neural tube defects in the bottom quartile of choline intakes was **17 times higher** than in the top quartile; among the median group the risk was **seven times higher.**[29]

That last statistic is worth pondering. Completely saturating the body with folate cuts the rate of neural tube defects in half. *Partially* relieving choline deficiency cuts the rate by a factor of 17. (Remember, most of the women in that top quartile were getting less than the U.S. Adequate Intake level of choline.) It seems likely that neural tube defects are a result of choline deficiency, and folic acid is a poor way to relieve choline deficiency.

Optimal Folate and Choline Levels

Except for women who are trying to conceive, we recommend obtaining folate **entirely from foods.** A wide array of foods have folate, but in general the highest levels are in the same foods that provide vitamin A: liver, giblets, egg yolks, seaweed, green leafy vegetables, and mushrooms.

Also, we recommend eliminating from the diet foods fortified with folic acid: commercial baked goods and cereal-grain products. For Perfect Health Dieters, this means rinsing enriched white rice before cooking to remove the enrichment coating that contains folic acid.

Women trying to conceive, and women in the first three months of pregnancy, should limit folic acid supplementation to at most 400 micrograms per day.

There are tremendous health benefits to high choline intake. Fortunately, it is easy to improve choline status by eating **egg yolks** and **liver.** We recommend that everyone eat three egg yolks per day and 115 grams of beef or lamb liver per week. These two steps alone will provide an average of 417 milligrams per day choline (348 milligrams from the egg yolks, 69 milligrams from the liver), roughly the adequate intake level for women — enough to ensure good choline status. Pregnant women and women trying to conceive should eat five to seven egg yolks per day or supplement choline.

36

Other Vitamins, Minerals, and Nutrients

· ·

- *Many nutrients may be beneficial to supplement occasionally —
  we recommend once a week — or in special circumstances, such
  as vitamin E during weight loss.*
- *Some nutrients shouldn't be supplemented at all — manganese,
  for example.*

· ·

L et's conclude our survey of micronutrition by quickly walking through
the other nutrients found in multivitamins.

B Vitamins

B vitamins are water-soluble and easily excreted in urine, which makes their
toxicity risk low:

- Some B vitamins are so non-toxic that the Food and Nutrition Board has not established a tolerable upper level (UL) of
  intake: thiamin (B1), riboflavin (B2), pantothenic acid (B5),
  biotin (B7), and vitamin B12.

Notes for this chapter may be found at www.perfecthealthdiet.com/notes/#Ch36.

- Vitamin B6 has a relatively high UL, 100 milligrams per day — more than 50 times the recommended daily allowance (RDA).
- Folic acid (UL of 1 milligram per day) and niacin (UL of 35 milligrams per day) are potentially more risky.

Deficiencies Are Fairly Common

Most Australians do not take a multivitamin and do consume a lot of 'empty-calorie' foods such as sugary beverages. As a result, they often develop B vitamin deficiencies. Some indicators of B vitamin deficiency rates:

- Thiamin deficiency was observed in 12 per cent of healthy persons and 33 per cent of heart failure patients.[1]
- Riboflavin deficiency afflicts somewhere between 25 and 75 per cent of the population, as evidenced by: (1) cataract rates in the bottom 20 per cent in riboflavin status are nearly double those in the top 20 per cent;[2] (2) 27 per cent of heart failure patients were found to have deficient red blood cell function due to riboflavin deficiency;[3] and (3) the bottom 25 per cent in riboflavin status is twice as likely to have advanced colorectal adenomas as the top 25 per cent.[4]
- Vitamin B6 deficiency was found in 38 per cent of heart-failure patients.[5]

On a whole-foods diet such as the Perfect Health Diet, B vitamin deficiencies will be rare. Still, given their low toxicity, there is a case for prophylactic supplementation.

Occasional Benefits from High-Dose Supplementation

Although there are few documented benefits to healthy people from B vitamin supplementation, high-dose B vitamins are therapeutic for some diseases. Here are a few instances:

- Thiamin reversed microalbuminuria in diabetics in a clinical trial.[6]
- Riboflavin reduced the frequency of migraines in a clinical trial.[7]

- Biotin and thiamin produced 'spectacular clinical and radiologic improvement' in two patients with brain disorders.[8]

Our Recommendation

The low toxicity of these vitamins means that they are safe to supplement. As deficiencies are dangerous and may possibly occur even on a whole-foods diet, we think it's prudent to supplement these — but not every day.

We suggest taking **a B-50 complex, 500 milligrams of pantothenic acid or pantethine, 5 milligrams of biotin, and 500 micrograms of vitamin B12** *once per week.* A B-50 complex contains 400 micrograms of folic acid, 50 micrograms of biotin, 50 micrograms of vitamin B12, and 50 milligrams of the other B vitamins.

Averaged over the week, these doses provide significantly more than the RDA and more than multivitamin doses for all but niacin and folic acid. Since deficiencies take longer than a week to develop, this will eliminate deficiency risk.

SCIENCE OF THE PHD
Why Weekly Supplementation May Be Best

The human body has sufficient stores of micronutrients to last a week or more. It doesn't need most micronutrients to be provided every day.

Microbes have much shorter life spans and need to be nourished more regularly.

Supplying nutrients intermittently on a schedule that works for humans can starve microbes long enough that they become vulnerable to the immune system or lose their ability to suppress immune defences.

Bacteria and other microbes are dependent mainly on B vitamins. Thus, supplying B vitamins once a week, in the form of a B-50 complex, may be optimal. Human cells can take up what they need, the remainder will depart in urine, and for most of the week bacteria will have low levels of B vitamins available to them.

Why We Don't Recommend Niacin

There is little need to supplement niacin, since it is ubiquitously present in foods — most meats have about 20 milligrams per 450 grams and most plant foods about 5 milligrams per 450 grams. The Perfect Health Diet therefore provides about 30 milligrams per day, which is double the RDA and triple the amount needed to prevent niacin deficiency.

There may be reasons to avoid an excess of niacin: (1) niacin is a nutrient for bacteria as well as humans; and (2) high doses can impair glycemic control, leading some to speculate that fortification of foods with niacin, which began in 1973, may have played a role in the obesity epidemic.[9]

Vitamin E

Vitamin E is the other fat-soluble vitamin, in addition to vitamins A, D, and K. Vitamin E's main role is to prevent peroxidation of polyunsaturated fats.

Vitamin E has not performed well in clinical trials. A meta-analysis of 19 vitamin E clinical trials covering 135,000 people, of whom 12,504 died, showed that supplemental vitamin E of more than 400 IU per day increased a person's risk of dying during the study period by 4 per cent.[10] In a later trial, death rates were the same in vitamin E and placebo groups.[11]

Two recent studies looked at vitamin E alone and in combination with vitamin C or selenium. In these studies, no benefit was seen:

- A clinical trial of almost 15,000 male doctors taking 200 IU per day of vitamin E and 500 milligrams per day of vitamin C for a decade found that the total mortality rate was 8 per cent higher in the vitamin E group and 7 per cent higher in the vitamin C group.[12] The differences were not considered significant.
- The SELECT trial (Selenium and Vitamin E Cancer Prevention Trial) studied supplementation of 400 IU per day of vitamin E and 200 micrograms of selenium in 35,000 men for five and a half years.[13] This time the placebo group had the highest mortality rate, but again the difference was not significant.

Though the evidence is hardly conclusive, it may be dangerous to supplement with more than 400 IU per day of alpha-tocopherol. This could be due to vitamin E toxicity at high doses, or it could be due to an imbalance in the different vitamin E types — since vitamin E in foods comes as a mix of various tocopherols and tocotrienols.

The case for vitamin E supplementation may be stronger during weight loss. Vitamin E is lost from tissue fairly quickly, while PUFA, which need vitamin E protection, may be released from adipose tissue for a period of years.[14] Therefore, it's plausible that vitamin E should be supplemented on weight-loss diets.

If supplements are taken, they should supply low doses of mixed tocopherols and tocotrienols, not alpha-tocopherol only. However, we recommend obtaining vitamin E from food; an excellent source is red palm oil. About 3 teaspoons per week of red palm oil, perhaps used as a spice in cooking, should ensure adequate vitamin E status in conjunction with a whole-foods diet.

Chromium

There is no good measure of bodily chromium status, and the chromium content of foods is not well characterised, so researchers have had difficulty coming up with a measure of chromium status. Since chromium deficiency is indetectable, it has been difficult to link chromium deficiency to health problems.

But although it is hard to characterise the chromium status of *living* humans, it is possible to precisely quantify the amount of chromium in tissue samples from *dead* people. Autopsies give a clue about the need for chromium.

Compared to the hearts of people who die from accidents, the hearts of people who die of heart attacks average 24 per cent less magnesium, 17 per cent less copper, 46 per cent less chromium, and 26 per cent *more* calcium. (Coronary calcification is a major risk factor for heart attacks and is largely attributable to vitamin D and K2 deficiencies.) The difference between the groups was eight standard deviations in the case of magnesium, four in the case of copper, and 3.3 in the case of chromium.[15]

These data strongly suggest that these three minerals — magnesium, copper, and chromium — are needed for heart health, and that deficiencies synergistically promote fatal heart attacks. It is quite remarkable that nearly everyone who died from a heart attack was deficient in all three minerals.

Another hint of chromium's importance comes from the days when chromium was not included in total parenteral (i.e., intravenous) nutrition. Patients on parenteral nutrition developed unexplained weight loss, impaired glucose utilisation, and peripheral neuropathy. Symptoms were cured by two weeks of chromium supplementation at 250 micrograms per day.[16]

Chromium's primary function is to assist in the entry of glucose into cells. With increased chromium, more glucose finds its way into cells from the blood; thus in a Chinese study a group of diabetics taking 1000 micrograms per day of chromium picolinate had blood glucose levels 15 to 19 per cent lower than those taking the placebo.[17]

Whether this is good for diabetics is unclear. Chromium doesn't eliminate glucose poisoning, it only moves it into cells. Whether it is better to poison the inside or the outside of cells is unknown.

The cells that most need to be able to take in glucose quickly are immune cells, which use glucose to generate reactive oxygen species for the killing of fungi and bacteria. Without chromium, their ability to kill is impaired.

Experiments in animals have confirmed the importance of chromium for immune defence against fungal infections. Depriving goats of chromium causes them to contract systemic fungal infections.[18] Chromium is also directly toxic to fungi.[19] It is likely that chromium also aids immune defence against bacterial infections.

Chromium deficiency is probably common. Chromium intake in the U.S. has been estimated at 23 to 29 micrograms per day for women and 39 to 54 micrograms per day for men.[20] These intakes are probably severely deficient.

Chromium doesn't seem to have much toxicity. Several studies have reported no ill effects from supplementation with 1000 micrograms per day for several months. On the other hand, there have been reports of kidney failure after use of 1200 to 2400 micrograms per day for four to five months and occasional reports of kidney failure on doses below 1000 micrograms per day.[21]

There is not enough information to identify a peak health range for chromium, but we believe that supplementation with **200 to 400 micrograms per week** is prudent.

Manganese

Manganese is included in multivitamins at 2.3 milligrams per day, which is the RDA, but we don't believe it should be supplemented at all.

First, *manganese deficiency rarely or never occurs on natural diets*, since fish, shellfish, and plant foods typically contain at least a few milligrams per 450 grams. Some plant foods contain much more: hazelnuts or filberts contain up to 60 milligrams per 450 grams, pine nuts contain 50 milligrams per 450 grams, many spices contain 40 milligrams per 450 grams, shellfish such as mussels may contain 30 milligrams per 450 grams, pecans and macadamia nuts contain 20 milligrams per 450 grams, blueberries, pineapple, and chocolate contain 10 milligrams per 450 grams, and potatoes, fish, seaweed, peas, onions, and many other foods contain close to 5 milligrams per 450 grams. It would be a rare implementation of the Perfect Health Diet that did not supply 5 milligrams of manganese per day.

Second, manganese is a neurotoxin. Manganese poisoning creates physical symptoms that closely resemble Parkinson's disease, plus behavioural effects similar to schizophrenia.[22]

It doesn't take much manganese to cause neurological symptoms.

- In Greece, there is a high prevalence of neurological symptoms in those exposed to water manganese levels of 2 milligrams per litre, which suggests that as little as 5 milligrams per day of manganese may be able to generate neurotoxicity.[23]
- Children whose drinking water contains 0.8 milligram per litre of manganese score lower on tests of intellectual function.[24] Children whose drinking water has 0.6 milligram per litre are prone to hyperactive behavioural disorders.[25]

It's not just water that's culpable. Those who have a high dietary intake of manganese or who supplement with a multivitamin are 70 per cent more likely to develop Parkinson's.[26] Iron is also a risk, so that those who have higher-than-median intakes of both iron and manganese are most likely to develop Parkinson's.

It appears that even normal dietary levels of manganese verge on toxicity. Supplementation at the level found in multivitamins has no known benefits and very real risks. Potential manganese toxicity appears to be a good reason not to take a multivitamin.

Iron

Iron is an essential nutrient, a component of hemoglobin and hundreds of proteins and enzymes.

Iron commonly becomes deficient in menstruating or pregnant women, vegetarians, those with *H. pylori* infections, and endurance athletes. The primary effect is anemia, and symptoms include fatigue, rapid heart rate, palpitations, rapid breathing on exertion, and impaired capacity for athletic performance and physical work.

The Perfect Health Diet has a substantial intake of iron-rich foods such as red meat, liver, and shellfish. Also, vitamin C supplementation enhances iron absorption. As a result, there is a low risk of iron deficiency.

We agree with standard recommendations that the only healthy persons who should consider iron supplements are menstruating and pregnant women. The RDA for pregnant women, in both Australia and the United States, is 27 milligrams per day, and supplements should not exceed 18 milligrams per day.

Other Trace Minerals

A few other minerals commonly found in multivitamins (or that should be) are the following.

- **Molybdenum** is essential for life and is extremely rare in soil. Although deficiencies are not known to occur in people with healthy digestive tracts, it's probably prudent to supplement 150 micrograms per week. Multivitamins typically provide 45 micrograms per day, or 315 micrograms per week.
- **Boron** is helpful for bone health,[27] brain function,[28] and possibly cancer prevention.[29] Multivitamins typically contain 150

micrograms, or 1 milligram per week. We suggest 3 milligrams once per week.

- **Nickel** is contained in multivitamins at 5 micrograms, but since it is abundant in Perfect Health Diet foods, we do not recommend supplementation.

- **Silicon** improves collagen formation, supporting wound healing and bone strength.[30] In the Framingham Offspring study, the subjects with the highest dietary silicon intakes (over 40 milligrams per day) had the strongest bones, and those with dietary silicon intakes below 14 milligrams per day had the weakest bones.[31] Multivitamins typically contain 2 milligrams, much lower than desirable dietary levels. We suggest supplementing 5 milligrams per day.

- **Vanadium** appears to be important for thyroid function and glycemic control.[32] Multivitamins typically contain 10 micrograms per day, a reasonable dose; the optimum dose is not known. Combination chromium-vanadium supplements are available.

- **Lithium** is a fascinating nutrient. Lithium intakes of Americans range from 0.65 milligram per day to 3 milligrams per day, depending mainly on vegetable consumption and lithium levels in local water. Lithium is essential to the health of rats: lithium-deficient rats have 20 to 30 per cent fewer pups per litter, and only half as many pups survive the first week. People with low lithium intake have higher rates of neurosis, schizophrenia, psychosis, psychiatric ward admissions, homicide, suicide, sexual assault, and burglary.[33] Moreover, the longevity of Japanese is related to the amount of lithium in their tap water: more lithium equals longer life span (a pattern that also holds in worms).[34] It looks as though low doses of lithium — around 3 milligrams per day — are highly beneficial. Note that these doses are far lower than the therapeutic doses given in bipolar disorder, which can range from 100 to several thousand milligrams per day; these doses distort immune function and damage thyroid function. Impairments to thyroid function may start at quite low doses. In a study of Peruvians with lithium intakes ranging from 2 to 30 milligrams per day, higher lithium intakes were associated with worse thyroid function.[35] In short, most Americans, and likely many Australians — especially those whose water is low in lithium — may benefit from low-dose lithium supplementation, but supplementation should probably not exceed 2.5 milligrams per day. Unfortunately, the lowest-dose lithium supplements we have seen for sale are 5 milligrams. As lithium influences circadian rhythms, it is best to take lithium daily in the morning. Therefore, a reasonable strategy would be to cut a 5-milligram tablet into halves of 2.5 milligrams each, and take one each morning.

Finally, not in most multivitamins but worth considering: **taurine.** This is the amino acid that Pottenger's cats needed so badly. Humans need it too: it is a crucial component in bile, which we need in abundance for optimal digestive health. Taurine is present in raw and rare meats, so those who like their meat well done should be especially careful to supplement taurine. It is readily available in 500-milligram doses, which may be taken weekly or daily. There is little data to guide us to the optimal amount.

37
Micronutrient Recommendations

There's every reason to believe that **optimising micronutrition will deliver substantial health and mortality benefits.** The leading causes of death in Australia are cancer and cardiovascular disease; and clinical trials and prospective studies have shown that *both diseases become far more frequent when nutrients are under- or overprovided.*

∙∙

READER REPORTS: micronutrition and sleep

After cutting back on coconut oil and adding all the supplements suggested by PHD I am sleeping 6 hours straight and can doze the next two hours, a ginormous improvement. Oh, and I upped my carbs! Delightful!
— Kathy, Burlington, Washington

∙∙

Some nutrients are best obtained from foods: especially fat-associated nutrients such as vitamin A, choline, folate, and vitamin E; electrolytes such as potassium and calcium; and minerals such as copper and selenium.

We consider the foods that provide these nutrients so crucial to health that they should be eaten habitually and routinely, as you would take a supplement. The following 'supplemental foods' should be eaten daily:

Notes for this chapter may be found at www.perfecthealthdiet.com/notes/#Ch37.

- three egg yolks (for choline, folate, vitamin A) — five egg yolks in pregnant women and women planning to conceive
- a bowl of bone and joint broth soup (for calcium, phosphorus, and collagen)
- vegetables such as tomato, avocado, potato, sweet potato, banana, green leafy vegetables, and seaweeds such as dulse (for potassium)
- dark chocolate (>70 per cent cocoa) (for magnesium and zinc)

The following supplemental foods should be eaten weekly:

- 115 grams of beef or lamb liver (copper, vitamin A, folate, choline)
- fish, shellfish, eggs, and kidneys (for selenium)
- three teaspoons red palm oil (vitamin E)

A few minerals are hard to get in optimal amounts from food, such as magnesium and zinc, and should be supplemented. Some are so crucial to health and safe that it's best to supplement: vitamins D and K2, vitamin C, iodine.

We therefore recommend the following supplements daily (optional nutrients, which may not be appropriate for everyone, are in parentheses):

- sunshine and vitamin D3 as needed to achieve a serum 25OHD level of 40 nanograms per millilitre
- vitamin K2: 100 micrograms or more
- vitamin C: 1 gram
- magnesium: 200 milligrams
- iodine: 1 milligram
- (lithium: 2.5 milligrams — a 5-milligram tablet cut into halves)
- (silicon: 5 milligrams)
- (if beef or lamb liver is not eaten, then copper: 2 milligrams)

And the following supplements once a week only:

- B-vitamins
    - For B1, B2, and B6, either: a B-50 complex which typically contains 50 milligrams each of thiamin (B1), riboflavin

(B2), and vitamin B6, as well as some niacinamide (B3), pantothenic acid (B5), folic acid and small amounts of biotin and vitamin B12; *or* individual supplements of 100 milligrams thiamin (B1), 100 milligrams riboflavin (B2), and 100 milligrams vitamin B6.

- biotin: 5 milligrams
- pantothenic acid or pantethine: 500 milligrams
- vitamin B12: 500 micrograms
- zinc: 50 milligrams
- through a mix of chromium and chromium vanadium supplements, obtain: chromium: 200 to 600 micrograms, and vanadium: 50 micrograms
- (molybdenum: 150 micrograms)
- (boron: 3 milligrams)
- (taurine: 500 milligrams)
- (if kidney is not eaten, and iodine is supplemented at 1 milligram per day or higher, then selenium: 200 to 400 micrograms)

Part V

. . . .

A Recipe for Healthful Living

. . . .

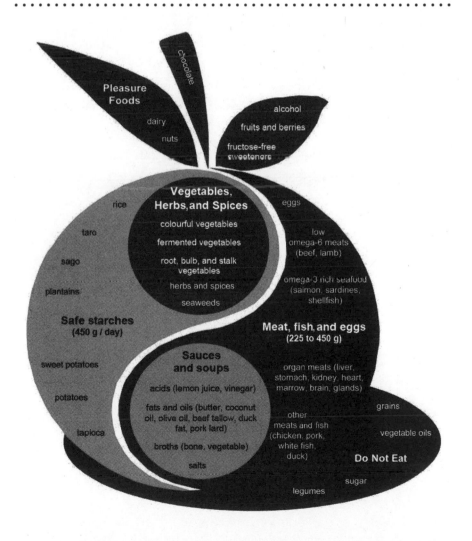

38

The Infectious Origins of Disease

. . . .

- *We all have chronic infections that become more severe as we age. If allowed to multiply, parasitic microbes will cause severe disease.*
- *It's desirable to improve your 'terrain' by helping your immune system control chronic infections.*

. . . .

Human beings are saturated with germs. Each person carries 100 trillion gut bacteria weighing 900 grams to 1.4 kilograms from over 1000 species.[1] Trillions more bacteria line the skin, sinuses, lungs, and every other body surface. These are mostly friendly or 'probiotic' bacteria.

Also inhabiting human beings are some not-so-friendly microbes: at least 300 species of pathogens are known to cause human disease.

Some infections are acute: they run their course and are cleared from the body in days or weeks. But many are chronic: the pathogens lodge in cells or biofilms, parasitise their hosts and steal glucose and nutrients for their own use, sabotage the immune system to ensure their survival, and gradually increase their numbers over decades.

At the start of the book, we said that disease and ill health are largely caused by three factors, all addressable by diet: nutrient deficiencies, toxins, and chronic infections. We've already considered how to eliminate nutrient deficiencies and food toxins. But how do we get rid of infections?

Notes for this chapter may be found at www.perfecthealthdiet.com/notes/#Ch38.

Exposure to Germs Is Inevitable

Eliminating exposure to germs is not an option. We're surrounded by them:

- With every breath of outdoor air, we take in 50,000 germs.[2]
- It's worse indoors: every hour, a person's body releases 37 million bacteria and seven million fungi into room air. These germs rapidly spread to every other person in the room.[3]
- There are 250 million viruses in every teaspoon of sea water. Each day, these viruses kill about 20 per cent of the ocean's microorganisms.[4]

Although most of these germs do not cause human disease, they do keep our immune systems busy. And exposure to environmental germs does increase the odds of becoming ill.[5]

Chronic Parasitic Infections

But the germs that do the most damage to our health are not found in sea water or air, but in our fellow human beings. Microbes that have evolved an ability to flourish inside human beings — to evade or block our immune defences and steal from our cells the resources they need to proliferate — are the greatest threats to our health.

It's common for germs that cause chronic infections to cause a mild illness at the time of infection, followed by an apparent recovery. But the recovery is often illusory; the germs persist in the body, causing a mild impairment of function and proliferate as parasites.

Some chronic infections are so common that nearly everyone acquires them. About 95 per cent of Americans and 57 per cent of Australians are infected with cytomegalovirus, for instance.

One way to estimate the prevalence of a given infection with a chronic pathogen is by measuring how many people have antibodies above a threshold titer. Antibody studies show that many infections are extremely common. One study of Alaskan Eskimos[6] found that:

- 94 per cent had antibodies to cytomegalovirus (CMV), 90 per cent to herpes simplex 1 (HSV1), 38 per cent to herpes simplex 2 (HSV2), 80 per cent to *H. pylori*, and 42 per cent to *C. pneumoniae*.
- 82.1 per cent had antibodies to at least three of the five pathogens tested.
- Seropositivity increased with age: at age 18, 16 per cent were infected by HSV2 and 27 per cent by *C. pneumoniae*, but by age 45, both rates were over 50 per cent.

People all over the world are infected with *C. pneumoniae* at similar rates:

- Among Finns, the prevalence of antibodies is 70 per cent in 15- to 19-year-olds and 100 per cent in elderly men.[7]
- Among Japanese, 59 to 73 per cent have antibodies, and there are recurrent epidemics every six years or so.[8] Dr Naoyuki Miyashita notes that '*C. pneumoniae* is widely distributed and nearly everybody is infected with the agent at some time'.[9]
- Among Israelis, 31 per cent of children and 74 per cent of adults are seropositive.[10]
- Among Italian schoolchildren, 29 per cent have antibodies, and the prevalence increases steadily with age.[11]
- In Singapore, antibody prevalence is 75 per cent in men and 65 per cent in women. By age group, it is 46.5 per cent at ages 18 to 29 and 78.9 per cent above age 40.[12]

Since many people infected with *C. pneumoniae* do not produce antibodies, these numbers suggest that by age 40 nearly everyone has been infected.

Infections with protozoa and fungi are also common. The protozoal parasite *Toxoplasma gondii* infects 20 to 60 per cent of the population in most countries, forms cysts throughout the body including the brain, and influences behaviour.

- -

READER REPORTS: fungal infection

I started PHD ten months ago after having previously pursued a low-carb paleo approach. At that time, I had a toe fungal infection which made the toenail of my right toe nearly black, plus it made my foot half-numb. It was getting so that I didn't even like to go for long walks, which I have done all my life. After six months of PHD eating, some of the fungus had receded and some feeling had returned to my foot. Recently, after a discussion or two on your blog mentioned Epsom Salts, I added a nightly foot soak in Epsom Salts. It seemed to me that almost immediately there was a reduction in both the visibility of the fungus as well as a reduction in the numbness. As of today, most (but not all) of the feeling has returned to my right foot. Although I suspect the most recent improvement resulted from Epsom Salts, it might also be due to other changes, including intermittent fasting and the PHD recommended supplements and nutrition.

— Kirk Condon

- -

Consequences for Human Health

Medicine is just beginning to uncover the links between chronic infection and human diseases.

In 2005, Barry Marshall and J. Robin Warren won the Nobel Prize in Medicine for showing that *H. pylori* bacteria cause stomach ulcers. The 2008 prize was awarded to Harald zur Hausen for linking human papilloma virus to cervical cancer. It's quite possible that infections may cause most human cancers.

C. pneumoniae is associated with a variety of diseases including atherosclerosis, stroke, Alzheimer's, multiple sclerosis, and arthritis. *C. pneumoniae* is found:

- in the central nervous system of 97 per cent of multiple sclerosis patients [13]

SCIENCE OF THE PHD
Infections as a Cause of Cancer

It has been argued that infections are likely to be a cause of most cancers.[14] Pathogens die when their host cell dies, and get to infect two cells instead of one when their host cell multiplies, so they benefit if they evolve an ability to suppress host cell death and promote host cell proliferation. But immortality and proliferation are precisely the characteristics of cancer cells!

A recent study found that just four pathogens — *Helicobacter pylori* (gastric cancer), hepatitis B and C viruses (liver cancer), and human papillomaviruses (cervical cancer) — are responsible for one-sixth of all cancers worldwide.[15]

It is certain that many more cancers are caused by infections, but the pathogens are not yet known. For instance, it is known that men with a mutation to RNase L, a molecule of the innate immune system that defends against viral infections, are much more likely to develop prostate cancer, indicating that a viral infection is responsible for many prostate cancers; but the virus or viruses at fault are currently unknown.[16]

- in the brains of 89 per cent of Alzheimer's patients, but only 5 per cent of non-Alzheimer's elderly[17]
- in 71 per cent of atheromatous arteries and 67 per cent of early atherosclerotic lesions, but only 9 per cent of nonatheromatous arteries[18]

People with *C. pneumoniae* antibodies have a 3.62 times higher risk of hemorrhagic stroke.[19]

People with cytomegalovirus infections are 12 times more likely to develop diabetes.[20] Parkinson's disease has been associated with the bacterium *Nocardia*.[21] Amyotrophic lateral sclerosis (ALS), also known as Lou Gehrig's disease, has been linked to cyanobacteria.[22] *Toxoplasma gondii* infection is associated with schizophrenia, mood disorders, and cognitive

READER REPORTS: juvenile rheumatoid arthritis

I muddled through 32 years of life on this drug or that, all in the hopes of ending my 'not-so in love affair' with Juvenile Rheumatoid Arthritis (RA). I was diagnosed at age 3 after a bout with what doctors thought to be a cold virus, and what followed was years upon years of aspirin (24 chewables daily, to be exact), gold salts, NSAIDs and DMARDs. Ugh!

Since beginning to uncover secrets of old three years ago, I have eaten a Weston Price, biblical, Paleo-ish diet and dabbled in various and sundry supplements. This part of my new-found health journey yielded results good enough to keep me off prescription meds, but something was still lurking in my body causing imbalances.

Thank God for my integrative MD, who ordered DNA testing of my stool, and lo and behold, found parasitic and fungal infections (imagine that, right?). I reluctantly gave in and started rounds of Flagyl (antibiotic) and Nystatin (antifungal), along with probiotics and a much lower carb/no sugar diet. The results have been nothing short of WOW!

I can sometimes feel the anger welling up inside me when I think of the years of my life this degenerative disease has robbed me of. But if it hadn't been for those nasty bugs that attacked that little three year old girl many years ago, I wouldn't be enrolled in a Naturopathic Doctor program now and my passion in life wouldn't be helping others with chronic, degenerative diseases.

Thank you kindly for joining the crusade and bringing your diet and this life-restoring information to light!

— Jenna L., Atlanta, Georgia

impairment.[23] *T. gondii* induces reckless behaviour; infected people are six times more likely to get into car accidents,[24] and seven times more likely to commit suicide.[25] Infected rats lose their fear of cats.[26]

Some isolated island populations have been remarkably disease-free:

- The Kitava Study found no evidence of stroke, diabetes, dementia, heart disease, obesity, hypertension, or acne among

SCIENCE OF THE PIID
Obesity Is Often an Infectious Disease

There is circumstantial evidence that infections cause obesity:

- Operations such as tonsillectomies that remove an immune-system organ are often followed by weight gain and obesity.[27]
- Medications that suppress immunity, given to transplant recipients and autoimmune disease sufferers, commonly lead to weight gain.[28]
- Chronic infections such as *C. pneumoniae* are associated with obesity.[29]

There is also direct evidence that:[30]

- Four viruses — canine distemper virus, Rous-associated virus type 7, Borna disease virus, scrapie agent — infect the central nervous system and induce obesity in chickens, mice, sheep, goats, dogs, rats, and hamsters through effects on the brain.
- An avian adenovirus, SMAM-1, infects humans and induces obesity in chickens. SMAM-1 acts directly on fat cells.
- Three human adenoviruses, AD-36, AD-37, and AD-5, act directly on human fat cells and are associated with human obesity. AD-36 has been shown to induce obesity when given to chickens, mice, and marmosets.

AD-36 is a major factor in human obesity. Twenty-two per cent of obese children, but only 7 per cent of non-obese, are infected with AD-36. Obese children infected with AD-36 are much fatter than other obese children.[31]

the 2300 residents of Kitava.[32] Were the Kitavans free of disease solely because of their healthful diet, or because the island lacked pathogens?

- There were no cases of multiple sclerosis in the Faeroe Islands until British troops were stationed there during World War II. After World War II, MS cases occurred in people who had lived as children in villages where the British were stationed.[33]

If chronic pathogens cause the diseases common in the elderly, much of what we consider 'ageing' is not a natural degeneration of the human body but increasing debilitation from chronic infections that build up over many years.

Cardiovascular disease, dementia and memory loss, neuropathy and lost balance and falls, 'grouchy old man' syndrome, cold intolerance, inflamed

---

READER REPORT: gut and joint infections, arthritis

A comprehensive stool test proved helpful to me. I found a fungal infection which I treated with two bottles of ProEnt-2. I found bacterial overgrowths, which I treated with Natren probiotics. The stool test showed gluten intolerance as well, and seeing the results on paper helped me to take the leap & kiss gluten goodbye.

I was also positive to toxoplasma, which I have not treated due to cost and efficacy of treatment. Maybe down the line?

I had a sudden severe arthritis flare and have been on low dose pulsing Doxy for it, successfully, since 2008.

My thyroid function has improved as I've gotten healthier. My guess is improving iodine status and other micronutrient status, plus knocking back infections are the major contributors.

I'm no longer anemic.

I can't tell you how empowering it felt to take steps, and to slowly see my labs improve. In my case, my labs tend to improve a bit ahead of symptoms.

— Michelle

and arthritic joints — these may all be symptoms, not of ageing, but of chronic infections.

When their host becomes sufficiently diseased, parasites may release poisons that help them spread to new carriers. Often they cause pneumonia, since sneezing is an effective way to spread. Acute diseases produced by chronic pathogens are a common cause of death in the elderly.

How Should We Respond to Chronic Infections?

Claude Bernard declared, 'The terrain is everything, the microbe is nothing.' Modern medicine has given us the ability to attack microbes. Should we treat infections with antibiotics? Or try to improve the 'terrain' — the quality of the body's immune defences?

SCIENCE OF THE PHD
Antibiotics and 'Terrain' in Acute and Chronic Diseases

Many antibiotics work by inhibiting bacterial protein synthesis. Since acute pathogens are in a race with the immune system, hobbling them with antibiotics is usually enough to guarantee victory for the immune system. Acute pathogens are visible to the immune system and rapidly killed by it, so if antibiotics limit their ability to reproduce, their numbers will rapidly dwindle.

But chronic pathogens follow a stealth strategy: they hide from the immune system and reproduce slowly, taking years or decades to generate overt disease. They hibernate through antibiotic treatment and return to activity when the treatment ends.

Since chronic pathogens aren't very active, inhibition of their activity may not hurt them much. Antibiotics also have downsides:

- Our mitochondria are relatives of bacteria, and antibiotics inhibit mitochondria from synthesising their own proteins. Antibiotic use can lead to mitochondrial damage.

(continued on next page)

- Antibiotics damage the gut flora, potentially creating a gut dysbiosis and enabling new pathogens to infect the body via the gut.

Strategies to improve the terrain, on the other hand, are relatively more effective in chronic than in acute infections. Chronic pathogens sacrifice their own growth in favour of subverting immune defences. It may take decades for chronic infections to progress to overt disease. So there is plenty of time for small, but steady, advantages to add up.

We may need to do both. But in chronic infections, improving the terrain is a critical step.

In most people, chronic pathogens multiply steadily and cause disease in the sixth, seventh, or eighth decade of life. If we can find a diet and lifestyle that slows microbial growth and enhances immunity, infections may take much longer — 20 or 30 decades — to generate disease.

But if it takes 20 decades for disease to appear, we'll die of old age without ever becoming sick!

39

A Strategy for Immunity

. . . .

- *The PHD strategy — a sufficiency of everything, an excess of nothing — is not only a good diet for losing kilos, it's the best diet for losing germs.*

. . . .

The most basic dietary strategy against infections is to nourish the immune system so that it functions at its best, while starving microbes so their ability to multiply is impaired.

Let's look at a few examples of nutrients that support immune function and nutrients that we might usefully restrict in order to starve microbes.

Nourishing the Immune System

Being well nourished is important for immune function. Some of the most important nutrients for immune function are the fat-soluble vitamins A and D, iodine, and antioxidant and pro-oxidant minerals.

Antimicrobial Secretions

In mucus, tears, and saliva, there are a number of compounds that kill pathogenic microbes. Two important kinds are:

- **Antimicrobial peptides (AMPs).** AMPs are small proteins that can disrupt microbial membranes, interfere with metabolism, and damage cell components. All sites where pathogens enter the body — such as the mouth, the gut, the skin, the sinuses, the lungs — secrete AMPs. The main human AMPs are *cathelicidin* and *defensin*.

- **Lysozymes.** Lysozymes are enzymes that damage bacterial cell walls by breaking down bonds in bacterial sugars. Lysozymes are abundant in tears, saliva, and mucus and in breast milk. Infants fed formula lacking lysozyme have three times more diarrhoeal disease.[1]

Secretion of these compounds is dependent upon adequate provision of certain nutrients:

- **Vitamin D.** The most important human AMPs, cathelicidin and defensins, are induced by vitamin D.[2]
- **Vitamin A.** In vitamin A deficiency, airway secretions are reduced 35 per cent and lysozyme concentration is decreased, greatly increasing susceptibility to infections.[3]
- **Water.** Dehydration decreases the amount of mucus and saliva and the number of AMPs released.[4]

Respiratory Bursts

Phagocytic white blood cells, such as monocytes and neutrophils, engulf extracellular pathogens and destroy them with respiratory bursts that generate reactive oxygen species (ROS).

The killing power of ROS-producing respiratory bursts begins with the generation of hydrogen peroxide using glucose by the enzyme glucose oxidase.[5] Next, myeloperoxidase, an iron-based enzyme, combines with a halide partner, preferably iodine, to turn the peroxide into a deadly acid.[6] This myeloperoxidase-halide-hydrogen peroxide system is especially important against fungi, extracellular bacteria, and cancers.

For immune cells to have a high killing capability, they need:

- **Antioxidants** for protection from their own respiratory bursts, especially glutathione, zinc-copper superoxide dismutase, and catalase. Glutathione status is supported by **selenium** and **vitamin C;** catalase by **iron;** zinc-copper SOD by **zinc** and **copper.**

- **Iodine,** the most effective halide for immune killing.[7] When immune cells employ phagocytosis against infections, they strip iodine from thyroid hormone.[8] Not surprisingly, chronic disease patients often develop iodine deficiency hypothyroidism. High-dose iodine often cures infectious conditions, as the old doctor's mnemonic, recalled by Albert Szent-Györgyi, suggests, 'If ye don't know where, what, and why/Prescribe ye then K and I.'[9] A typical prescribed dose of iodine for acute infections in Szent-Györgyi's time was 770 milligrams. We suggest 1 milligram daily for healthy people and 12 milligrams daily for chronic infections.
- Adequate **carbohydrate intake.** Perhaps because of the need to conserve glucose, low-carbohydrate ketogenic diets inhibit immune cells from using the glucose-myeloperoxidase pathway to kill pathogens.[10] Avoidance of glucose deficiency and ketosis is therefore important in many infections, especially fungal infections.[11]

Starving the Microbes

Sequestering or destroying nutrients in order to starve pathogens is a primary immune defence. Two examples are tryptophan destruction and iron sequestration.

Tryptophan and Niacin Starvation

Bacteria such as *C. pneumoniae* and protozoa such as *T. gondii* are highly dependent on certain amino acids, such as tryptophan, tyrosine, and phenylalanine, to grow.[12] Tryptophan, for instance, is required for protein synthesis and manufacture of niacin, the vitamin that is essential to bacterial energy metabolism.

The human immune response to intracellular infections generates high levels of interferon and induces a compound called indoleamine 2,3-dioxygenase (IDO). The function of IDO is to strip the cell of as much tryptophan as possible, thereby preventing bacteria from reproducing and from synthesising niacin or proteins.[13] It works.[14]

This has side effects for the human cell, of course — notably, deficiencies of serotonin and melatonin, which are made from tryptophan. This is why people with brain infections get symptoms of serotonin and melatonin deficiency, such as depression and insomnia. However, overall the benefits of depriving bacteria of tryptophan far outweigh the costs.

We can assist this immune defence by:

- eating a moderate-, not high-, protein diet
- engaging in resistance exercise to direct protein toward our muscles
- avoiding routine niacin supplementation

Iron Starvation

Iron is an essential mineral for nearly all life, including microbes. Iron's natural forms are poorly soluble in water, so the human body has a variety of ways to transport or store iron.

The human immune system takes advantage of this situation by trying to starve pathogens of iron. Within hours of infection, concentrations of iron in extracellular fluid and blood drop dramatically. Cells that recycle iron from red blood cells cease releasing recycled iron; infected cells store their iron in ferritin, an iron storage protein that is inaccessible to most pathogens; neutrophils in infected tissue secrete proteins such as lactoferrin that chelate iron.[15]

This immune strategy can be defeated by excessive iron intake:

- Iron supplementation or elevated iron levels make tuberculosis far more severe.[16]
- Iron overload exacerbates some viral infections, including HIV and hepatitis C.[17]
- Blood iron levels predict mortality in people with HIV infection — the higher the ferritin, transferritin, and other iron markers, the higher the mortality rate.[18]
- People with hemochromatosis, an iron overload disorder, have more infections.[19]

Iron deficiency, meanwhile, is protective against many infections, including malaria.[20]

For optimal immunity, then, it's desirable to keep iron stores at low levels. To achieve that, most people should **avoid iron supplementation** and **give blood regularly.** Menstruating and pregnant women, who are at higher risk of iron deficiency, are possible exceptions.

READER REPORTS:
stomach problems, fatigue, weight gain, anemia

About 5 years ago, I started having horrible stomach problems (pain, bloating, etc.), extreme fatigue, weight gain of about 15 lbs [6.8 kilograms], and anemia. After many useless visits to traditional doctors, I finally went to see a naturopath who put me on a restricted diet: no sugar (or fruit), no grains other than rice, no cow dairy, no legumes, no nuts. It was actually pretty much a PHD diet.

Within 4 months on this diet I felt 80% better; the fatigue was gone, I lost the weight, and the anemia went away (with some help from iron supplements), and my stomach pain was intermittent and brief when it did occur. I went on like this for about 2 years.

Then, about 2 years ago, I discovered the paleo diet. It was already similar to the way I was eating with some minor tweaks: upping the fat content of my diet, eliminating rice and sweet potatoes, adding back some moderate fruit. Within a year of eating this way, I began experiencing some additional stomach discomfort, more bloating and pain. I went to see a doctor for some help. Unfortunately, she just made the situation worse.

Well, I adopted the PHD in October 2010 and I am happy to say that my stomach issues are almost completely gone. I would definitely recommend PHD to anyone looking for a healthy way of eating. I would also recommend it for anyone who is still experiencing stomach issues while on a Paleo diet.

— J. Spencer

A Strategy for Improving the Terrain

Let's generalise this idea of nourishing immune function and starving pathogens.

To have a well-functioning immune system, we need to get all of our nutrients into their peak health range, so that additional nutrition provides no further benefit.

To starve pathogens, we need to avoid an excess of any nutrient. So we need to get all of our nutrients into their peak health range simultaneously — and at the low end of their peak health ranges, so that we're eating the minimum amount of each nutrient consistent with peak health.

But this is exactly the strategy of the Perfect Health Diet! It is, in fact, nearly the same as the strategy we identified for avoiding obesity and losing weight, which sought to get all nutrients into their peak health range simultaneously while avoiding an excess of any macronutrient.

It is the strategy of having a balanced, nourishing diet that avoids overnutrition.

A Diet for Losing Germs?

Russ Farris, the author of *The Potbelly Syndrome,* has called the Perfect Health Diet 'a diet for getting rid of germs, not pounds'.[21] We agree with the first part but not the second. The same strategy that is optimal for getting rid of germs is also optimal for getting rid of excess weight!

We're not the first to recognise that this is a good approach for avoiding infectious disease. A review of nutritional immunology states, 'Optimum but balanced food intake maintains healthy growth and disease-free life span. However, imbalanced and over-nutrition promotes . . . infectious diseases.'[22]

40
Fasting

- *Daily intermittent fasting helps kill many pathogens and is likely to extend life span and improve health.*

Some pathogens live outside human cells: they circulate in the blood or in extracellular fluids. Such extracellular pathogens are killed by white blood cells.

But how do we kill pathogens that live inside human cells? White blood cells can and do go inside human cells — for instance, they pass through the endothelial cells that line blood vessels on their way to infected or injured tissue — but white blood cells are not the primary way our bodies kill intracellular microbes.

The main killing mechanism for intracellular pathogens is a process called 'autophagy' or 'self-eating'. Every cell has organelles called **lysosomes** that are devoted to the recycling of cellular junk — damaged proteins and organelles, and bacteria, viruses, and other germs. Lysosomes digest the junk to its constituent parts — fatty acids, amino acids, sugars, and the like — which are then reused by the cell to make useful proteins and organelles.

Cells try to keep levels of fatty acids, amino acids, and sugars constant, so when these are available — say, after a meal — autophagy is suppressed. When they become scarce — say, after a fast — autophagy is turned on.

This means that after a meal, *most cells are not killing germs.* They wait until a period of fasting to hunt germs and other junk and turn them into cellular food.

Notes for this chapter may be found at www.perfecthealthdiet.com/notes/#Ch40.

This suggests an idea: fasting protects us from intracellular infections.

Let's look a little closer at how autophagy protects us and then see how we can induce it.

Autophagy and Infections

Autophagy is a sophisticated immune defence mechanism. It can[1]:

- recognise, capture, and destroy intracellular pathogens
- deliver antimicrobial molecules to pathogens hiding in inaccessible locations
- engage in immune surveillance, detecting the presence of foreign pathogens, and present microbial compounds for antibody generation

Autophagy thus doubles as a pathogen-killing mechanism, and a sentinel that brings the rest of the immune system to bear against infections.

Autophagy has been shown to be highly effective against many infections. *Streptococcus* is rapidly destroyed by autophagy but readily survives inside cells when autophagy is blocked. *Mycobacteria, Listeria, Salmonella, Francisella tularensis,* and *Toxoplasma gondii* are other pathogens that are targeted by autophagy.[2]

SCIENCE OF THE PHD
When Pathogens Fight Back

Evolution is a two-sided race, and pathogens have evolved ways to fight back against autophagy.

It's possible that only microbes that can obstruct human autophagy can cause infections. A much-cited review in *Nature* noted:

> [S]uccessful intracellular pathogens modulate the signalling pathways that regulate autophagy or block the membrane trafficking events required for autophagy-mediated pathogen

delivery to the lysosome . . . [M]icrobial evasion of autophagy
may be essential for microbial pathogenesis.[3]

Pathogens known to suppress autophagy include herpes simplex
virus type 1 (HSV-1), Epstein-Barr virus,[4] and cytomegalovirus.[5]

Autophagy suppression by HSV-1 not only prevents its own
eradication, it also prevents infected cells from clearing protein tangles
— the amyloid plaques and neurofibrillary tangles that are common in
Alzheimer's.[6] HSV-1 is strongly associated with Alzheimer's, right down
to the very plaques and tangles: 90 per cent of all amyloid plaques in
Alzheimer's disease brains contain HSV-1, and 72 per cent of HSV-1
DNA is located within amyloid plaques.[7]

Sometimes pathogens promote aspects of autophagy in order to
release amino acids and fatty acids for their own growth. Viruses that
promote autophagy include poliovirus, hepatitis B and C viruses, and
dengue virus.[8] Picornavirus can both upregulate aspects of autophagy
that support its replication and subvert aspects of autophagy that lead to
its degradation.[9]

If autophagy is impaired so that intracellular threats are not
successfully eliminated, the result may be continued infection
accompanied by excessive inflammation as other parts of the immune
system try to make up for insufficient autophagy. This is what happens
in Crohn's, an inflammatory bowel disease. Crohn's patients have low
levels of autophagy; many have mutations in autophagy genes.[10]

Dysfunctions in autophagy lead to a host of diseases: cancer, neurodegenerative diseases, infections, and early ageing.[11] A key autophagy gene is
deleted in 40 to 75 per cent of cancers.[12]

If genetic suppression of autophagy promotes cancer, microbes that suppress autophagy, such as cytomegalovirus, probably promote cancer. There
are, indeed, strong associations between these infections and cancer.[13]

Fasting for Autophagy: how long?

Autophagy is turned on fairly quickly in response to a scarcity of macronutrients. Newborn babies turn on autophagy within 30 minutes of birth to make up for the loss of nourishment from the placenta. In adults, autophagy has a strong diurnal rhythm, peaking at the end of the overnight fast and lowest just after breakfast.[14]

A 24-hour fast in mice, equivalent to a fast of several days in humans, induces autophagy throughout the body, including 'profound neuronal autophagy' in the brain.[15] Many of the benefits of fasting appear to be triggered as the liver starts to run short of glycogen. The liver's glycogen store is 70 to 100 grams, or about 300 to 400 calories. Since the body consumes 500 to 600 glucose calories per day, liver glycogen stores become low about 12 to 16 hours into a fast. This suggests that *a 16-hour fast is sufficiently long to trigger autophagy.*

Long fasts do not upregulate autophagy more than short fasts do. In mice, autophagy peaks within the first 24 hours of a fast and then drops back to normal levels within 48 hours of fasting. Possibly after 24 hours of fasting, cells become depleted of proteins, and continued high levels of autophagy would impair cellular function.[16]

Although long fasts do not upregulate autophagy, they do lead to a more exaggerated drop in autophagy upon resumption of feeding. Mice starved for 48 hours experience complete suppression of autophagy when feeding is resumed.[17] In rats starved for five days, autophagy is completely eliminated throughout the first day of refeeding and takes several more days to return to normal.[18]

This period of autophagy suppression allows cells to restore normal levels of proteins and normal cell size. However, with autophagy suppressed, pathogens are free to multiply.

A study of famine victims who had lost 25 per cent of body weight during a famine and then were given unlimited food found that only 4.9 per cent had detectable infections when refeeding began, but 29.1 per cent had overt infections two weeks later. The infections that flared up were all intracellular infections — the kind that are fought by autophagy. The infection that flared the most was malaria, caused by the intracellular protozoal parasite *Plasmodium falciparum.*[19]

READER REPORTS:
borderline personality disorder, mood, cravings, Raynaud's

I have Borderline Personality Disorder (BPD) and am taking a very low dose of risperdal (same drug in higher doses used to treat schizophrenia).

Following the PHD diet has greatly reduced my symptoms. I feel like a new person.

Better mood
I have found that following the PHD diet (in particular, getting enough Omega 3 and not excessive Omega 6 and eating PHD 'safe starches', etc., eliminating toxins (grains, legumes, vegetable oils, soy, etc.), taking the recommended supplements, and doing the optional intermittent fasting) has helped me tremendously. I feel so much better now: better mood, more energy, more patient, clearer thinking, happier, calmer, less emotional, less anxiety, and better able to cope with issues such as difficult people.

Very nutritious, no cravings
This diet is superhealthful and does allow plenty of choices: meat, fish, vegetables (peas & green beans are fine), nuts (not peanuts which are a legume), fruit, 'safe starches' (rice pasta, sweet/white potatoes and white rice), wine (which I like but don't drink due to Rx), healthful fat like lard, butter, cream, olive oil and coconut oil, dairy, chocolate, eggs, fermented vegetables and some safe sweeteners such as rice syrup. A benefit of eating a variety of healthful foods including 'safe starches': no cravings.

Intermittent fasting — easy
This is optional, but I'm so happy I discovered this. Fasting sounds difficult and you'd think it would involve hunger and suffering and a strong

(continued on next page)

will power, but not so. No need to go hungry. And I'm not even hungry
and don't suffer but feel great and clearer thinking/more energy in the
morning (even with my risperdal which for years had made me lethargic
in the morning) during my daily intermittent fasting (16 hour fast with
coconut oil during the fast with 8 hours feeding). When the fast is over,
I eat normally: usually 2 meals and a snack during the 8 hour feeding
window, sometimes just 2 meals. I'm not ravenous when it's time to eat,
surprisingly. Sure, I'm a little hungry, but in no hurry to eat and sometimes the fast lasts longer than 16 hours just because of circumstances.
And I exercise during the fast — no problem with a lack of energy. No
longer am I anxious about eating every 4 hours like I used to be while
doing low carb. In fact, I think I have a much healthier relationship with
food — it's not so important and I know I can go without it if I need to.
Food doesn't control me anymore. It has really simplified my life.

Raynaud's

Another benefit of the PHD is that my Raynaud's is much better now
and I'm not as cold as I used to be. I think this was helped by eating
more healthy fat and Omega 3.

So give PHD a try if you want to feel better and be healthy too.
I highly recommend it — it really has worked for me.

— Anonymous

The authors concluded:

> Severe undernutrition can suppress certain infections, mostly those
> due to intracellular pathogens and especially *P. falciparum*. Refeeding
> reactivates suppressed infection and can increase vulnerability to
> certain new infections especially of viral origin.

What this tells us is that in order to maximise immunity, we want our
fasts to be *shorter than 24 hours*. Such short fasts are long enough to induce
the highest rates of autophagy — thus maximising immunity. Longer fasts
would not increase autophagy, but would increase the period of immune suppression after the fast ends. *Long fasts make infections worse, not better.*

There is another argument for fasts that are shorter than 24 hours. Autophagy follows a strong diurnal rhythm and may be coordinated with the circadian clock. Disruption of the circadian clock leads to impaired immunity, faster ageing and shortened life span, and high rates of diseases such as osteoporosis, sarcopenia, cataracts, neurodegenerative diseases, and cancer. A review of links between autophagy and circadian rhythms concludes: 'Diurnal rhythms of autophagy may be required to . . . [prevent] neurodegeneration . . . metabolic disease . . . DNA damage and accelerated aging.'[20]

Fasting, then, should maintain a normal diurnal rhythm: a long overnight fast followed by daily feeding.

Foods for Autophagy

Food choice can also influence the rate of autophagy:

1. Reduced protein intake promotes lysosomal autophagy,[21] which kills bacteria and viruses.
2. Ketosis, which is induced by eating MCT oil or coconut oil, also promotes autophagy.[22]

Ketogenic diets have been successfully tested as Alzheimer's therapies. A placebo-controlled study found that those receiving supplemental coconut oil fats performed significantly better on a standard test for cognitive function.[23] Another randomised placebo-controlled trial also found substantially improved cognition on a ketogenic diet.[24] This success may be due to an antimicrobial effect, or to increased clearance of plaques by autophagy.

Coffee may make a fast more comfortable. Adding coconut oil or MCT oil to the coffee will promote ketosis, which may relieve hunger and increase autophagy.

Also, it's healthful to replace fluids and electrolytes during a fast. A bone broth, tomato, and seaweed or spinach soup, lightly salted, will provide potassium, sodium, calcium, and other minerals.

Fasting and Healthy Longevity

Compelling evidence from worms and flies shows that any method that induces autophagy, such as fasting, extends life span.[25]

In lab animals, calorie restriction stimulates autophagy and extends life span. But it has unfortunately side effects, such as stunting of growth. In general, sustained calorie restriction makes animals fragile and vulnerable to disease.

It turns out that regular fasts of duration less than 24 hours can deliver similar life span extension to rats without restricting calories, without stunting growth, and without promoting disease.[26]

Alternate-day fasting, which typically involves 24-hour fasts, has an excellent record of life extension and disease prevention in animal trials.[27]

Short fasts can also prevent obesity in mice. On an obesogenic high-fat diet, mice that could eat whenever they wanted became obese, but mice that could eat only in an eight-hour window did not gain weight. This happened even though calorie intake was the same between the two groups![28]

It looks as though regular short fasts give us all the benefits of elevated autophagy but without the downsides of long fasts.

- -

READER REPORTS: fasting for weight loss

I bought your book in June last year and have been 99% PHD-compliant since then, complete with intermittent fasting (restricting eating to 6 hour window each day), supplements and a lot of exercise.

I've lost a substantial amount of body mass and I am doing well, health wise.

— Ulf Benjaminsson

- -

Overfeeding Shortens Life Span

If fasting is good, its opposite, overfeeding or regular feeding, should be bad.

In critically ill patients in hospital beds, regular feeding combined with lack of exercise leads to a reduction in autophagy. In one study, critically ill hospital patients had a 62 per cent reduction in autophagic vacuoles and proteins normally degraded by autophagy reached up to 97 times normal concentrations. Lack of autophagy was associated with organ failure in these patients.[29]

Size-and-strength athletes, who overfeed for muscle gain, offer another case in point: they exercise and are healthy, yet their life spans are shortened by overfeeding. The average age of death among NFL players is less than 60 years, and each year in the NFL takes three years off a player's life span. Life span is shortest for the largest, strongest men — the linemen.[30]

When to Avoid Fasting

Some infections are best attacked by eating.

An old wives' tale advises us to 'feed a cold, starve a fever'. There's scientific support for this advice. Food restriction increases the severity of flu, a viral infection with coldlike symptoms.[31] It also appears to accelerate the progression of Amyotrophic Lateral Sclerosis (ALS, Lou Gehrig's disease).[32] When calorie restriction pioneer Dr Roy Walford died of ALS at age 79, it was a warning: every extreme dietary strategy will eventually meet a pathogen that can exploit it.

In general, healthful fasting is easy and free of stress. Anyone who feels unwell or who becomes hungry during a fast should eat.

Takeaway

Fasting is an effective way to enhance immunity against intracellular pathogens.

But fasts should be short — less than 24 hours. It is better to fast frequently but briefly. Long fasts actually promote intracellular infections by suppressing autophagy during the refeeding period. Long fasts may also interfere with circadian rhythms, which are supported by daily food consumption.

We believe 16 hours is the optimal length for fasts. This is short enough that it is possible to repeat the fast daily but long enough to induce elevated levels of autophagy. In animals, daily fasting for 16 hours with an eight-hour feeding window delivers significant health benefits.

Populations that fast are noted for their good health and longevity.[33] Indeed, early studies of the Mediterranean diet, which found it to be extremely healthy, were done mostly in populations of Orthodox Christians, who frequently fasted; it was probably the fasting, not the diet, that accounted for the result.[34]

Another population that fasts daily is the Kitavans, who are noted for their absence of disease. An ethnographic atlas describes their dietary practice:

> The main and only cooked meal is at sunset, after the gardening has been completed, and generally consists of yams, taro, and occasionally fish, wild fowl, pork, or sea fowl eggs. During the day, mangoes, breadfruit, bananas, and green coconuts and their milk may be eaten while working.[35]

As the Kitavan practices suggest, it's quite reasonable to snack during a fast. The benefits of fasting are greatest from routine short fasts, not from arduous self-denial.

A fast should be terminated if it generates hunger or other signs of nutrient deprivation, such as dry mouth, dry eyes, irritability, anger, or anxiety.

41
Blood Lipids

• •

*The Perfect Health Diet commonly optimises blood lipids, but
a few additional dietary steps can increase HDL levels
further, enhancing immunity.*

• •

Most people know the names of the blood lipids — LDL, HDL, triglycerides, total cholesterol — that doctors test during checkups. But most people don't know their functions. To judge by pharmaceutical company advertisements, the function of serum cholesterol is to give us heart attacks!

In fact, these fatty blood particles have two functions. They transport fats and cholesterol; and they are a critical part of our immune defence.

Optimal HDL Levels

HDL particles, for instance, carry 24 different immune molecules, including apolipoproteins such as clusterin (apoJ), coagulation factors, and complement factors.[1]

To pathogens that can metabolise fat — protozoa, fungi, and worms — an HDL particle looks like food. These pathogens engulf HDL particles and try to eat them. But they are engulfing a Trojan horse; once inside the pathogen, the immune molecules that were hidden amongst the fat and cholesterol are able to kill it or attract white blood cells that can finish the job.

Notes for this chapter may be found at www.perfecthealthdiet.com/notes/#Ch41.

For instance, some HDL particles carry molecules, apolipoprotein L-1 and haptoglobin-related protein, that are deadly to trypanosomes — the protozoal parasites that cause sleeping sickness and Chagas disease. Many trypanosomes that cause disease in animals are not dangerous to humans because they are destroyed by HDL. The trypanosomes that do generate human disease have evolved an ability to recognise HDL particles carrying the antitrypanosome molecules and refuse to eat them.[2]

In addition to killing pathogens, HDL clears toxins in the following ways:

- It binds bacterial endotoxins, especially lipopolysaccharide (LPS), and neutralises their toxicity. As a result, people with high HDL levels have substantially less inflammation during infections.[3] Injecting reconstituted HDL into humans relieves endotoxemia and LPS-induced inflammation.[4]
- It picks up circulating toxins, such as oxidised cholesterol, and carries the toxins back to the liver for detoxification. HDL particles carrying toxins are much more likely to be taken up by the liver than HDL particles that lack toxins.[5]

Most Americans and many Australians have too little HDL, resulting in impaired immunity and insufficient clearance of toxins. It's beneficial to have high HDL levels:

- People with high HDL levels are only one-sixth as likely to develop pneumonia,[6] and in the Leiden 85-Plus study, those with high HDL levels experienced a 35 per cent lower mortality rate from infection.[7]
- Each rise of 16.6 milligrams per decilitre in HDL levels reduced the risk of bowel cancer by 22 per cent in the EPIC study.[8]
- In the VA Normative Aging Study, 'Each 10-mg/dl increment in HDL cholesterol was associated with a 14% [decrease] in risk of mortality before 85 years of age.'[9]

The optimal HDL level is around 70 milligrams per decilitre. Americans average 50 milligrams per decilitre, and in 2011 Australia's largest study of cholesterol levels found that one in three GP patients had 'less than ideal' HDL levels.

How to Raise HDL Levels

Fortunately, it is easy to get HDL levels into the optimal range. Here's how:

- **Eat more saturated fat.** The Perfect Health Diet macronutrient ratios are just right. The reason this works is that dietary fat is packaged into particles called chylomicrons; after chylomicrons deliver their fat to adipose tissue, they are often turned into HDL.[10] Butter and cream are great for increasing HDL levels.[11]
- **Do intermittent fasting, and eat coconut oil.** These two steps are ketogenic, meaning they cause the liver to create ketones. Ketones stimulate a receptor that causes the liver to make more HDL.[12] (Niacin metabolism stimulates the same receptor, which is why doctors prescribe niacin to raise HDL levels. But niacin is toxic to the liver, so it's better to use coconut oil.)
- **Exercise.** In one 12-week trial, HDL levels were raised by 24.8 per cent on a moderate-intensity walking program and by 20.9 per cent on a high-intensity walking program.[13] Resistance training also works.[14] If you take a break, don't make it too lengthy: 20 days of bed rest leads to a 20 per cent reduction in HDL levels.[15]
- **Drink alcohol in moderation.**[16] A beer per day raises HDL levels by 4.4 per cent;[17] a half bottle of wine per day raises HDL levels by 17 per cent.[18]

The Immune Functions of LDL

Like HDL particles, LDL particles are part of the immune system. But they have a different role. Whereas HDL fights pathogens and clears toxins from the body, LDL acts as a scout to detect the presence of invaders.

LDL lipoproteins are, by design, fragile. They are easily damaged by oxidation, and the compounds that oxidise them most readily are bacterial cell wall components such as lipopolysaccharide (LPS). In the process of being oxidised, LDL binds the LPS, helping to clear it from the body.

Oxidised LDL ('oxLDL') particles have a different fate from that of normal LDL. Whereas normal LDL particles are taken up by cells throughout the body when they need fat or cholesterol, oxLDL is taken up by white blood cells called macrophages. This has several effects:[19]

- Macrophages begin to seek out and kill the specific pathogens that oxidised the LDL.
- Macrophages extract the LPS or other compound that oxidised the LDL and present it for antibody formation, stimulating formation of antibodies against invading pathogens.

So LDL is an important part of immune defence.

On bad diets, however, the sentinel function of LDL can become a liability. Fructose and omega-6 fats can oxidise LDL directly, or create a metabolic endotoxemia so that LPS from gut bacteria oxidises LDL. High levels of oxLDL create chronic, systemic inflammation and turn macrophages into 'foam cells' that form atherosclerotic lesions. As macrophages start to refuse oxLDL, their levels build up in the blood, creating dyslipidemia.

Optimal Blood Lipid Levels

The ideal serum lipid profile — the one that produces the best health and minimises mortality — looks like this:[20]

- **total cholesterol level** between 200 and 260 milligrams per decilitre
- **LDL cholesterol level** above 100 milligrams per decilitre
- **HDL cholesterol level** above 60 milligrams per decilitre
- **triglyceride level** around 50 to 60 milligrams per decilitre

Most people's triglyceride levels are too high and HDL levels too low.

Low triglyceride levels[21] and high HDL levels[22] are strongly associated with longevity. In the elderly, high HDL levels are associated with faster walking speed and better balance[23] and with improved cognitive function.[24]

Total cholesterol below 200 milligrams per decilitre indicates impaired immune function. A good illustration is provided by infants. At the moment of birth, infants have extremely low LDL levels and a total serum cholesterol level of about 72 milligrams per decilitre.[25] (Low LDL levels prevent babies in the womb from forming antibodies against their mum.) As a result of low LDL levels, infants have a limited ability to form antibodies and their immunity is impaired.

In breast-fed infants, serum cholesterol rises rapidly, reaching 163 milligrams per decilitre at age one month and 194 milligrams per decilitre at age six months.[26] This serum cholesterol level, around 200 milligrams per decilitre, is where immune function is normal.

Cholesterol rises more slowly in formula-fed infants, reaching only 140 milligrams per decilitre at age six months[27] — one reason formula-fed infants suffer more frequent infections.

Troubleshooting Blood Lipids

Blood lipids have diagnostic value. When blood lipids deviate from optimal despite a good diet, this indicates specific problems that doctors may be able to treat.

When total cholesterol is low (below 200 milligrams per decilitre), possible causes include:

- A lipid-deficient diet, such as a macrobiotic diet. If this is your problem, eat more fat!
- Hyperthyroidism, which can be relieved by lithium supplements.
- An infection with a eukaryotic pathogen — protozoa, fungi, or parasitic worms — that eats lipoprotein particles.[28]

If you eat a healthful diet and still have a low serum cholesterol level, ask your doctor to test your blood and stool for protozoal and worm infections.

When total and LDL cholesterol levels are high, it usually indicates reduced clearance of LDL particles from the blood. Possible causes include:

- Hypothyroidism or iodine or selenium deficiency. Thyroid hormone is needed to activate the LDL receptor, allowing cells to pull LDL from the blood. Iodine supplementation significantly lowers total cholesterol, LDL, and triglyceride levels.[29]
- Insufficient exposure to sun, preventing the body's manufacture of vitamin D and other sterols from serum cholesterol.[30]
- Excessive oxidation of LDL beyond the ability of macrophages to clear oxLDL. This can have several causes:
  - Deficiency of copper or zinc, the ingredients of zinc-copper superoxide dismutase, which is the main extracellular antioxidant (it binds to extracellular matrix and the lining of blood vessels to clear reactive oxygen species). Copper deficiency is a common cause of high LDL levels.[31]
  - Endotoxemia from gut dysbiosis or systemic bacterial infection leading to high levels of LPS and other oxidants in the body.

Doctors can help diagnose and treat these conditions. It is generally better to ferret out and fix the root cause of dyslipidemia than to artificially alter cholesterol levels with drugs such as statins.

42

Circadian Rhythm Enhancement

· ·

For optimal health, strengthen and synchronise circadian rhythms by:

- *Getting sun exposure during the day and avoiding bright light at night.*
- *Sleeping in a darkened room and waking naturally.*
- *Timing food intake and carbohydrate consumption for maximum circadian rhythm benefit.*
- *Doing light outdoor activity in the early morning and afternoon.*

· ·

The human body runs on a daily cycle. Some bodily functions happen at night, while we sleep; others during the day. Every cell has an internal clock telling it the time of day. When one is in good health, all these clocks are in sync, so that the body's activities will be properly coordinated.

When circadian rhythms are disrupted, disease often results. For instance, night-shift workers, whose bodies are in a perpetual state of jet lag, are at greater risk of developing cancer,[1] heart disease,[2] metabolic syndrome and diabetes,[3] hypothyroidism,[4] and a host of other diseases.

Infertility may often be due to disrupted circadian rhythms. Mice whose circadian rhythms are altered have difficulty conceiving and carrying pregnancies to term.[5]

Obesity, too, may be a circadian rhythm disorder. In mice, impairment

Notes for this chapter may be found at www.perfecthealthdiet.com/notes/#Ch42.

of circadian clocks in liver and adipose tissue precedes metabolic abnormalities and obesity.[6] Butter causes obesity in rodents when they eat it at all hours, disrupting their circadian rhythms.[7] But if they are allowed to eat it only in an eight-hour feeding window that conforms with their normal circadian feeding period, they do not become obese.[8]

Immune function follows a circadian rhythm: white blood cells involved in antibody generation circulate at night, while inflammation is tamped down during the day.[9] This is why sound sleep is so important for immunity: poor sleep depresses antibody formation.[10]

When circadian rhythms are disrupted, immune function is impaired. Mice suffering from the equivalent of jet lag are more likely to die from infection or endotoxemia.[11]

Time of infection matters: mice infected while immune function is at the low point of the daily cycle are more likely to die than mice infected at other times.[12] The high point of immunity to new infections is in the evening, when mosquitoes come out.

A number of factors help set our circadian rhythms, but the most important are **light** and **food; sleep** and **physical activity** are extremely important too.

Let's see how we can manage light exposure, meal timing, sleep, and activity to enhance our circadian rhythms and immune function.

Light Exposure

Light exposure is the most powerful factor setting our circadian rhythms. The brighter the light, and the longer we are exposed to it, the stronger its ability to shift circadian rhythms. *Blue and ultraviolet light* have the strongest effect; much lower intensities of blue than red light are sufficient to shift rhythms. Sunlight, which is up to 100 times more intense than room light in the blue and ultraviolet spectrum, is by far the most effective at setting circadian rhythms.

Sunlight affects circadian rhythm primarily via neural input from the eyes — not from vitamin D levels or other changes to the skin or blood. Lesions to the suprachiasmatic nucleus (SCN), a part of the brain that receives neural input from the eyes, destroy the influence of light upon circadian rhythms. The SCN, among other functions, controls melatonin release at night and cortisol release in the morning.

Damage to the SCN can have large effects on mortality, especially in wild animals. Chipmunks whose circadian rhythms are no longer sensitive to light, thanks to SCN lesions, are likely to be eaten by weasels.[13]

One reason the elderly have poor circadian rhythms is that ageing eyes filter out blue and ultraviolet light. This loss of light on the eyes, even if the elderly go outdoors, leads to such disorders as memory loss, slower reaction times, insomnia, and depression.[14] Cataracts, which block blue light, may be extremely dangerous to health.

Seek Bright Light by Day

For best health, we need to 'nudge' our internal clocks by *exposing our eyes to bright blue light every day*.[15]

It's possible that ultraviolet light, not just blue light, is helpful. If so, it would be beneficial to spend time outdoors without glasses or contact lenses, which block ultraviolet light. Beneficial compounds created by the action of sunlight on skin and blood, such as vitamin D, beta-endorphin, and nitric oxide, are additional reasons to get daytime sun exposure.[16]

We think it's best to get sun exposure several times per day, but *at least one of those times should be early in the morning*. There are two reasons for this:

- **The morning is the safest time for sun exposure.** Our DNA repair mechanisms follow a circadian rhythm, with peak activity about 7.00 A.M. In mice, UV light exposure is least likely to cause skin cancer if it comes when DNA repair mechanisms are most active. The inference is that 'humans . . . would be less prone to the carcinogenic effect of UV radiation in the morning hours and it might be advisable for humans, to the extent possible, to restrict their occupational, therapeutic, recreational, and cosmetic UVR exposure to the morning hours'.[17]
- **Morning sunshine is best for our circadian clock.** Experiments with vitamin D reported by psychologist Seth Roberts show that vitamin D taken at night can result in insomnia, while vitamin D taken early in the morning results in better sleep and mood.[18] It's likely that exposure to the sun, which

generates vitamin D, is also most healthful from early morning to midday.

While indoors during daylight hours, lights should be as bright as possible. It's a good idea to turn your computer monitor up to maximum brightness and turn on many lights during the day.

Avoid Light at Night

Our eyelids are translucent, and even a small amount of light at night, perceived through closed eyelids, can disrupt circadian rhythms and sleep quality.[19]

Light exposure before bedtime suppresses melatonin release and disrupts circadian rhythms. Worse, the presence of light in the room during sleep suppresses melatonin by greater than 50 per cent in most trials.[20] What's more, the amount of light needed to suppress melatonin release is small. Dim light will do it.[21]

Because blue light is most effective at disrupting circadian rhythms, wearing goggles that filter out blue light can help preserve normal melatonin rhythms.[22]

To optimise circadian rhythms, it's a good idea to sleep in a darkened room: get opaque drapes for your windows, and turn clocks face down so that their light is hidden. Just one pulse of sufficiently intense artificial light at night impairs cell division in mice brains and promotes patterns of gene expression associated with cancer.[23]

Blue or bright light from computer monitors and TVs suppresses melatonin rhythms.[24] It's not a bad idea to install the program f.lux, which reddens and dims computer displays after sunset, on your computer.

We're not aware of similar programs for televisions, but those would be helpful too. In epidemiological studies, television watching has a huge negative effect on health:

- Adults age 50 to 71 who watch the most television each day have a 61 per cent higher risk of dying than those who watch the least, even after adjustment for amount of exercise. The most vigorous athletes, who exercise more than an hour per day, still have a 47 per cent higher risk of dying with greater television viewing.[25]

- An Australian study found that every hour spent watching television reduces life expectancy by 22 minutes.[26]

The negative effects of television viewing are often blamed on inactivity (by 'couch potatoes'), but we believe it's more likely that the problem is that television watching disrupts circadian rhythms when it occurs at night. There's no similarly large effect from sitting in a chair at work; sedentary office workers have good health if they get a little exercise.

Circadian rhythm disruption by nighttime television viewing is probably driven by brightly lit screens, and by engagement with human faces and dialogue. (Social interactions probably promote daytime rhythms, even if the interactions are only with fictional characters on a television screen.) Ways to reduce the health impact of night-time television viewing include:

- Minimise blue light exposure by wearing orange goggles that filter out blue light, or dimming and reddening the screen and room lights at night.
- Refrain from watching programs with human social interaction at night; instead, nature images and relaxing music would be appropriate for nighttime television viewing.

If we're right that viewing human social interactions promotes daytime circadian rhythms, then television viewing during the daytime should be health-improving, especially for those (such as the solitary elderly) who have limited social interactions.

. . . .

READER REPORTS: lyme/bartonella-induced autism

My ten-year-old daughter is being treated for a lyme/bartonella infection and lyme induced autism and immune dysregulation. My daughter is responding well to treatment; her speech, executive function, handwriting, sound/light sensitivities have improved greatly with antibiotics and supplementation, and the ~80% implementation of your diet. Thank you so much for your hard work, you are helping so many.

— Louise Stanley, Ontario, Canada

. . . .

Sleep and Melatonin

The sleep scientist William Dement has argued that sleep is 'the most important predictor of how long you will live — perhaps more important than smoking, exercise or high blood pressure'.[27] One paper states, '[I]n the long run [lack of sleep] makes us sick. An increasing amount of scientific data indicate that sleep deprivation has detrimental effects on immune function.'[28]

The negative effects of sleep loss are significant:

- People getting less than six hours of sleep per night were 12 per cent more likely to die over a 25-year period than people getting six to eight hours per night.[29]
- Insomnia causes a progressive loss of grey matter from the brain.[30]
- People with sleep apnoea experience shortened telomeres, a sign of premature ageing; are more likely to develop high blood pressure, stroke, and heart attack, and have higher all-cause mortality.[31] Over a 22-year follow-up in the Wisconsin Sleep Cohort study, people with severe apnoea were 4.8 times more likely to die of cancer than normal sleepers.[32]

Negative effects from sleep loss show up immediately:

- One week of sleep curtailment in young men induces the hormonal profile of a diabetic elderly person: insulin resistance, high levels of stress hormones, low levels of testosterone and growth hormone.[33]
- One week of sleep restriction cuts antibody formation in response to an immune challenge in half.[34]
- Sleep curtailment in healthy young men increases hunger and appetite and promotes obesity.[35]

Conditions that impair sleep quality, such as apnoea, should be treated. Continuous positive airway pressure (CPAP) treatment can relieve much of the mortality risk associated with apnoea.[36]

Some of the ill effects of lost sleep or a shortened daily darkness window may result from deficient production of the hormone melatonin and may be addressable through supplementation.

The Hormone of Darkness

If vitamin D is the daylight hormone, melatonin is the nighttime hormone. Generated during sleep, its production normally peaks at about 2.00 A.M.

Centenarians are noted for their successful maintenance of rhythmic melatonin secretion throughout life.[37]

Melatonin is an antimicrobial hormone that has many benefits:

- It increases levels of growth hormone and amplifies the effects of resistance exercise, promoting muscle growth.[38]
- It kills tumour cells and prevents tumour growth.[39] It also extends cancer patient survival. In a trial of metastatic lung cancer, no patient survived two years on chemotherapy alone, but 6 per cent of patients on melatonin plus chemotherapy were still alive after five years.[40]
- Its anticancer effect is confirmed by higher-than-normal cancer rates among people who work at night and lower-than-normal cancer rates among the blind.[41]
- It has antimicrobial functions and protects against infections by the parasitic bacterium *Chlamydia*.[42]
- It is effective against diseases such as irritable bowel syndrome, high blood pressure, macular degeneration, glaucoma, and diabetes.[43]

In chronic infections and other inflammatory conditions of the brain, the intracellular immune response sequesters tryptophan. This prevents melatonin manufacture.

Since melatonin is so important for health and immune function, melatonin supplementation should be considered in such cases. Time-release melatonin tablets can maintain a relatively even level of melatonin through the night, preventing early waking from a drop in melatonin levels. Melatonin is non-toxic.[44]

Food Timing

Circadian rhythm is also influenced by the timing of meals. If you regularly eat food or drink caloric beverages such as alcohol at night and fast during the day, the body will start treating night as day and day as night.[45]

Following the general principle that we should always try to synchronise our circadian rhythms, our goal is to coordinate food intake with light exposure. That suggests that we should try to *eat food primarily during daylight hours* or at least several hours before a normal bedtime.

Carbohydrates seem to have an especially strong influence upon circadian rhythm, but it is opposite to that of food in general: they promote night rhythm and sleep.

For example, the hormone leptin follows a strong circadian rhythm. Leptin levels are low in the morning and rise over the course of the day, peaking in the middle of the night.[46] Food also affects leptin: eating fat has hardly any effect on leptin levels, but eating carbohydrates increases leptin for four to nine hours postmeal.[47] This suggests that, to enhance leptin rhythm, we should *eat most of our carbs around sunset.*

This hypothesis was supported by an Israeli study that tested two weight-loss diets; the diets were identical except that one concentrated the carbohydrates mostly at dinner. Those who had their carbs at dinner lost more fat and inches from their waist and had less hunger, lower blood glucose and insulin levels, less inflammation, and higher HDL levels.[48]

It looks as though fat and protein in the morning, starches and fat at dinner is a recipe for enhanced circadian rhythm. It's not bad to have coffee, bacon, and eggs for breakfast!

Timing of micronutrient intake can also impact circadian rhythm.

- Vitamin D3 may be best taken in the morning.[49] It's conceivable that vitamin D's effect on circadian rhythms may be of comparable importance to its nourishing effects. One of the puzzles of vitamin D science is that most populations on earth benefit from relatively high levels of vitamin D, but Scandinavians are consistently found to have the lowest mortality at low vitamin D intakes.[50] Scandinavians obtain much of their vitamin D from cod liver oil, which is often taken late in the day with dinner. Perhaps vitamin D taken in the morning is health-improving, while vitamin D taken in the evening is not. Or perhaps vitamin D needs to be accompanied by light on the eyes for its effects to be beneficial and Scandinavians get too little sunlight.

- Lithium upregulates circadian clock genes in a similar fashion to sunlight[51] and is best taken in the morning. Lithium's enhancement of circadian rhythm may be why it is helpful in bipolar disorder, a disease of disrupted circadian rhythm.[52] Any enhancement of circadian rhythm is therapeutic for bipolar disorder; simply looking at pictures of human faces in the morning helps.[53]
- Many people find magnesium, which has a calming effect, most helpful when taken at night. Its calming effect can promote sleep and nighttime rhythm. Magnesium, by the way, is essential to proper function of circadian clocks.[54]

Exercise and Rest

- -

The sovereign invigorator of the body is exercise, and of all the exercises walking is the best.

— Thomas Jefferson

- -

Physical activity has a huge impact on health and life span.

Moderate Exercise Has Tremendous Benefits
But there's something curious about it: the benefits of regular exercise are significant *even if the exercise isn't making the exerciser very fit.*

This shows up most clearly in studies of how much exercise is needed to obtain benefits. Not much!

- A study of 52,656 Americans over 31 years found that runners had a 19 per cent lower risk of death than nonrunners. Those who ran between one and 20 miles [1.6 and 32 kilometres] per week at a jogger's pace of ten or 11 minutes per mile reduced their risk of dying as much as those who ran more than 20 miles a week or who ran faster.[55]

- In the Copenhagen City Heart Study, the mortality rate of Danes who exercised two or three times per week for a total of one to two and a half hours was reduced by 44 per cent and their life span was extended by 6.2 years for men and 5.6 years for women. Those who exercised either more or less had less benefit.[56]

- A study of 416,175 Taiwanese adults found that an hour and a half of moderate exercise per week (13 minutes per day) reduced their mortality rate by 14 per cent and extended life span by three years. An additional 15 minutes per day reduced their mortality rate by only another 4 per cent. Benefits peaked at 50 minutes of exercise per day.[57]

Based on these studies, running 3.2 kilometres a day at a slow pace will extend life span by three to six years. Additional exercise improves fitness but has little effect on life span.

Low doses of exercise provide the greatest immune benefits. When aged rats ran just 0.8 of a kilometre per week, they were able to reverse infection-induced impairments in memory and brain function.[58] A comparable exercise dose in humans would be to run 9 kilometres per week — say, to run 3 kilometres three times per week.

Now, there are very real benefits to being fit. But the great life extension that comes from physical activity may be in large part due to circadian rhythm enhancement. To get in sync, circadian clocks require a small 'nudge' from physical activity to inform them that it is daytime, not night. It is this 'nudge' that extends life.

An indication that daytime exercise promotes good circadian rhythms is its effect on sleep quality. For every additional hour of physical activity during the day, children fall asleep three minutes more quickly and sleep 20 minutes longer.[59] The same pattern holds in adults.[60]

Support for this view comes from another curious fact: *health benefits are greatest when exercise is performed in natural settings.* For instance, those who exercise in natural settings are only half as likely to have poor mental health as those who exercise indoors or in urban settings.[61]

This is interesting, because we know from animal studies that living in a natural setting improves circadian rhythms. For instance, flies with certain mutations have disrupted circadian rhythms when living indoors, but healthy rhythms when living outdoors in a natural setting.[62]

Moderate exercise has a powerful anticancer effect — cancer patients who engage in moderate exercise live longer[63] and are less fatigued[64] — but so do other circadian rhythm enhancers, such as sun exposure and vitamin D. Exercise in natural settings may have the greatest anticancer effect. It seems to have helped John Matzke, who was terminally ill with melanoma metastasised to his lungs but recovered without treatment after long hikes in the mountains.[65]

Such spontaneous regressions of cancer might be common. Up to a quarter of the breast cancers revealed by mammography screening will spontaneously regress without treatment, according to a Norwegian study.[66]

SCIENCE OF THE PHD
Is Exercise Always Beneficial?

Almost everyone benefits from moderate exercise. But there may be a few exceptions.

A recent study looked at how metabolic markers such as blood pressure and HDL, triglyceride, and fasting insulin levels respond to exercise. In about 90 per cent of people, exercise improves these markers — a very impressive result, we think. But about 7 per cent of exercisers have an adverse change in two or more markers.[67] This could be due to chance — some people will pick up infections and suffer worsened health even if they do everything right — but could also indicate that some people are engaging in exercise that is inappropriately intense for their health condition.

Some illnesses do call for rest. Our advice: listen to your body. If your body is telling you to take it easy, tone it down. But nearly everyone will benefit from walking.

It's Easy to Underexercise

Evolutionary evidence confirms that only a small amount of exercise is necessary for human health. How so? Evolution neglected to build a *liking* and *wanting* for activity into the reward system of the human brain.

Many people are quite content to live completely sedentary lives. Forty-three per cent of Americans and 31 per cent of people worldwide do no exercise and walk less than 20 minutes per day.[68]

Daily physical activity is crucial to our health, and if there had been any opportunity to evade it in the Paleolithic, a desire for activity would have been built into our brains. That we lack an innate desire to exercise us tells us that Paleolithic activity levels were probably higher than is necessary for good health.

Hunter-gatherers walk eight to 16 kilometres every day, often carrying food, water, and wood. About two days a week, they would engage in more strenuous activity, including running (as during a hunt) and pushing or pulling objects (as in the construction or repair of shelters).[69] This activity level would be a very healthful one for us; but, as evolution didn't see fit to prompt a desire for more, it may be more than we need.

It's Easy to Overexercise

Moderate exercise is almost always beneficial, but strenuous exercise is more risky.

There is an increase in white blood cells during and immediately after exercise, followed by a drop below preexercise levels and a return to normal within 24 hours.[70] As long as there is an adequate period of rest between bouts of exercise, these changes to immune function seem to be beneficial. It has been proposed that exercise causes senescent white blood cells from tissue to enter the blood, where they can be cleared; over time this leads to higher white blood cell quality and improved immune function and may delay ageing.[71]

However, overtraining — regular intense exercise with inadequate rest — leads to depressed immune function. The immune response to strenuous exercise resembles that to sepsis and trauma.[72] If intense exercise is repeated daily, white blood cell functions are continuously depressed. Immune depression is greatest when exercise is 'continuous, prolonged, strenuous and performed without food intake'.[73] Endurance athletes are at the greatest risk of immune depression.

Recreationally competitive athletes get sick only half as much as sedentary people. But highly trained elite athletes get sick 4.5 times more often than recreational athletes.[74] Exercise is a stress on the body, and the dose makes the poison. Give yourself the right dose of exercise, a dose that strengthens your body. Listen to your body, and let how you feel be your guide.

If one's goal is an Olympic medal or a professional sports career, it is necessary to train at a very high volume, which may sacrifice health for fitness. But even Olympians have to avoid overtraining. The Olympic high jumper Amy Acuff has ceased weight lifting and considers it counterproductive. Instead, she jumps two days a week and on the other five does sprints and Pilates.[75]

Toward a Health-Optimising Exercise Program

So what should we do to be healthy in the modern world? The Paleolithic practice of walking eight to 16 kilometres a day would require two to three hours a day, and most people don't have the time.

If good health is your goal, the crucial step is to stimulate circadian rhythms with light early morning and afternoon activity.

- Every day early in the morning, go outdoors and spend ten to 20 minutes in light activity. Some possible activities: walking, jogging, bicycling, yoga, calisthenics, dancing, jumping rope, or track-and-field warm-up exercises. This should be light and easy; you should feel refreshed and awakened, not tired.
- At midday, afternoon, or early evening, whatever is convenient, go outside again for another ten to 20 minutes of activity. Again, it can be any activity you like, but it must not be exhausting. The purpose is twofold: to reinforce daytime circadian rhythms and get some sun exposure on bare skin.

If you do this for a while, you will probably start getting pleasure from exercise and will want to do more. If you decide to invest more time and seek a high level of fitness, one good strategy is to expand the afternoon or evening session.

- One day a week, engage in **vigorous cardiovascular exercise** such as running 5 or 6 kilometres. Exertion is good for the heart, and shear stress from fast-flowing blood along the sides of blood vessels stimulates healing of vascular injuries. Start by alternating walking and jogging; gradually add in intervals of sprinting. If you prefer, bicycling or any other exercise that elevates your heart rate is fine.

- One day a week, engage in **intense strength-building exercise.** This should exercise major muscle groups — for the lower body, a hip-hinging exercise such as deadlifts or kettlebell swings and a bent-knee exercise such as squats or leg presses; for the upper body, pressing and pulling exercises, such as push-ups or bench presses and pull-ups or rows; for the core, a plank. 'Intense' means that the exercise should push muscles to failure or near failure.

- On the other five days a week, engage in activity that is **actively restful.** Walk, jog, play sports, dance, hike, or engage in mobility-enhancing exercises such as yoga, tai chi, qi gong, or pilates. These activities should be refreshing and meditative, not intense. If possible, do these activities in a natural setting with your skin exposed to the sun.

What do we mean by activity that is actively restful? Mobility exercises should encompass most of the movements included in the fitness-developing workouts, but without weights or intensity. For instance, some yoga sun salutations keep a straight back and straight legs with a hip-hinging movement, similar to a deadlift. Such similar but low-intensity movements assist recovery, prevent muscle damage, and enhance strength gains.[76]

To further promote recovery and fitness gains, separate the two intense workouts by three days, and follow each workout immediately with a meal and over the next 24 hours with overfeeding — about 25 per cent more food than normal.

Avoid Stress and Be of Good Cheer

Chronic stress increases the risk of nearly every health problem. It accelerates ageing and suppresses immune function.

Mice that are stressed and anxious, as indicated by a greater desire to hide in dark corridors or hidden passageways, have impaired immunity. They develop aggressive forms of cancer; their immune systems fail to attack the cancers; and they have higher levels of stress hormones.[77]

The major stress hormones, such as cortisol, follow a circadian rhythm. One of the problems of chronic stress is that it disrupts that rhythm. In chronic stress, the hormone cortisol becomes continuously elevated, and this causes the body's cellular clocks to fall out of synchrony.[78] Elevation of cortisol and disruption of circadian rhythms are early stages in the development of depression.[79]

Sleep disruption affects cortisol, inducing the pattern of chronic stress. Cortisol levels follow a circadian rhythm, high during the day and low at night. When sleep is impaired, cortisol levels rise.[80] Cortisol levels are higher in insomniacs than in normal sleepers.[81]

One effect of elevated cortisol: it prevents telomeres, a stabilising end cap on DNA, from being maintained. Shorter telomeres bring impaired cellular function, unstable DNA, and shortened life span. Immune cells with shortened telomeres lose their effectiveness against viral infections.[82]

We mentioned earlier that lithium taken in the morning improves circadian rhythms. It turns out that elevated cortisol depresses circadian rhythms by the same molecular pathways lithium uses, so that low doses of lithium taken in the morning might help relieve chronic stress.[83]

In fact, almost any circadian rhythm–enhancing step will relieve chronic stress — including exercise, sun exposure, darkness at night, and proper food timing.

Here are a few additional steps.

- **Breathe slowly and deeply.** Diaphragmatic breathing — slow, relaxed, deep breaths, as practiced in many yoga disciplines — is a proven method for reducing cortisol and increasing melatonin.[84] Breathing deeply and slowly throughout the day can significantly reduce stress.

- **Be sociable.** One of the most consistent findings of centenarian studies is that they are extraverted and sociable.[85] Those who regularly attend church live longer,[86] perhaps because of the social connections they make there. But to restore circadian rhythms and improve mood, it seems we don't even need genuine friends: looking at pictures and videos of human faces can fool the brain into thinking we have friends! Psychologist Seth Roberts has found 'morning faces therapy' — looking at photos of human faces in the morning — to be mood-enhancing, stress-relieving, and therapeutic for depression and bipolar disorder.[87]

- **Be grateful.** Gratitude relieves depression and improves sleep.[88] Frequently recalling in prayer the many things we have to be grateful for may be another reason the religious live longer.

- **Be of good cheer.** People who are cheerful and optimistic live longer.
  - The Nun Study compared the emotional content of handwritten autobiographies 180 Catholic nuns had written in their youth to their life outcomes 60 years later. The nuns whose autobiographies were the most positive had a 2.5-fold lower mortality rate between ages 75 and 95. Youthful good spirits, it seems, are associated with longevity six decades later.[89]
  - Studies of centenarians and near centenarians have found that they are relaxed, friendly, conscientious, and upbeat about life; they have an easy laugh and an active social life.[90]

Good health certainly causes good spirits. We believe that a healthy body and brain naturally generate a cheerful, optimistic mood. So perhaps the nun and centenarian studies tell us only that those who are healthier are happier and that those who are healthy in their youth are more likely to be healthy 60 years later.

But we believe causality runs both ways — that good cheer promotes good health.

Norman Cousins, in *Anatomy of an Illness,* described how he suffered from heart disease and arthritis. He claimed his arthritis was cured with megadoses of vitamin C and laughter induced by watching Marx Brothers movies. Ten minutes of laughter, he said, gave him two hours of pain-free sleep.[91]

But remember — an hour of the Marx Brothers may take 22 minutes off your life, if you watch at night!

READER REPORT: good health and good cheer

Have been on PHD for only about 3 weeks and I am amazed by my new outlook on life. I was not 'unhealthy' before (by modern standards) — but I feel so much more able to see the positive now. Thanks a million.

— P.C., San Jose, California

Takeaway: a suite of circadian rhythm therapies

Not only what we do but *when we do it* has a big effect on our health.

Modern life makes it difficult to maintain healthful circadian rhythms. Office workers are stuck indoors most of the day, missing sunshine. Meals and exercise are pushed into nighttime hours, where they disrupt circadian rhythms.

Yet healthful circadian rhythms are essential to immune function. Cancer and a host of infectious and autoimmune diseases become more prevalent when circadian rhythms are not maintained.

Fortunately, the investment of time and effort needed to entrain circadian rhythms is small:

- ten to 15 minutes of sun exposure and physical activity in the early morning
- another 15 minutes of sun exposure and physical activity in the afternoon
- concentration of food consumption in the daytime and early evening

- avoidance of bright light at night, especially white and blue light, and darkening of the bedroom during sleep
- adoption of a bed time that allows a full night's rest, is consistent from night to night, and ends by waking naturally

It's well worth making the investment!

43
Healthful Weight Loss

lthough we have avoided discussing specific diseases in this book, we will make an exception for obesity. So many overweight people follow misguided weight-loss strategies that it seems important to provide some guidance.

The modern obesity epidemic does not arise from overeating or lack of exercise. Gluttony and sloth have always been with us, but obesity has not.

The Invention of Obesity

In the 1880s and 1890s, every circus had a fat man; crowds paid good money to see them because they were so rare.

You might search online for a photo of Chauncy Morlan, the fat man of the Barnum & Bailey Circus.[1] In the 1800s, he was a sideshow freak; today no one would give him a second glance.

In the 20th century, we invented a lot of new foods: vegetable oils extracted from poisonous seeds, high-fructose corn syrup, and chemically processed industrial foods manufactured from purified nutrients. At the same time, we invented obesity.

Over the course of this book, we've mentioned a number of factors that contribute to obesity.

Notes for this chapter may be found at www.perfecthealthdiet.com/notes/#Ch43.

- **Toxins.** Fructose and omega-6 fats readily induce obesity in lab animals by poisoning the liver and causing metabolic endotoxemia. Wheat toxins also promote obesity, as do various toxins generated in industrial processing of food.
- **Malnourishment.** Obesity can be induced in mice and rats via choline-deficient diets[2] and mineral-deficient, sugar-rich diets.[3] The obese are generally malnourished in a wide range of micronutrients. This malnourishment generates hunger and increases food consumption, creating an excess of energy that the obese can't dispose of.
- **Infection.** The level of bacterial endotoxins in the liver predicts metabolic syndrome and obesity. Any number of infections can cause generalised inflammation that promotes obesity. Recently, researchers have connected viruses to obesity. The adenovirus AD-36 causes fat cells to proliferate; people infected with AD-36 are three times more likely to become obese and obese people infected with AD-36 are much fatter than noninfected obese.[4]
- **Circadian rhythm disruption.** A little bit of exercise, sun exposure, and nighttime light and food avoidance can maintain healthful circadian rhythms. Yet many people don't get any exercise, work indoors with dim light during the day, and eat, drink, and watch television at night, disrupting their circadian rhythms and promoting obesity.

These factors — toxins, malnutrition, infections, and disruption to the circadian immune and healing functions of the body — are the same factors behind all other diseases. Obesity, like other diseases, is **polycausal** and the causes are mostly dietary and lifestyle factors.

Except for some infections, the causes of obesity are not, for the most part, amenable to medical treatment. The solution lies in a more healthful diet and lifestyle.

Calorie Restriction Is Dangerous

Most people think of a 'weight-loss diet' as a calorie-restricted diet. They think the recipe for weight loss is temporary starvation.

But that is a dangerous strategy. Malnourishment is one of the causes of obesity, and *reduced food intake aggravates malnourishment.* So **a starvation diet may cause more obesity.**

Experience bears this out:

- People who lose weight through starvation diets usually end up *more obese than when they started.* UCLA researchers analysed 31 long-term diet studies and found that a majority of people who dieted to lose weight subsequently regained even more weight than they had lost.[5]
- When we look at countries that have suffered famines, we find that *people become obese once the famine is over.* Malnourished people tend to become obese as soon as they have sufficient calories.[6]

Since starvation continued long enough results in death, the period of calorie restriction must come to an end. If enough damage was done by malnourishment during the 'diet', **the obesity will become even more severe and intractable.**

Now, it is true that a caloric deficit is necessary for weight loss. But that does not mean tiny portion sizes. If food quality is improved, a hunger-free caloric deficit is usually easy to generate.

Calorie Restriction to the Point of Hunger Is Unnecessary

Weight can be lost and body shape normalised *without ever reducing calories below a normal person's intake.*

The reason is that caloric expenditure increases with body weight. The obese burn more calories per day than the slender. It's a lot of work to carry that extra weight around, and extra surface area means more energy lost as heat.

In one study, slender persons (average weight 66.2 kilograms) used 2481 calories per day, while obese persons (average weight 130.6 kilograms) used 3162 calories per day.[7]

So an obese person can eat a normal, 2481-calorie-per-day diet and still lose weight at a steady pace. At an expenditure of 3162 calories per day and consumption of 2481 calories per day, fat loss would be about 75 grams per day, 540 grams per week, 27.2 kilograms per year.

READER REPORTS: weight loss without cravings

I am a 65 year old woman who has fought weight control all my adult life. January 2011 I started following the Perfect Health Diet. I am maintaining my 40 pound [18 kilogram] weight loss without cravings or white knuckling and feel great. Thank you! Thank you! I have printed out so much from your blog and share with all who ask — and they do ask. My husband is also on board and is doing great. Perfect Health Diet is now our way of life — no more yo-yo dieting.

— Nancy

The Best Weight Loss Diet Is a Diet for Life

Some diet gurus advocate different diets for weight loss and maintenance.

This is unnecessary. Since it's possible to lose weight eating the same calories as a normal person, it's not necessary to eat a diet different than a normal person's to lose weight.

We think it's also a mistake. After all, an obese person got that way by being inclined toward an unhealthy diet. Adopting a new diet is hard. Making an obese person learn *two* new diets — a 'weight-loss' diet and a 'maintenance' diet — imposes an unnecessary burden.

We think it's much better to train yourself in healthful eating from the beginning, while the motivation to lose weight is strong. Use the Perfect Health Diet for weight loss from the beginning, and the odds of long-term success will be higher.

....

READER REPORTS: diabetes and obesity

I am down from 341lbs [154.7 kilograms] to 272lbs [123 kilograms] doing mostly Paleo, but modified with some safe starches per your book. Just so you know this is not just about weight loss for me, I was a type 2 diabetic with full metabolic syndrome and most importantly, I had popping capillaries in my retinas that were leading to blindness. All is better now, no pills etc.

— J. Hippman

....

Key Steps for Weight Loss

Here are the most important steps in any weight loss program.

1. Eliminate omega-6-containing oils, replacing them with butter and coconut oil; reduce omega-6 fats by getting protein from beef, lamb, and seafood; cut fructose intake by eliminating added sugars and getting carbs from safe starches.

Excessive intake of omega-6 fats may be the primary cause of the obesity epidemic, and fructose from added sugars and toxins from grains are contributing factors. Eliminating these foods will go a long way toward fixing any weight problem.

In their place, eat:

- Meats: beef, lamb, salmon, shellfish.
- Oils: coconut milk, butter.
- Safe starches: white rice, potatoes, sweet potatoes, taro.

2. Eat normal PHD amounts of carbohydrates and protein; restrict fat.

Carbs and protein are nutrients and they are not stored in the body, so eating less of them will lead to malnourishment. Fats are stored in the body — it's all that stored fat that you're trying to get rid of! — so you don't need to eat much fat. If your diet is fat-deficient, any needed fats will be pulled from adipose tissue. As long as you continue eating some seafood for omega-3 fats and liver and egg yolks for fat-soluble vitamins and choline, you can reduce fat quite a bit with no risk of malnourishment.

Therefore, the weight loss version of PHD is very similar to the regular version, only tweaked slightly to reduce fat:

- Instead of using 6 to 12 teaspoons of fat or oil in cooking and sauces, use at most 3 teaspoons per day. Instead of a large dollop of butter or sour cream on a baked potato, flavour it with a small pat of butter plus vinegar and salt.
- Replace fatty meats with somewhat leaner meats. When you have ribeye steak, instead of eating attached fat, trim excess fat.

You're still eating the same PHD foods, and they should still taste delicious. Quantities shouldn't be much different than a normal diet, since you still need the same amount of carbs and protein. A diet with 500 calories from carbs, 300 calories from protein, and 500 calories from fats (primarily via egg yolks, liver, seafood, beef or lamb, and coconut milk) is the minimum caloric intake consistent with proper nourishment.

3. Be well nourished. Eat all the supplemental foods we recommend, plus our supplemental vitamins and minerals.

When you are hungry, eat. Malnourishment is a cause of obesity. Nutrition must be sufficient to enable all bodily tissues to heal and function properly.

A nutrient-dense diet reduces appetite. So for good health and rapid weight loss, be sure to make nutrient-rich foods such as eggs, bone broth, liver, shellfish, potatoes, tomatoes, and green leafy vegetables a part of your diet. Get every major nutrient into its plateau range.

4. Do intermittent fasting.

Every day, confine your food intake to an eight-hour feeding window. Inducing autophagy by fasting will help defeat any obesity-inducing bacterial and viral infections and will also promote beneficial metabolic adaptations. To support circadian rhythms, the feeding window should conclude around sunset.

During the 16-hour fasting window, allowable foods are:

- a spoonful of coconut oil or MCT oil when hungry
- a bowl of tomatoes and greens in bone broth, lightly salted or vinegared
- calorie-free beverages such as water and coffee

Coffee can be flavoured with a spoon of coconut oil. The MCT oil or coconut oil is ketogenic and supports autophagy during the fast. It also applies the Shangri-La Diet idea of eating tasteless calories during a fast to lower appetite. The soup provides nourishment with few calories.

5. Enhance your circadian rhythms.
Go out every morning about 7.00 A.M. for ten to 20 minutes of light activity in the morning sun. In the afternoon, get some sun on bare skin and more light activity. The goal isn't to burn calories: it's to reset circadian rhythms. So have fun.

At night, avoid exposure to bright light. Sleep in a darkened room; invest in opaque drapes.

6. Normalise your thyroid function.
It is impossible to be healthy and difficult to lose weight with a malfunctioning thyroid. Hypothyroidism is underdiagnosed and undertreated.

The first step toward normalising thyroid function is toxin removal and supplementation of iodine, magnesium, and vitamins C and D, along with consumption of selenium-rich and copper-rich foods. If these are not sufficient to restore thyroid function, supplemental thyroid hormone (obtainable with a doctor's prescription) should be considered. Aim for a TSH of 1.0 or below.

. . . .

READER REPORTS: 30 kilograms lost

My friend introduced me to the Perfect Health Diet over 14 months ago. When I first switched I weighed 284 lbs [129 kilograms]. I am at the lowest weight of my adult life — I weigh 218 lbs [99 kilograms] now. I want to lose even more now that I am seeing it work.

— Roxy Rocker, Boston, MA

. . . .

Be Patient

In cases of obesity, it's essential to **optimise health, not speed of weight loss.** Rapid weight loss from excessive calorie restriction leads to malnourishment and yo-yo weight loss and regain.

Rapid, healthful weight loss *is* possible for many people — many Perfect Health Dieters report rapid, easy, lasting weight loss of 900 grams per week — but not for everyone. Everyone has a different mix of health problems causing their obesity, and those with infectious causes will have slower weight loss than those merely suffering from an omega-6 excess. Another common pattern is an initial period of weight gain followed by a steady, sustainable weight loss. (See Connie's reader report on p. 185 for an example.) This pattern may be due to malnourishment, which stimulates appetite upon starting the Perfect Health Diet, leading to an initial weight gain as the brain seeks to replenish hitherto missing nutrients. Once a healthy nutritional status is obtained, preferably by intake of nutrient-dense foods like egg yolks, liver, and shellfish, appetite lessens and weight loss begins.

A few markers will show that you're on the right track:

- **Absence of hunger.** Hunger indicates malnourishment, so if you're hungry you're doing something wrong. Calorie restriction may bring a mild appetite, but it should be easy to resist, and it should go away with some exercise or a spoon of coconut oil. If it's more than that, figure out what nutrients you are missing, and eat foods that contain them.
- **Increasing pleasure in physical activity.** As your health improves, exercise and movement will become more enjoyable. It should become easier to gain muscle.
- **Improved sleep.** Sleep is a marker of circadian rhythms. If your sleep is better, you're improving your rhythms.

As these markers improve, odds are the weight on the scale will drop.

44
Meal Plans

Now that we've covered all the bases — we know **what to eat** and **when to eat it** — we can plan our meals.

Meal Planning Principles

Here are the basic principles of meal planning.

Weekly Preparation

On the weekend, prepare a large quantity of soup stock from **bones,** joint-rich tissue such as **chicken feet** or **ox hooves,** or **vegetables.** This stock will let you quickly make soups throughout the week.

Try to do the bulk of your shopping on weekends, but make frequent stops on the way home from work to get fresh ingredients. If you have access to a farmer's market, visit it on the weekends and stock up on organic meats, bones for stock, organ meats, and organic vegetables. If you don't have a local farmer's market, many supermarkets carry a range of organic products. Talk to your butcher or stockist for guidance. Meat can be divided into suitable sizes for a day's cooking (e.g., 0.6 to 0.9 kilograms for a household of two people) and frozen until ready for use. Seafood or shellfish is best purchased the day it is eaten.

Notes for this chapter may be found at www.perfecthealthdiet.com/notes/#Ch44.

Dinner

Dinner consists of meat or seafood; a safe starch; another plant food; and a vegetable soup, perhaps with a glass of wine.

It's nice to prepare enough food at dinner so that leftovers can provide the next day's lunch. To supply enough for both dinner and lunch, buy 340 to 450 grams of meat or seafood per person per day.

- **Meat and seafood** choices should consist of beef, lamb, salmon, or sardines, and other fish and shellfish *at least* five days a week. The other two days can be anything: birds (duck or naturally raised pastured chickens), pork, eggs, and cheese or other protein-rich dairy products can provide alternatives to the usual beef, lamb, fish, and shellfish.

    What if you're a vegetarian for moral reasons? We hope you're a lacto-ovo vegetarian, because eggs and dairy products are better protein sources than plants. If so, it's easy: add cheese and eggs to meals to get adequate protein; use coconut milk or oil and butter or sour cream as your fats. Most vegetarian recipes can be made PHD-compatible simply by substituting ingredients — white rice and potatoes for grains and beans; coconut milk or butter for vegetable oils.

- **Safe starches** include white potatoes, sweet potatoes, taro, and white rice. About 450 grams per day is desirable. They should be flavoured with butter, sour cream, or coconut milk; vinegar; and a bit of salt.

- **Other plant foods** should vary, but good choices include beets, carrots, onions, and mushrooms, squash, avocado with tomato, and any vegetables you like. It's possible to mix in some of our pleasure foods — such as cheese and crackers, mozzarella and tomato slices drizzled in olive oil, or macadamia nuts — if you like.

- **Soups** are simple; just add a plant food to stock. Good choices are: (1) tomatoes and green leafy vegetables, (2) seaweed, and (3) puréed pumpkin or squash.

Lunch

Lunch consists of leftovers plus our supplemental food of three egg yolks daily, possibly with vegetables and flavourings (usually vinegar or lemon or lime juice) added.

How can you prepare leftovers? Here are three basic recipes:

- **Bibimbap.** In a bowl, mix a safe starch (diced into pieces), meat (cut into pieces), and other leftover plants and vegetables with egg yolks and vinegar, lemon juice, or lime juice. Add tomato slices or spinach or seaweed to taste. Add a bit of stock if it needs moisture. Heat the mixture in a microwave.
- **Fried rice (or fried potato mix).** In a pan oiled with coconut oil or butter, add day-old rice (or a diced starch such as potato), meat (cut into pieces), and other plants and vegetables with eggs or egg yolks and vinegar, lemon juice, or lime juice. Add tomato slices or spinach or seaweed to taste. Stir-fry in the pan and eat warm.
- **Pho.** To a bowl of soup stock, add leftover starch, meat, and vegetables cut into pieces. Add egg yolks and vinegar, lemon juice, or lime juice, plus vegetables such as tomato slices and spinach to taste. Heat in a microwave.

These have three very different tastes, but they are made from the same ingredients and all are quite easy to prepare. Of course, leftovers can also be eaten in the same style in which they were originally prepared.

By varying the choice of meat or seafood, the vegetable, the safe starch, the cooking or flavouring fat, the flavouring acid, the soup stock, and the spices, you can create a fair amount of variety in the taste of your leftovers.

Breakfast

If you're doing intermittent fasting, you won't be eating much breakfast. Acceptable fasting foods are:

- a spoonful of MCT oil or coconut oil, to assuage hunger
- a bowl of vegetable soup; add tomatoes, spinach, and salt to a bowl of soup stock, and heat in the microwave

- coffee, tea, and water; coffee may be flavoured with coconut oil or cream

If you're eating breakfast, some choices include:

- leftovers (see 'Lunch')
- fried eggs, plantains, and tomatoes; or fried eggs, potatoes, and spinach with butter and vinegar on the potatoes
- boiled eggs and fruit (say, a banana)
- plain whole milk yogurt and berries
- cream of rice with cream and berries, perhaps some leftover meat for protein
- puffed rice cereal with milk
- berries, nuts, and cream
- cheese, nuts, and fruit
- cheese and rice crackers

But be creative. As long as the ingredients are healthful, the breakfast will be healthful.

Snacks and Desserts

Snacks and desserts will consist mostly of cheese, fruit, nuts, chocolate, dairy products, and vegetables dipped in a fatty dip.

Often, we'll make a liver pâté as our dip. It's essential to eat 115 grams of beef or lamb liver every week. Liver can be made one of the dinner entrées (e.g., liver and onions) or prepared as a pâté, which makes a convenient dip for raw vegetables such as carrots or cauliflower. We make the pâté on the weekend at the same time as our stock.

Drinks

Drinks should be calorie-free; water, tea, and coffee are good choices.

The exception are alcoholic beverages, which we support in moderation. We recommend wine, but beer and mixed drinks are also acceptable.

A Sample Meal Plan

This meal plan is a blueprint. As long as you are eating according to PHD principles, feel free to adapt the menu to your preferences and what foods are in season. Note that we've listed three options for dinner each day. Choose from one and serve with the side dishes, listed in italics.

Day	Breakfast	Lunch	Dinner
Sunday	Fasting	Omelette (eggs, cream, onions, cheese, tomato, mushroom)	**Ground Beef and Organ Meats Entrée (choose one):** • Spaghetti (liver and ground beef sauce over rice noodles) • Lasagna (liver and ground beef sauce, rice noodles and cabbage leaves) • Shepherd's pie (mashed potatoes, ground beef and liver, vegetables) *Vegetable soup*
Monday	Boiled egg(s) and bowl of raspberries	Leftovers — Bibimbap	**Beef 1 Entrée (choose one):** • Beef stew (beef cooked in potatoes, tomatoes, peas, onions, stock, and flavourings) • Beef bourguignon • Beef stroganoff *Served over white rice* *Vegetable soup*
Tuesday	Fasting	Leftovers — Bibimbap	**Oily fish Entrée (choose one):** • Bengali salmon curry • Poached salmon • Salmon casserole *Potato mashed with butter* *Roast beets* *Butternut squash soup with a dollop of sour cream*
Wednesday	Soup with seaweed, rice, and eggs	Leftovers — Pho-style meat and starch soup	**Bird Entrée (choose one):** • Chicken tikka masala with sour cream • Roast duck • Thai chicken coconut milk curry *Sweet potato with butter* *Steamed cauliflower with parmesan cheese* *Vegetable soup*

(continued on next page)

Day	Breakfast	Lunch	Dinner
Thursday	Fasting	Leftovers — Bibimbap	**Beef 2 Entrée (choose one):** • Ribeye steak • Rack of lamb • Roast beef *Baked potato with butter or sour cream and vinegar* *Shiitake mushrooms, roast beets, and greens* *Pumpkin soup with a dollop of sour cream*
Friday	Fried eggs, fried plantains, and tomatoes	Leftovers — Bibimbap	**Shellfish Entrée (choose one):** • Broiled scallops • Steamed mussels or clams in a coconut milk sauce • Pho (noodle soup) with shrimp, scallops, and egg yolks *Taro corms with sour cream and fig spread* *Salad*
Saturday	Plain whole milk yogurt with blackberries	Leftovers: Fried rice	**Miscellaneous Meat or Vegetarian Entrée (choose one):** • Pizza (gluten-free crust, cheese, tomato sauce, choice of meat and vegetables) • Dong Po's pork with white rice and seaweed • Chicken cacciatore over white rice • Mutter paneer *Taro and coconut cream soup* *Salad*

A large number of recipes and meal suggestions can be found on our blog. Visit www.perfecthealthdiet.com and click the Recipes tab for more ideas.

Perfect Health — for Life

There is disturbing evidence that the health of people in much of the Western world has taken a turn for the worse. It's not just obesity; a recent analysis found that in 2006, men and women of all ages were becoming diseased or disabled at higher rates and earlier ages than they had been eight years earlier.[1]

Modern medicine has failed to cure chronic diseases. Doctors regard most diseases as incurable and are content to palliate symptoms.

Drugs and medical care do little to halt disease or extend life span. Perhaps they shorten life span: research based on the Dartmouth Atlas of Health Care found that chronically ill patients who receive the most intensive treatments fare worse than those who receive minimal care.[2]

We believe that:

- Nearly all diseases can be cured if they are attacked at their root causes: toxic foods, malnutrition, and chronic infections.
- Nearly everyone can achieve a healthy weight and a long, healthy life by eating as they were meant to eat.

If we're right, there should be people who have stumbled upon the right way of eating and achieved exceptionally long, healthy lives. Do such people exist?

Notes for this chapter may be found at www.perfecthealthdiet.com/notes/#PHDforLife.

The Diets of the Oldest Old

We've taken to reading the obituaries of centenarians. One pattern repeats: *centenarians love to cook.*[3]

This is probably the single most important step to good health. Home cooking starts with real food — plants and animals — and uses gentle heat that doesn't generate many toxins. It is almost a prerequisite for a long, disease-free life.

To reach age 105 or older, usually something more is required: a high-fat, low-sugar, low-omega-6 diet, often supported by intermittent fasting.

Here are a few stories from the oldest old:

- Gertrude Baines 'lived to be the world's oldest person on a steady diet of crispy bacon, fried chicken and ice cream'. She died at age 115 in 2009.[4]
- Edna Parker, an Indiana schoolteacher, was the world's oldest person when she died at age 115 in November 2008. Her diet was dominated by eggs, sausage, bacon, and fried chicken.[5]
- Jeanne Calment, who lived to age 122, 'ascribed her longevity and relatively youthful appearance for her age to olive oil, which she said she poured on all her food and rubbed onto her skin'. She also drank wine and ate chocolate — both recommended PHD foods.[6]
- Dr Leila Denmark was the world's oldest active pediatrician when she retired at the age of 103; she recently died at age 114. She counselled avoidance of sugary drinks, including fruit juice; whole fruits were the only source of sugar she supported. At her 100th birthday she refused cake because it had sugar in it, and at her 103rd birthday party, when she again refused cake, she explained that she hadn't eaten any food made with sugar for 70 years.[7]
- Larry Haubner of Fredericksburg, Virginia, passed away at age 108 in 2010. On his 107th birthday he complained that he had been served an unhealthy food — cake — for his birthday.[8] A visitor recalled the hostile reception she received when she took him candy; thereafter she took fruit.[9]

- Walter Breuning of Great Falls, Montana, was the world's oldest man when he died at age 114. He practiced a daily 16-hour fast, eating only breakfast and lunch. On his 114th birthday, he celebrated with his favourite food: **liver and onions.**[10]

A Grand Experiment

We consider the Perfect Health Diet the beginning of a grand experiment — a start toward a medical revolution, a shift toward natural healing. In adopting the Perfect Health Diet, you are helping to test whether we are right and whether those who 'eat the way we are meant to eat' can cure their diseases, improve their fitness, and live to become healthy centenarians.

If you do try the Perfect Health Diet, please share your experiences, good or bad, with us and our readers at www.perfecthealthdiet.com. By sharing experiences, we can learn from one another and hasten the arrival of that happy day when chronic disease will be a thing of the past and good health and long life everyone's birthright.

Thank you, dear reader, for your time with us. We wish you a long life, free of disease, and the best of health always!

Acknowledgements

This book is the fruit of a long journey: five years seeking to improve our own health, and more years helping others improve theirs.

It has been said that 'the best way to learn is to teach', and so it has been with us. We were blessed to gain readers quickly — intelligent, kind, and curious readers — and they have taught us as much as we have taught them. We have also learned much from our fellow bloggers and scholars in the ancestral health and natural healing movements. In many cases, we have been able to credit in the footnotes those who introduced us to ideas or papers. Credited or uncredited, we are grateful to all from whom we have learned.

We're grateful beyond words to the many readers who have tried our diet and reported their results, and above all to those who gave permission for their stories to be shared in this book. Thank you!

Many have made specific contributions to this edition. We're grateful to scholars who provided data in support of figures: Stephan Guyenet of the University of Washington; Steve Simpson of the University of Sydney, Australia; and Tony Hulbert of the University of Wollongong, Australia. We're grateful to Mark Sisson for his foreword; Chris Kresser, Dallas and Melissa Hartwig, Seth Roberts, Court Wing, and Aaron Blaisdell for blurbs; Dan Pardi, Stephan Guyenet, Sally Fallon Morell, and J. Stanton for critical comments on the manuscript; Monika Chas, for our yinyang apple; Doug Abrams, our agent; Shannon Welch, our editor; and everyone at Scribner in the U.S. and Scribe in Australia for their support of the book.

It seems fitting to close by expressing our gratitude to the two to whom we dedicated the book: Paul's mother, Annette Marie Jaminet, and Shou-Ching's father, Tei-Kuang Shih.

Annette befriended a deaf neighbour as a child and became a teacher of the deaf. At age 22, just a few months after marriage and while pregnant with Paul and his twin sister Linda, her first tumour was discovered; she died of cancer 11 years later. She did much that we now know to be mistaken in her fight against cancer: though sun exposure and physical activity are crucial, she avoided the sun and would rest during the day in a darkened bedroom; and she gave the best food to her children, reserving burnt portions — rich in cancer-promoting amines — for herself. Yet if she lacked knowledge of how to be healthy, she had no peer in courage, kindness, or love. Even as she lost her hair to chemotherapy and her belly bloated with ascites, she smiled and spread good cheer. Paul remembers her laughter — like the time she brought a root beer float to his dad, who was working on the oft-broken family car; and when Paul cried, 'What's that?' she joked, 'A laxative.' Paul had no idea what a laxative was, but he knew he wanted one. She made root beer laxatives for everyone, and they were very satisfying.

Tei-Kuang was an architect and artist who fled Shandong, China, during the civil war of 1948 and settled in Korea in time for the Korean War. In Korea he became a restaurateur. He imparted his love for food, Chinese culture, and art to Shou-Ching; as a young girl she would carry her pillow and blanket to his bed upon waking, and they would trade stories, hers made up. He cooked for the family, and his food was delicious; dinner was the best time of every day. Though impoverished, he became the patron of the small Chinese community of Yeongwol, and created a Chinese school for 40 local children. He was very sociable, had many friends, and was always their first resource in times of trouble. At age 62 he suffered two strokes and, after the second, fell into a coma for six months. The family fed him liquid food through a tube and massaged and turned him every few hours. Shou-Ching was at his bedside when he died. She vowed then to become a biomedical scientist and, if she could, help others avoid a similar fate. She also gave up animal fat, which she blamed for his stroke, and wondered why her food never tasted as good as his, and why her skin and hair were never as healthy as when she was a girl — until they recovered on our diet.

Some will scoff, but we suspect that Annette and Tei-Kuang have been united and are now friends; and that their prayers sustain us. If this work has power to heal, it may be because by the grace of Love, they have helped lead us to Truth.

— Paul and Shou-Ching Jaminet, September 2012

Index